Communication and
Relational Maintenance

Communication and

Relational Maintenance

Edited by

Daniel J. Canary
School of Interpersonal Communication
Ohio University
Athens, Ohio

Laura Stafford
Department of Communication
Ohio State University
Columbus, Ohio

Academic Press, Inc.
A Division of Harcourt Brace & Company
San Diego   New York   Boston   London   Sydney   Tokyo   Toronto

at

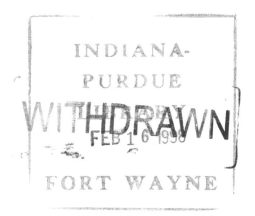
This book is printed on acid-free paper. ∞

Academic Press, Inc.
525 B Street, Suite 1900, San Diego, California 92101-4495

United Kingdom Edition published by
Academic Press Limited
24–28 Oval Road, London NW1 7DX

Library of Congress Cataloging-in-Publication Data

Communication and relational maintenance / edited by Daniel J. Canary,
   Laura Stafford.
        p.   cm.
     Includes bibliographical references (p,   ) and index.
     ISBN 0-12-158430-5
     1. Interpersonal relations.   2. Interpersonal communication.
   3. Conflict management.   I. Canary, Daniel J.   II. Stafford, Laura.
   HM132.C6247   1993   93-11326
    302.2--dc20   CIP
PRINTED IN THE UNITED STATES OF AMERICA
94   95   96   97   98   99   BB   9   8   7   6   5   4   3   2   1

Contents

PART I

Communication Action Approaches

1. Maintaining Relationships through Strategic and Routine Interaction

Daniel J. Canary and Laura Stafford

2. When Partners Transgress: Maintaining Violated Relationships

Michael E. Roloff and Denise H. Cloven

3. Steady as (S)he Goes: Relational Maintenance as a Shared Meaning System
Steve Duck

4. A Social Skills Approach to Relationship Maintenance: How Individual Differences in Communication Skills Affect the Achievement of Relationship Functions
Brant R. Burleson and Wendy Samter

5. A Multiphasic View of Relationship Maintenance Strategies
Kathryn Dindia

PART II
Social Psychological Approaches

9. Love Ways: An Elaboration and Application to Relational Maintenance

Peter J. Marston and Michael L. Hecht

10. Why Can't Men and Women Get Along? Developmental Roots and Marital Inequities

John M. Gottman and Sybil Carrère

PART III

Dialectical Approaches

11. A Dialogic Approach to Relationship Maintenance

Leslie A. Baxter

12. Relationship Rejuvenation

William W. Wilmot

13. Being There and Growing Apart: Sustaining Friendships during Adulthood

William K. Rawlins

PART IV

Epilogue

14. Tracing the Threads of Spider Webs

Laura Stafford

Contributors

Numbers in parentheses indicate the pages on which the authors' contributions begin.

Mark Attridge (141), Department of Psychology, University of Minnesota, Minneapolis, Minnesota 55455

Leslie A. Baxter (233), Department of Rhetoric and Communication, University of California, Davis, Davis, California 95616

Brant R. Burleson (61), Department of Communication, Purdue University, West Lafayette, Indiana 47907

Daniel J. Canary (3), School of Interpersonal Communication, Ohio University, Athens, Ohio 45701

Sybil Carrère (203), Department of Psychology, University of Puget Sound, Tacoma, Washington 98416

Denise H. Cloven (23), Department of Communication Arts, University of Wisconsin, Madison, Madison, Wisconsin 53706

Kathryn Dindia (91), Department of Communication, University of Wisconsin, Milwaukee, Milwaukee, Wisconsin 53201

Stephen M. Drigotas (115), Department of Psychology, University of North Carolina at Chapel Hill, Chapel Hill, North Carolina 27599

Steve Duck (45), Departments of Communication Studies and Psychology, University of Iowa, Iowa City, Iowa 52242

John M. Gottman (203), Department of Psychology, University of Washington, Seattle, Washington 98195

Michael L. Hecht (187), Department of Communication, Arizona State University, Tempe, Arizona 85287

Ted L. Huston (165), Department of Human Ecology, The University of Texas at Austin, Austin, Texas 78712

Peter J. Marston (187), Department of Speech Communication, California State University, Northridge, Northridge, California 91330

William K. Rawlins (275), Department of Communication, Purdue University, West Lafayette, Indiana 47907

Michael E. Roloff (23), Department of Communication Studies, Northwestern University, Evanston, Illinois 60201

Caryl E. Rusbult (115), Department of Psychology, University of North Carolina at Chapel Hill, Chapel Hill, North Carolina 27599

Wendy Samter (61), Department of Communication, University of Delaware, Newark, Delaware 19716

Laura Stafford (3, 297), Department of Communication, Ohio State University, Columbus, Ohio 43210

Anita L. Vangelisti (165), Department of Speech Communication, The University of Texas at Austin, Austin, Texas 78712

Julie Verette (115), Department of Psychology, University of North Carolina at Chapel Hill, Chapel Hill, North Carolina 27599

William W. Wilmot (255), Department of Communication Studies, University of Montana, Missoula, Montana 59812

Preface

This book addresses the issue of how people maintain their personal involvements. We see *maintenance* as a valuable metaphor to stimulate diverse approaches in the examination of the thoughts and actions people undertake to sustain their relationships. More specifically, as the title suggests, this book highlights the role of communication in the maintenance of relationships. Although all contributors share the belief that communication is important in maintaining personal relationships, the precise manner in which communication is seen to serve maintenance functions varies from chapter to chapter. Indeed, whereas some authors focus exclusively on communication processes, others examine communication in conjunction with factors such as cognitions and contexts.

These chapters are not the first to examine relational maintenance phenomena. However, they do constitute the first volume to explore the manner in which relationships are sustained through communication. The research histories of most of the contributors indicate that they have something of importance to say on the topic. The recent research of other contributors provides a new perspective on maintenance activities. Whether established or emerging, all the contributors turned their attention to the task at hand: to offer their position in regard to communication and relational maintenance. Moreover, all authors were asked to address four issues. In addressing the same issues, they provide a sense of coherence, although their perspectives may differ radically.

The first of the four issues concerned basic definitions. That is, each author was asked to articulate a conceptualization of relational maintenance. No scope parameters or limitations were placed upon these definitions. In addition, the definitions demonstrate a range of styles (e.g., from informal to formal, from indirect to direct). Second, contributors were asked to provide a theoretical orientation or a set of research assumptions. Such orientations help the reader understand how relationships are maintained from the authors' points of view. Third, we asked each author to offer empirical support for the statements made. Empirical support could be drawn from their own research or from a synthesis of other research efforts. Finally, we asked each author to indicate promising directions for future research. Although we asked the contributors to address these four issues, we did not impose any organizational requirements; an imposition of the same structure was not tenable and would lead to a set of fairly predictable chapters.

This book is divided into four major parts. Each of these parts reflects a different perspective on the topic of communication and relational maintenance. Part I, "Communication Action Approaches," contains chapters that examine relational maintenance processes from a communication action point of view. That is, these chapters stress how people use symbolic action to sustain their relationships. In other words, more than anything else, communication is seen as the primary means of maintaining relationships. Part II, "Social Psychological Approaches," focuses on sociological and psychological factors that sustain relationships. In Part II communication is contextualized by such factors as barriers to leaving the relationship, equity in doing household chores, and cognitive appraisals of the relationship as valuable. Part III, "Dialectical Approaches," concerns the experience of tensions that occur as the result of contradictory, but mutually necessary terms. For example, people experience tensions that arise from their needs for connection and their needs for autonomy, because the dialectic of connection–autonomy is a commonly cited one. In Part IV, "Epilogue," Stafford concludes the book by offering a retrospective analysis of the chapters' themes and by presenting a prospective view on how maintenance can be studied in the future.

We stress that these divisions do not necessarily reflect the contributors' "home" disciplines, and the labels we use to name these parts are not useful in depicting the fields of communication or psychology. Instead these part titles indicate differences in *emphasis* among the chapters. Because our divisions concern matters of degree and not kind, the reader may see how a chapter in one part could also be placed in another part. For example, Marston and Hecht's chapter on "love ways" has a strong social psychological basis; hence it is placed in "Social Psychological Approaches." However, it is also compatible with the dialectical chapters, as it stresses the *nexus* of love ways as an existential experience. Also, several of the chapters in "Communication Action Approaches" rely on research that is clearly social psychological, and they could also have been placed there. In short, the placement of chapters reflects their primary emphasis, with the part titles emerging from the chapters more than from the authors' fields of study.

As stated earlier, Part I, "Communication Action Approaches," focuses on communication behaviors as they function to maintain relationships. In Chapter 1, we (Canary & Stafford) present our conceptual framework for studying relationship maintenance, which then provides a background for our report of research on strategic and routine relational maintenance behaviors. Next, Roloff and Cloven (Chapter 2) offer an understanding of how and why people in transgressed relationships (e.g., verbally or physically abused women) maintain these involvements. Roloff and Cloven provide a new taxonomy of "approaches" partners enact to maintain these relationships. In Chapter 3, Duck emphasizes the everyday, taken-for-granted aspects of communication. It is the routine practice of talk that recreates the partners' understanding of their relationship, according to Duck. In Chapter 4, Burleson and Samter stress the kinds of communicative skills people need to engage and maintain friendships. Burleson and Samter stress such factors as comforting and conflict behaviors, and they argue that partners' similarity of such skills may be more important than partners' individual prowess at these skills. To conclude this part, Dindia offers a specific analysis of the communication strategies reported across the life span of relational development. Dindia notes that the strategies used to escalate relationships are similar to those used to maintain relationships; thus Dindia argues for a "multiphasic" view on relationship strategies.

Part II, "Social Psychological Approaches," emphasizes the psychological and sociological factors that keep relationships intact. In Chapter 6, Rusbult, Drigotas, and Verette see commitment as a central "macromotive" feature of relationships. That is, commitment leads to such relationship-enhancing activities as deciding to remain in the relationship, accommodating the partner, and derogating alternatives to the relationship, among others. Whereas commitment is primary for Rusbult and colleagues, the notion of barriers is crucial for Attridge. In Chapter 7, Attridge discusses how couples could use both internal and external barriers to maintain the relationship. This chapter makes explicit many factors most people do not acknowledge as reasons for being in relationships; that is, it presents a variety of factors that may actually prevent people from exiting their relationships. Next, Vangelisti and Huston (Chapter 8) examine relational maintenance as a function of different "domains" of marriage. That is, Vangelisti and Huston examine how changes in marital partners' love and relational satisfaction over a two-year period are associated with interaction (e.g., communication, sex), behavioral organization activities (e.g., household labor), and contextual factors (e.g., finances). Their findings reveal several intriguing gender differences, showing the ways that men and women differ in their valued maintenance activities. Marston and Hecht (Chapter 9) also focus on love. Specifically, they discuss various experiences of love, or "love ways," showing how the existential experience of love varies. More precisely, these authors present their theory of love ways, demonstrating how the functional and structural relations of these various love ways affect what is meant by "maintaining" a loveship. In the last chapter in this part, Gottman and Carrère explore differences between men's and women's interaction styles as a function of their social development. More specifically, they examine how the sexes are segregated until marriage and how such segregation may lead to differences in interaction. Gottman and Carrère then report the results of an eight-year longitudinal study that investigates the effects of verbal and nonverbal communication, physiological factors, and several self-report measures (e.g., satisfaction and intention to separate) on couples' long-term stability and satisfaction.

Part III, "Dialectical Approaches," examines the ontological experiences of relating. In Chapter 11, Baxter presents a dialogical account of relational maintenance, relying on Bakhtin's theory of dialectics. This theory provides a general framework for viewing dialectics as responses to complementary, and not necessarily opposite, poles. Wilmot (Chapter 12) then entertains the issue of relational rejuvenation. For Wilmot the critical question is, How do couples go about rejuvenating their relationships? By examining different relational prototypes, Wilmot implies that acceptance of a particular proto-typical model may help or impede an individual's ability to maintain relation-ships. In Chapter 13, Rawlins reports a study that is guided by the assump-tions of dialectical theory. In particular, Rawlins is interested in the accounts of middle-aged people as they relate their experiences of friendship. Through use of interview segments and personal insights gained during this study, Rawlins shows how long-distance friendships are sustained.

We would like to express our appreciation to a trio of editors at Academic Press. Jean Mayer was most helpful in supervising the production of this project. And Linda Shapiro did an excellent job in designing the book. Of course, we are grateful to Nikki Fine, who has shown great flexibility from the acquisition of the book to its distribution.

We would also like to mention that all of the contributors not only met but exceeded our expectations and requests. They were unanimously enthusiastic about undertaking this project. Importantly, all contributors submitted excel-lent initial drafts and received our critiques with a willingness to revise their chapters. Such professionalism makes editing a pleasurable experience. We are proud of this collection of papers, for it represents first-rate scholarly thinking on the topic of relational maintenance. Each chapter says something important and different about maintaining relationships. We sincerely hope you find this book as informative and interesting as we have.

Daniel J. Canary
Laura Stafford

PART

I

Communication
Action
Approaches

1

Maintaining Relationships through Strategic and Routine Interaction

Daniel J. Canary
School of Interpersonal Communication
Ohio University
Athens, Ohio

Laura Stafford
Department of Communication
Ohio State University
Columbus, Ohio

Introduction

For several reasons, *maintenance* is a useful metaphor for the examination of personal relationships. First, maintenance focuses attention on relational stability, satisfaction, and important characteristics, such as commitment, that are critical to personal involvements (Dindia & Canary, 1993). Second, maintenance connotes both a stage of relational development and the dynamic processes involved in relating. Maintenance is often seen as a stage of relational development that follows escalation and precedes de-escalation (Dindia, this volume).[1] As such, maintenance may be seen as a goal for people;

[1]We should mention that, as editors, we had access to all the chapters contained in this book as we were completing our own chapter. We would be foolish if we did not use these fine works; we would be dead if we did not cite them.

that is, most people desire long-term, stable, and satisfying relationships. Moreover, it appears that people spend more time maintaining their relationships than entering or exiting them (Duck, 1988). We also realize that maintenance is a *process*; that is, relational maintenance involves dynamic activities. Although some think maintenance entails a lifeless constant, we see the term connoting change necessary to relating.

In addition, maintenance is a heuristic metaphor because it prompts us to consider communication behaviors people use to sustain their relationships. In this vein, several researchers have offered taxonomies of communication strategies people use to maintain relationships (e.g., Ayres, 1983; Bell, Daly, & Gonzalez, 1987; Dindia & Baxter, 1987; Stafford & Canary, 1991). Finally, the term maintenance serves a pragmatic coordinating function. Theorists and researchers have spent considerable energy examining maintenance, as the contributors to this volume document. For example, Gottman's (1979) research on couples' interaction behaviors and patterns implicitly concerns maintenance when those behaviors are tied to relational stability and satisfaction. There have been hundreds of studies on relational stability and satisfaction; each of these likely has something to say about relational maintenance as a stage or process. But the term has only recently been used as a rallying point for research on communication and personal relationships.

Conceptualizations of what it means to maintain a personal relationship are diverse. Braiker and Kelly (1979), for example, researched maintenance activities as direct discussions about the relationship. Ayres (1983) conceived of maintenance behaviors as actions taken to keep a relationship at a satisfactory level, once patterns of exchange stabilized. According to Ayres, maintenance strategies function to keep a relationship from decreasing or increasing its level of intimacy. Bell et al. (1987), however, conceptualized maintenance activities as affinity-enhancing actions, which could maintain or increase, but not prevent from increasing, the level of relational satisfaction. From still a different perspective, Dindia and Baxter (1987) conceptualized maintenance and relational repair as similar processes, wherein maintenance strategies prevent trouble from occurring and repair strategies restore the relationship to a previous satisfactory state. Duck (1988, this volume) has argued that routine behaviors do as much as strategies do to keep relationships going. In brief, the recent interest in how communication functions to maintain relationships has materialized in different conceptual forms.

We do not believe that alternative conceptualizations of maintenance can or should be made uniform; a variety of approaches increases knowledge and understanding on the topic. Nevertheless, we do believe that the links between communication and maintenance should be theoretically based, represent a broad array of activities, and provide direction for continued research.

In light of these assumptions, our objective in this chapter is to summarize strategic and routine maintenance behaviors, given our conceptualization of maintenance. To accomplish this goal, we first present our conceptualization of maintenance behaviors. Our definition and conceptual framework guide the analyses we report later. Following that, we present findings from several studies that focus on the simple question, What do people do to sustain their relationships? Finally, we conclude by articulating what we feel are important future research directions.

Conceptualization of Maintenance

Definition

As every college student learns, definitions are important because they indicate the nature of, and imply boundaries for, the phenomenon under investigation. Our definition of maintenance behaviors functions in the same manner. Specifically, we define *relational maintenance behaviors* as actions and activities used to sustain desired relational definitions (Canary & Stafford, 1992, 1993a; Stafford & Canary, 1991).

First, people engage in "actions and activities" to maintain their relationships. These terms are meant to imply that strategic and routine behaviors are in operation, and these strategies and routine practices involve both interactive and noninteractive behaviors. Later in this chapter we develop more completely the concepts of strategic and routine interactive approaches. Second, by use of the verb "sustain" we mean to imply that maintenance behaviors function not only to keep a dyad together but also to uphold desired relational definitions, and that relational properties erode without the benefit of maintenance behaviors. Third, by "desired relational definitions" we refer to important features that indicate the character of the relationship. There exists a number of factors that could be interpreted as relevant to "desired relational definitions." For example, Burgoon and Hale (1984) presented a dozen characteristics that have been considered central to relationships and interpersonal communication. We assume that some relational properties are universal to all relationships: *control mutuality, trust,* and *liking* (for a similar taxonomy, see Millar & Rogers, 1987). In addition, we believe *commitment* is vital to romantic relationships (see also Rusbult, Drigotas, & Verette, this volume). In other words, the features of control mutuality, trust, liking, and commitment are critical components of personal relationships that portray the nature of relationships and indicate relational stability; without mutuality of control, trust, liking, or commitment the relationship lacks substance. Because of their importance to our research, we briefly review each of these characteristics.

Control mutuality refers to the extent to which couples agree on who has the right to influence the other and establish relational goals. This concept is similar to Morton, Alexander, and Altman's (1976) mutuality of control construct. Control mutuality also implies bilateral agreement over who controls interdependent goals and behaviors, elements Kelley (1979) described as mutual fate control and mutual behavioral control. Hence, control mutuality refers to consensus or agreement on who takes control, not necessarily whether only one or both parties have control. To illustrate, a measure of control mutuality includes the following items: "Both of us are satisfied with the way we handle decisions between us"; "We agree on what we can expect from each other"; and "We are attentive to each other's comments" (Canary, Weger, & Stafford, 1991). Research has revealed that lack of control mutuality, or unilateral control, is displayed in domineering behaviors inimical to relational satisfaction (e.g., Courtright, Millar, & Rogers-Millar, 1979).

Trust is a second feature universal to relationships. Trust refers to the degree to which someone is willing to risk him- or herself to the partner because the partner is seen as honest and dependable (Johnson-George & Swap, 1983; Rempel, Holmes, & Zanna, 1985). Trust has been positively associated with several positive relational outcomes, including love (Larzelere & Huston, 1980) and confidence in the partner (Johnson-George & Swap, 1982). A lack of trust may been easily witnessed in suspicious behaviors and jealousy (e.g., Buunk & Bringle, 1987).

Liking is also fundamental to close relationships. Bell et al. (1987) even presume that increasing the partner's liking for self is sufficient for maintaining the relationship. Likewise, Dickens and Perlman (1981) indicated that liking is a premise of ongoing friendships. Rubin (1979) has stated that liking is primarily composed of affection and respect for the partner and that relationships have little future without liking. It would appear difficult at best to sustain a relationship characterized by lack of affection and respect.

Finally, commitment concerns the degree to which one wants to continue in a relationship indefinitely—a property of particular importance to romantic involvements. Sabatelli and Cecil-Pigo (1985) noted that commitment is critical to relational stability. These authors conceptualized commitment as a barrier against relational alternatives, whereby dyadic cohesion is ensured. Similarly, Lund (1985) found that the barriers of investment in the relationship and commitment were better predictors of relational stability than were love or rewards gained from the relationship.

In sum, we define maintenance behaviors as actions and activities used to sustain desired relational definitions. Relational definitions are seen in the characteristics of control mutuality, trust, liking, and (in romantic relationships) commitment. There are, of course, other important relational features, such as satisfaction and love (see also Marston & Hecht, this volume; Vangelisti & Huston, this volume); however, the properties just reviewed provide concrete, varied, and important dimensions of personal relationships.

Conceptual Framework

Elsewhere we have presented our theoretical commitments (Canary & Stafford, 1993a) and research assumptions (Stafford & Canary, 1991). Here, we want to synthesize and extend these statements in a series of propositions.

Proposition 1: All relationships require maintenance behaviors or else they deteriorate. In other words, without maintenance efforts, desired characteristics of a relationship decay like any system that has been neglected. In Duck's (1988) language, we ascribe to a centrifugal (vs. a centripetal) analogue; that is, relationships fall apart unless people invest the energy to keep them together. Without maintenance behaviors, the forces pulling dyads apart are generally more powerful than the barriers keeping dyads together (cf. Attridge, this volume). Even dating relationships require maintenance or else they deteriorate. In their study of dating couples, Guerrero, Eloy, and Wabnik (1993) found that maintenance strategies were reported less frequently in declining relationships than in escalating or stable relationships.

Proposition 2: People are more motivated to maintain equitable relationships than inequitable relationships. The assumptions of an equity theory have been articulated (e.g., Hatfield, Traupmann, Sprecher, Utne, & Hay, 1985; Walster (Hatfield), Berscheid, & Walster, 1983). In a word, *equity theory* predicts that people are content in relationships where both persons have equal ratios of inputs to outcomes, that people are distressed when involved in an inequitable relationship, and that people try to restore and maintain equity. Equity theory has generated much research to support it (e.g., Hatfield et al., 1985; Van Yperen & Buunk, 1990). In particular, the research supports the premise that people are more satisfied in equitable relationships than inequitable relationships.

People appear to be distressed by inequity. There are two types of inequity: *underbenefitedness*, where one's partner receives more outcomes relative to his or her inputs; and *overbenefitedness*, where one person receives more outcomes relative to his or her inputs than does the partner. Equity theory suggests that the more disturbing type is underbenefitedness, because the overbenefited at least have the comfort of enjoying their relative benefits. Sprecher (1986) directly examined men's and women's emotional reactions to inequity and found support for the prediction that underbenefitedness is more distressing. Sprecher found that men tended to react to inequity with feelings of resentment and anger, whereas women turned inward, with feelings of depression, sadness, and frustration. In addition, Sprecher found that underbenefitedness was more predictive than overbenefitedness of attitudes toward the partner.

Research also supports the contention that equitable relationships are more stable than inequitable ones (Van Yperen & Buunk, 1990). For example, Prins, Buunk, and Van Yperen (1993) found that among women (but not men) inequity was positively related to having an extramarital affair. Our own research indicates that inequity affects the relational features of control mutuality, trust, liking, and commitment directly as well as indirectly. More precisely, underbenefitedness directly and negatively affects these relational features, as two studies have found (Canary & Stafford, 1992, 1993a). Additionally and indirectly, inequity, especially underbenefitedness, negatively affects maintenance behaviors which then affect the relational characteristics. We found that both husbands and wives who were classified by the wives as underbenefited were less likely than those in equitable marriages to engage in relational maintenance behaviors of positivity, assurance, and openness (Canary & Stafford, 1992).

Some researchers argue that people who keep account of equity may be undermining their relationships; attending to equity reflects an "exchange orientation," which may be less functional than a "communal orientation" (Mills & Clark, 1982). However, the rigidity implied by an exchange orientation may be overstated. Roloff (1987) noted that people are adaptable in counting rewards and costs; that is, considerations of equity are not limited to identical or immediate reciprocation of outcomes. The potential adverse effects due to an exchange orientation are probably moderated by flexibility in people's assessments of outcomes and inputs.

Proposition 3: Maintenance activities vary according to the development and type of the relationship. Braiker and Kelley (1979) have shown that both conflict and maintenance activities increase as couples become more interdependent over time. Using an experimental design, Ayers (1983) found that maintenance strategies varied according to escalating, de-escalating, or stable relationship conditions. Ayres found that persons whose hypothetical partner wanted to de-escalate the relationship were more likely to use balance than those in the escalation condition (i.e., keep emotions consistent, remind partner of decisions made in the past, etc.). Similarly, using a survey design, Stafford and Canary (1991) found that engaged and married people perceived more assurances than those in dating relationships. Stafford and Canary also found that engaged and seriously dating couples perceived more openness in their relationships than either married people or people in newly formed dating relationships. That maintenance activities vary as the relationship develops appears clear (see also Guerrero et al., 1993).

Maintenance strategies also vary among different types of relationships.

We expect different maintenance activities without broad relational types as well as between different types. For example, the research on relational trajectories by Huston, Surra, Fitzgerald, and Cate (1981) shows that dating couples vary qualitatively in their experiences of conflict and commitment. Similarly, the research on marital couple types by Fitzpatrick (1988) shows that married couples vary in their ways of relating to one another. For example, Witteman and Fitzpatrick (1986) found that "Separates," who prize limited emotional involvement, are vigilant in defending their autonomy. But "Traditionals," who rely on traditional role expectations and who are interdependent, engage one another and appeal to the nature of their relationships when seeking compliance. Also, "Independents," who are egalitarian and seem to negotiate everything, seek information from the partner. Accordingly, we would anticipate that Separates engage in fewer maintenance behaviors than do Traditionals and Independents. This hypothesis remains to be tested. Nevertheless, the evidence shows that within relationships, experiences are anything but uniform. These different experiences likely require different kinds of maintenance strategies and routines.

One study (Canary, Stafford, Hause, & Wallace, 1993) has found that particular maintenance strategies varied according to *different* relationship types. Specifically, positivity, openness, assurances, sharing tasks, and use of mediated messages (i.e., "cards/letters/calls") all varied according to relationship type (we describe these strategies in full later). Positivity, openness, and assurances were used less than expected in friendships, but more than expected in romantic involvements. Assurances, sharing tasks, and cards/letters/calls were used more than expected by chance among relatives, and less frequently than expected in friendships.

Proposition 4: Maintenance behaviors may be used in isolation or in combination with other maintenance behaviors to variously affect the nature of the relationship. The reader of this volume will find a range of strategies that potentially may be used to sustain relationships. Roloff and Cloven (this volume) discuss the various approaches people use to maintain transgressed relationships, including minimization of the transgression, attempts to prevent future transgressions, and even retribution. Sampling more functional relationships, Dindia has been involved in several research studies associating various maintenance strategies to relational satisfaction (1989; this volume; Dindia & Baxter, 1987; see also Baxter & Dindia, 1990). For example, Dindia (1989) found that husbands' antisocial maintenance behaviors are negatively associated with wives' satisfaction. These findings suggest that although antisocial strategies are ineffective in functional relationships, they may be more effective in sustaining less functional relationships, perhaps even to the dismay of the communicator.

Our own attempts to associate maintenance strategies to relational characteristics have presented a few consistent findings (Canary & Stafford, 1992, 1993a, 1993b; Stafford & Canary, 1991). First, positivity has consistently emerged as an important predictor of control mutuality and liking. In addition, sharing tasks, reliance on social networks, and use of assurances also contribute to explaining control mutuality and liking. Use of assurances has been found to be most effective in sustaining commitment (Canary & Stafford, 1992, 1993a; Stafford & Canary, 1991). Finally, positivity and assurances have been the primary maintenance behaviors predicting trust (Canary & Stafford, 1993a; Stafford & Canary, 1991). These results show that maintenance strategies have *varying functional utility;* that is, people use maintenance strategies alternately to sustain the relational features deemed most salient.

Proposition 5: Maintenance actions and activities involve both interactive and noninteractive behaviors. Interactive behaviors are communication based; that is, they involve some type of symbolic exchange between parties. Noninteractive behaviors do not involve symbolic exchanges between participants. For example, sharing tasks does not necessitate an exchange of symbols, although it is feasible that by doing a fair share of the household responsibilities, a partner is "communicating" his or her good intentions to the other partner. Other contributors to this volume also investigate interactive and noninteractive factors. In this light, the exit–voice–loyalty–neglect behaviors discussed by Rusbult et al. (this volume) are primarily interactive, but other factors in their model are more psychological than communicative: derogation of alternatives, willingness to sacrifice, and relationship-enhancing illusion. Likewise, Vangelisti and Huston (this volume) separate interaction (e.g., communication, sex) from other maintenance activities of behavioral organization (e.g., spending time together, leisure activities) and contextual factors (e.g., finances, social network activities).

Proposition 6: People use both strategic and routine interactions to maintain their relationships. Maintenance behaviors are further distinguished into strategic and routine categories (Duck, 1988). That is, people maintain their relationships both by using approaches they believe will function to sustain their involvements and, through the practices of daily living, by enacting particular routines which become part of the dyad. The next section explores more completely maintenance strategies and routines.

Strategic and Routine Maintenance Behaviors

Communication researchers often study strategies that people use in relationships (e.g., Cody & McLaughlin, 1990). *Strategies* are often understood as approaches used to obtain desired goals, and *tactics* indicate the specific procedures taken to achieve the goal (e.g., Newton & Burgoon, 1990). Accordingly, for purposes of this chapter, we define a strategy as the general approach someone takes to maintain their relationship, whereas tactics refer to the specific behavioral moves that institute the strategy.

We find it useful to distinguish strategic from routine communication. In our view, both types of communication function to achieve goals, but in doing so, routine patterns are less mindful and more habituated. In other words, whereas social actors select different strategies for their functional utility in achieving particular goals, people engage in routine behaviors without concern for achieving particular goals. In addition, routine behaviors occur at a lower level of consciousness (Greene, 1984). People are less mindful of their routines, until those routines become inefficient or otherwise dysfunctional (Langer, 1989). Even when people enact routines at a conscious level, they may do so without attending to the goal such routines serve (Motley, 1986). In short, people probably often engage in routine behaviors that both reflect and affect their relationships until such routines are called into question. When the goal of maintaining their relationship does become salient, people then choose to enact particular strategies. We have attempted first to make sense of the literature on relational maintenance strategies and then to identify the more routine behaviors people perform less consciously which have as a by-product the maintenance of their relationships.

Deriving Proactive and Constructive Strategies

In Stafford and Canary (1991), we surveyed the empirical research on maintenance strategies and found much disparity in terms of definitions and operationalizations. In order to identify the domain of maintenance strategies, we collated published items that operationally defined the strategies. Additionally, a sample of married and dating couples indicated in an open-ended format what they did to maintain their relationships to their satisfaction. Nominated behaviors that were not in the literature were added to those derived from the literature. For example, several participants mentioned that sharing tasks was an important maintenance activity, a type of behavior not found in the published literature. Once the deductively derived and open-ended responses were collated, factor analyses were performed on a separate sample of dating and married participants, which reduced the pool of eighty items into five strategies.

Positivity was the first strategy. This strategy consists of such behaviors as acting cheerful, being courteous and polite in conversation, and avoiding criticism of the partner. Positivity has been associated at moderate levels with all the relational factors and it has been the primary predictor in regression models of control mutuality and liking, as previously mentioned. The second strategy was *openness*. Openness refers to direct discussions about the nature of the relationship and setting aside times for talks about the relationship. *Assurances* was the next strategy and it was composed of items referencing behaviors that imply a future and expressions of love. As mentioned before, assurances has been the primary predictor of commitment in regression analyses. Use of *social networks* was the fourth strategy. It means surrounding the relationship with valued friends and/or family who support the relationship, spending time with one another's family and friends, and similar activity. Other researchers (e.g., Milardo, 1986) have also noted the importance of social networks to a couple's stability. Finally, *sharing tasks* refers to doing a fair share of the household chores, performing responsibilities, and so on. We would have missed this strategy had it not been nominated in the open-ended responses, although other researchers have commented on the importance of sharing tasks to relational satisfaction (e.g., Gottman, this volume; Huston, McHale, & Crouter, 1986; Vangelisti & Huston, this volume; Wilmot & Sillars, 1989).

Do couples consistently report these strategies? This question is important to determine which maintenance activities are part of people's everyday life. To begin answering this question, Canary and Stafford (1993b) asked 165 married couples to indicate the extent to which their spouse enacted each of the five strategies (i.e., positivity, openness, assurances, social networks, and sharing tasks) at three points in time, with each point separated by 3–4 weeks. Couples indicated the extent to which their spouse enacted each of these strategies on 7-point Likert scales, ranging from *strongly agree* (1) and *strongly disagree* (7). The means and medians (and standard deviations) for each of the strategies for the three time points are reported in Table 1.

As Table 1 indicates, both husbands and wives tended to agree that the other spouse enacted each of the maintenance behaviors, although wives perceived significantly less openness and sharing of tasks than the husbands. In addition, correlations computed across each of the time points indicated a moderate level of consistency in reports of strategy use. For wives, the average intercorrelation was .60; for husbands the average intercorrelation was .61. Accordingly, approximately 36% of the variance in perceptions of spouses' maintenance behaviors overlap with previously reported perceptions of the same maintenance behaviors. In short, there appears to be moderate consistency in the extent to which maintenance strategies are perceived.

It is important to note there were several differences between Stafford and Canary's (1991) set of strategies and other sets. In a similar effort, for example, Dindia (1989) factor analyzed items she found in the literature and found three factors: *prosocial, romantic,* and *antisocial* behavior. We did not share in Dindia's discovery of an antisocial strategy, probably because we had a differ-

Table 1

Means, Medians, and Standard Deviations of Reports of Spouses' Maintenance Strategies[a]

Strategy	Husbands' reports			Wives' reports		
	M	Md	SD	M	Md	SD
Positivity 1	2.2	1.9	1.1	2.2	1.9	1.1
Positivity 2	2.2	1.9	1.1	2.2	1.9	1.1
Positivity 3	2.3	2.1	1.2	2.2	1.9	1.1
Openness 1*	2.8	2.6	1.2	3.2	3.0	1.5
Openness 2*	2.7	2.5	1.2	3.2	3.0	1.5
Openness 3	2.9	2.5	3.2	3.1	2.8	1.5
Assurances 1	1.8	1.5	1.0	1.8	1.4	1.0
Assurances 2	1.8	1.5	1.0	1.8	1.5	0.9
Assurances 3	1.9	1.5	1.1	1.8	1.3	1.1
Tasks 1*	1.8	1.4	1.1	2.2	1.7	1.3
Tasks 2*	1.6	1.2	2.0	2.0	1.6	1.2
Tasks 3*	1.8	1.4	1.0	2.2	1.3	1.8
Networks 1	2.8	2.4	1.0	2.9	2.6	1.1
Networks 2	2.8	2.6	1.1	2.9	2.6	1.1
Networks 3	2.9	2.6	1.1	2.9	2.6	1.1

[a]Adapted from Canary and Stafford (1993b); the lower the number the greater the perceived use of each strategy. Tasks = Sharing Tasks; Networks = Social Networks.

*Husband and wife means differ according to paired t tests ($p < .05$).

ent pool of items to begin with. As Guerrero et al. (1993) correctly noted, positivity, openness, assurances, social networks, and sharing tasks are all proactive and constructive maintenance actions. Still, not finding an antisocial strategy through data reduction techniques lead us to question whether our typology was as exhaustive as we first hoped. The answer to this question would probably not be found in a replication of the same procedures (i.e., literature search and factor analysis).

Two decisions were made. First, we decided to sample a variety of relationships, in addition to romantic couples. Stafford and Canary (1991) only sampled romantic couples. We expected that a broader array of strategies would be offered by people in various kinds of personal relationships (i.e., friends, family members, and others in addition to romantic partners). Second, we sought to use an inductive approach, rather than starting with the literature. Inductive analyses of participant responses can reveal information not found in deductive approaches. Also, inductive analyses of open-ended data are relatively unobtrusive (Lolas, 1986) and allow content categories to emerge from the participants' point of view (Viney, 1983).

Inductive Analyses of Strategies and Routines

In this study (Canary, Stafford, Hause, & Wallace, 1993) we arranged for students in multiple section communication courses at two universities to write a paper in which they detailed how they maintained three different personal relationships over the course of the term. Of course, separate from the course requirement, voluntary consent was sought for research purposes. Students addressed the question, "What are the communication behaviors that I use to maintain my various relationships?" To prevent any systematic biases from the literature, students were instructed not to refer to texts or any outside sources but instead to nominate both positive and negative behaviors they in fact used over the course of the term. The students were required to title each behavior and to list these titles on summary sheets. These summary sheets provided the data for the inductive analysis. The research team inspected each of the behaviors from the summary sheets (transferred to index cards). We used the Stafford and Canary (1991) typology as a start, and then we relied on other labels found in the research (to avoid reinventing the wheel). After several passes through the cards, which involved constructing categories and subcategories, the taxonomy reported in Table 2 was derived. Moreover, independent coder agreement was satisfactory at 81% and Cohen's kappa = .80.

Of interest is the scope of behaviors offered by this sample. For example, *joint activities* included such behaviors as "share time together" (e.g., "I spend free time with my Dad"), "routine events and places" (e.g., "We play softball together"), "rituals" (e.g., "We go to church together every Sunday"), and "antirituals" (e.g., "We do things sporadically"). Although joint activities appeared to be nonstrategic, about 45% of the sample indicated these behaviors were used purposefully to maintain their relationships. In terms of their frequency, openness was the most commonly nominated strategy (52.7% mentioned this), with self-disclosure as the most frequently used behavior in that category. In addition to joint activities, assurances was nominated by approximately 45% of the sample. Positivity, cards/letters/calls, and avoidance were listed by approximately 33% of the sample. The strategies of humor, antisocial behavior, social networks, and sharing tasks were infrequently mentioned (i.e., nominated by fewer than 10% of the participants). In addition, several of the strategies varied according to relationship type, as mentioned earlier.

Although the behaviors in Table 2 indicate a variety of maintenance activities and actions, the task of identifying routine behaviors that incidentally function to maintain relationships still needed to be addressed. Toward that end, Dainton and Stafford (1993) asked romantic couples to relate the behaviors they used to maintain their relationships, just as Stafford and Canary

Table 2
Inductively Derived Maintenance Strategies with Examples[a]

Strategy	Example
I. Positivity: Attempts to make interactions pleasant.	
a. Nice and cheerful	"I try to be upbeat and positive around her."
b. Favors	"We do nice favors for each other to show we care."
c. Prosocial behaviors	
1. Proactive	"I act excited to do things even if I am not."
2. Reactive	"I give in a lot to keep her happy."
d. Show affection	"We hold hands and hug a lot."
II. Openness: Direct discussions, offering and listening to one another.	
a. Self-Disclosure	"We share things with each other that no one else knows."
b. Meta-Relational communication	
1. Problems and feelings	"We discuss our problems in the relationship."
2. History	"We often talk about how things used to be."
c. Advice	
1. Advice-Giving	"I try to provide advice through past experience."
2. Advice-Seeking	"I rely on her for advice."
d. Conflict	"When something he does angers me, I let him know."
e. Empathic behavior	"We listen to each other without judging."
III. Assurances: covertly and overtly assuring each other.	
a. Supportiveness	"I encourage his personal achievement and goals."
b. Comfort	"We comfort and stand behind each other."
c. Need satisfaction	"I try to fulfill her need."
d. Overt expressions	"I express an unconditional love for my sister."
IV. Social Networks: Relying on friends and family.	"I try to accept her other friends that I do not know."
V. Sharing Tasks: Performing routine tasks and chores in a relationship.	"We share the cleaning responsibilities."

(*continues*)

Table 2   (*Continued*)

Strategy	Example
VI. Joint Activities: How interactants choose to spend time with one another to maintain their relationship.	
a. Share time together	"We spend time hanging out."
b. Routine events and places	"We like to go to the same bars together."
c. Rituals	"We attend Saturday football games."
d. Anti-Rituals	"Once in a while, as a surprise, I'll take her away for the weekend."
e. Talk time	"We designate time when just the two of us can talk."
f. Occasional visits/road trips	"I visit my brother when he is away at school."
VII. Cards, letters, and calls: Use of various channels to keep contact in relationships.	
a. Cards and letters	"We write letters to each other."
b. Phone calls	"We keep in frequent contact by phone when apart."
c. Combination	"We communicate on the phone and through letters when we are at school."
VIII. Avoidance: Evasion of partner or issues.	
a. Topic avoidance	"I avoid discussing her husband."
b. Person avoidance	"I avoid him."
c. Alternate associations	"We plan separate activities to enjoy time with our friends."
d. Negotiated autonomy	"We respect each other's privacy and need to be alone."
IX. Antisocial: Behaviors which seem unfriendly.	
a. Indirect	"I act moody so he will not want to get closer."
b. Direct	"I am rude to his friends."
X. Humor: Jokes and sarcasm.	
a. Positive	"We have funny nicknames for one another."
b. Negative	"I tease him about his nose."

*a*Adapted from Canary, Stafford, Hause, & Wallace (1993).

(1991) had asked. In addition, however, Dainton and Stafford used the follow-up probe, "Much of maintaining a relationship can involve mundane or routine aspects of day-to-day life. These are things you may not have thought of above because they might seem too trivial. Please try to describe the routine things you do to maintain your relationship."

Dainton and Stafford used the previous literature and Canary et al. (1993) in particular as starting points for naming content categories. Dainton and Stafford's typology of maintenance behaviors that purposefully probed for routine actions included the following categories: positivity, openness, assurances, social networks, sharing tasks, joint activities, talk, mediated communication (calls/letters/cards in Canary et al.), avoidance, antisocial, affection, and focus on self (e.g., keeping in shape). Talk, affection, and focus on self were three additions to the Canary et al. (1993) categories.

Three observations concerning Dainton and Stafford's (1993) study are offered. First, there was a high degree of overlap in the behaviors identified by Canary et al. (1993) and Dainton and Stafford (1993). Likewise, Dainton, Stafford, and McNeilis (1992) found that although most of the categories tended to be reported by participants as more frequently routine or strategic, all of the behaviors were indeed listed in both categories. This overlap suggests that strategic and routine actions may not differ in the *kind* of behavior as much as the *planning* involved in executing the behavior, with strategic behavior requiring more planning. For example, people probably consciously share activities to maintain the relationship and also as part of a daily or weekly routine. In a similar vein, two individuals may engage in shared activities, with one person more conscious than the other about the relational implications (i.e., strategic importance) of doing things together. This example suggests that individual differences in mindfulness affect maintenance behaviors, a possibility that requires future research.

Second, task sharing was more frequently mentioned in the Dainton and Stafford study. This was probably because sharing tasks is more common in romantic dyads (especially marriage) than in the friendships and sibling relationships which were also sampled in the Canary et al. study. Finally, Dainton and Stafford reported several sex differences. In general, women reported greater use of positivity, openness, use of talk, and antisocial behaviors. Married women specifically reported greater use of these strategies and greater use of avoidance, and single women reported a greater use of affection to maintain their romantic relationships. These findings also replicate and extend the results reported by Canary and Stafford (1992, 1993b), who did not hypothesize any sex differences in strategy use but incidentally found weak effects linked to gender.

In sum, our research efforts at discovering strategic and routine maintenance behaviors have led to two sets of typologies. The first set (Stafford & Canary, 1991) was anchored by the literature published through 1989. The second set (Canary et al. 1993; Dainton & Stafford, 1993) reflects participants' accounts of what they view as maintenance strategies and routines, although many of the terms used to label the major categories were also previously represented in the literature.

Future Directions

We conclude this chapter by offering our assessment of future research needs. We believe that future efforts should be directed at continued exploration of routine as well as strategic maintenance behaviors, at combining interactive and noninteractive factors to determine the relative importance of each, and at proceeding systematically with applications of this research so that relational partners may benefit.

We have learned that it is one thing to criticize art and quite another to attempt to paint a portrait. In retrospect, we recognize several shortcomings of our efforts. Some of these shortcomings arise because the research on relational maintenance is relatively new (vs. relational development) and because in these first attempts we relied on survey approaches. Accordingly, the list of behaviors in Table 2 (and the subsequent findings of Dainton and Stafford, 1993) should not be taken as completed works. Nor are the theoretical propositions we offer necessarily complete; instead, we see these as early sketches.

To be sure, we want to use these sketches to study further the link between maintenance activities and relational outcomes. For example, one issue concerns the degree to which each of the 10 supraordinate behaviors presented in Table 2 is associated with interdependence. It appears obvious that sharing tasks, sharing activities, and openness function primarily to increase the extent to which partners are interdependent. But antisocial and avoidance strategies probably work against interdependence, or at least keep partners at a distance. In addition, we hope to collect observational data on couples interacting. Perhaps through role playing their routine conversations, couples may reveal additional microscopic behaviors that serve to sustain the relationship (see also Gottman, 1979; Gottman and Carrère, this volume). Moreover, using observational analyses, we may see how maintenance behaviors occur at the tactical level—that is, how people's general approaches unfold behaviorally and sequentially.

Future research should also be directed at comparing strategies and routines, as well as interactive and noninteractive actions, to determine how these types variously affect relational characteristics. Such efforts would inform us about the relative importance of communication strategies, routines, and noninteractive maintenance behaviors. For example, positivity has been found to be the most significant predictor of control mutuality in three studies (Canary & Stafford, 1992, 1993a; Stafford & Canary, 1991). But these studies did not include measures of sharing activities. It is possible that control mutuality arises as much (if not more) from day-to-day sharing of activities. Also, we do not presuppose that we have identified all the noninteractive factors that compel people to maintain their relationships. Accordingly, future comparisons of interactive and noninteractive factors must include a representative set of noninteractive factors.

Finally, future research should proceed systematically and carefully toward applications. What is said in this text will very likely be applied, if only in the diffusion of information. At some point researchers will come to ask, What should we *do* with this information? Certainly, our own research implies that positivity, sharing tasks, and offering assurances help sustain control mutuality, trust, liking, and commitment. But the findings must be qualified further before they are applied to clinical settings. One qualification is that not all relationships may benefit from these strategies, simply because these strategies would not "work" in them. For example, the transgressed relational partner may find positivity too naive or even ludicrous (see Roloff & Cloven, this volume). Accordingly, an important future direction is to discover under what conditions and in which relational types partners successfully employ maintenance strategies and routines. A second qualification concerns how these strategies are enacted at the relational, or dyadic level. As Fincham and Bradbury (1987) observed, behavior in personal relationships is "less concerned simply with levels of performance than with issues such as affective exchange, collaborations, and commitment" (p. 1117). In other words, we want to study how people respond *in situ* to these maintenance behaviors. Once these issues are explored, then we may offer with greater confidence prescriptions regarding the use of maintenance behaviors.

Maintenance is a useful metaphor. It brings coherence to the study of how communication and relationships are linked. Given the recentness of research explicitly concerned with relational maintenance processes, there are many areas open for research. Insights about the role of communication in relational maintenance will continue to come forth as the result of continued efforts to build theory and conduct research on the topic.

References

Ayres, J. (1983). Strategies to maintain relationships: Their identification and perceived usage. *Communication Quarterly, 31*, 62–67.

Baxter, L. A., & Dindia, K. (1990). Marital partners' perceptions of maintenance strategies. *Journal of Social and Personal Relationships, 7*, 187–209.

Bell, R. A., Daly, J. A., & Gonzalez, C. (1987). Affinity-maintenance in marriage and its relationship to women's marital satisfaction. *Journal of Marriage and the Family, 49*, 445–454.

Braiker, H. B., & Kelley, H. H. (1979). Conflict in the development of close relationships. In R. L. Burgess & T. L. Huston (Eds.), *Social exchange in developing relationships*. New York: Academic Press.

Burgoon, J. K., & Hale, J. L. (1984). The fundamental topoi of relational communication. *Communication Monographs, 51,* 19–41.

Buunk, B., & Bringle, R. G. (1987). Jealousy in love relationships. In D. Perlman & S. Duck (Eds.), *Intimate relationships: Development, dynamics, and deterioration* (pp. 123–147). Newbury Park, CA: Sage.

Canary, D. J., & Stafford, L. (1992). Relational maintenance strategies and equity in marriage. *Communication Monographs, 59,* 239–267.

Canary, D. J., & Stafford, L. (1993a). Preservation of relational characteristics: Maintenance strategies, equity, and locus of control. In P. J. Kalbfleisch (Ed.), *Interpersonal communication: Evolving interpersonal relationships* (pp. 237–259). Hillsdale, NJ: Lawrence Erlbaum.

Canary, D. J., & Stafford, L. (1993b). Continuity of maintenance strategies and relational characteristics. Unpublished manuscript, School of Interpersonal Communication, Ohio University.

Canary, D. J., Stafford, L., Hause, K. S., & Wallace, L. A. (1993). An inductive analysis of relational maintenance strategies: A comparison among lovers, relatives, friends, and others. *Communication Research Reports, 10,* 5–14.

Canary, D. J., Weger, H., Jr., & Stafford, L. (1991). Couples' argument sequences and their associations with relational characteristics. *Western Journal of Speech Communication, 55,* 159–179.

Cody, M. J., & McLaughlin, M. L. (1990). *The psychology of tactical communication.* New Clevendon, England: Multilingual Matters.

Courtright, J. A., Millar, F. E., & Rogers-Millar, L. E. (1979). Domineeringness and dominance: Replication and extension. *Communication Monographs, 46,* 179–192.

Dainton, M., & Stafford, L. (1993). Routine maintenance behaviors: A comparison of relationship type, partner similarity and sex differences. *Journal of Social and Personal Relationships, 10,* 255–271.

Dainton, M., Stafford, L., & McNeilis, K. S. (1992, November). *The maintenance of relationships through routine behavior.* Paper presented at the Speech Communication Association convention, Chicago.

Dickens, W. J., & Perlman, D. (1981). Friendship over the life-cycle. In S. Duck & R. Gilmour (Eds.), *Personal relationships: Vol. 2. Developing personal relationships* (pp. 91–122). New York: Academic Press.

Dindia, K. (1989, May). *Toward the development of a measure of marital maintenance strategies.* Paper presented at the International Communication Association conference, San Francisco.

Dindia, K., & Baxter, L. A. (1987). Strategies for maintaining and repairing marital relationships. *Journal of Social and Personal Relationships, 4,* 143–158.

Dindia, K., & Canary, D. J. (1993). Definitions and theoretical perspectives on relational maintenance. *Journal of Social and Personal Relationships, 10,* 163–173.

Duck, S. W. (1988). *Relating to others.* Chicago: Dorsey.

Fincham, F. D., & Bradbury, T. N. (1987). Cognitive processes and conflict in close relationships: An attribution-efficacy model. *Journal of Personality and Social Psychology, 53,* 1106–1118.

Fitzpatrick, M. A. (1988). *Between husbands and wives: Communication in marriage.* Newbury Park, CA: Sage.

Gottman, J. M. (1979). *Marital interaction.* New York: Academic Press.

Greene, J. O. (1984). A cognitive approach to human communication: An action assembly theory. *Communication Monographs, 51,* 289–306.

Guerrero, L. K., Eloy, S. V., & Wabnik, A. L. (1993). Linking maintenance strategies to relationship development and disengagement: A reconceptualization. *Journal of Social and Personal Relationships, 10,* 273–283.

Hatfield, E., Traupmann, J., Sprecher, S., Utne, M., & Hay, J. (1985). Equity and intimate relationships: Recent research. I. W. Ickes (Ed.), *Compatible and incompatible relationships* (pp. 91–117). New York: Springer-Verlag.

Huston, T. L., McHale, S., & Crouter, A. (1986). When the honeymoon's over: Changes in the marriage relationship over the first year. In R. Gilmour & S. Duck (Eds.), *The emerging field of personal relationships* (pp. 109–132). Hillsdale, NJ: Lawrence Erlbaum.

Huston, T. L., Surra, C., Fitzgerald, N. M., & Cate, R. (1981). From courtship to marriage: Mate selection as an interpersonal process. In S. Duck & R. Gilmour (Eds.), *Personal relationships: Vol. 2. Developing personal relationships* (pp. 53–88). New York: Academic Press.

Johnson-George, C., & Swap, W. C. (1982). Measurement of specific interpersonal trust: Construction and validation of a scale to assess trust in a specific other. *Journal of Personality and Social Psychology, 43*, 1306–1317.

Kelley, H. H. (1979). *Personal relationships: Their structure and processes.* Hillsdale, NJ: Lawrence Erlbaum.

Langer, E. J. (1989). *Mindfulness.* Reading, MA: Addison-Wesley.

Larzelere, R. E., & Huston, T. L. (1980). The dyadic trust scale: Toward understanding interpersonal trust in close relationships. *Journal of Marriage and the Family, 42*, 595–604.

Lolas, F. (1986). Behavioral text and psychological context: On pragmatic verbal and behavior analysis. In L. A. Gottschalk, F. Lolas, & L. L. Viney (Eds.), *Content and analysis of verbal behavior.* Berlin: Springer-Verlag.

Lund, M. (1985). The development of investment and commitment scales for predicting continuity of personal relationships. *Journal of Social and Personal Relationships, 2*, 3–23.

Milardo, R. M. (1986). Personal choice and social constraint in close relationships: Application of network analysis. In V. J. Derlega & B. A. Winstead (Eds.), *Friendship and social interaction* (pp. 145–166). New York: Springer-Verlag.

Millar, F. E., & Rogers, L. E. (1987). Relational dimensions of interpersonal dynamics. In M. E. Roloff & G. R. Miller (Eds.), *Interpersonal processes: New directions in communication research* (pp. 117–139). Newbury Park, CA: Sage.

Mills, J., & Clark, M. S. (1982). Exchange and communal relationships. In L. Wheeler (Ed.), *Review of personality and social psychology* (pp. 121–144). Beverly Hills, CA: Sage.

Morton, T. C., Alexander, J. F., & Altman, I. (1976). Communication and relationship definition. In G. R. Miller (Ed.), *Explorations in the interpersonal communication* (pp. 105–126). Beverly Hills, CA: Sage.

Motley, M. T. (1986). Consciousness and intention in communication: A preliminary model and methodological approaches. *Western Journal of Speech Communication, 50*, 3–23.

Newton, D. A., & Burgoon, J. K. (1990). Nonverbal conflict behaviors: Functions, strategies, and tactics. In D. D. Cahn (Ed.), *Intimates in conflict: A communication perspective* (pp. 77–104). Hillsdale, NJ: Lawrence Erlbaum.

Prins, K. S., Buunk, B. P., & VanYperen, N. W. (1993). Equity, normative disapproval, and extramarital relationships. *Journal of Social and Personal Relationships, 10*, 39–53.

Rempel, J. J., Holmes, J. G., & Zanna, M. P. (1985). Trust in close relationships. *Journal of Personality and Social Psychology, 49*, 95–112.

Roloff, M. E. (1987). Communication and reciprocity within intimate relationships. In M. E. Roloff & G. R. Miller (Eds.), *Interpersonal processes: New directions in communication research* (pp. 11–38). Newbury Park, CA: Sage.

Rubin, Z. (1979). *Liking and loving.* New York: Holt, Rinehart, & Winston.

Sabatelli, R. M., & Cecil-Pigo, E. F. (1985). Relational interdependence and commitment in marriage. *Journal of Marriage and the Family, 47*, 931–937.

Sprecher, S. (1986). The relation between equity and emotions in close relationships. *Social Psychology Bulletin, 49*, 309–321.

Stafford, L., & Canary, D. J. (1991). Maintenance strategies and romantic relationship type, gender, and relational characteristics. *Journal of Social and Personal Relationships, 8,* 217–242.

Van Yperen, N. W., & Buunk, B. P. (1990). A longitudinal study of equity and satisfaction in intimate relationships. *European Journal of Social Psychology, 20,* 287–309.

Viney, L. L. (1983). The assessment of psychological states through content analysis of verbal communications. *Psychological Bulletin, 94,* 542–563.

Walster (Hatfield), E., Berscheid, E., & Walster, G. W. (1983). New directions in equity research. *Journal of Personality and Social Psychology, 25,* 151–176.

Wilmot, W. W., & Sillars, A. L. (1989). Developmental issues in personal relationships. In J. F. Nussbaum (Ed.), *Life-span communication: Normative processes* (pp. 119–135). Hillsdale, NJ: Lawrence Erlbaum.

Witteman, H., & Fitzpatrick, M. A. (1986). Compliance-gaining in marital interaction: Power bases, processes, and outcomes. *Communication Monographs, 53,* 130–143.

When Partners Transgress

Maintaining Violated Relationships

Michael E. Roloff

Department of Communication Studies
Northwestern University
Evanston, Illinois

Denise H. Cloven

Department of Communication Arts
University of Wisconsin, Madison
Madison, Wisconsin

Introduction

Intimate relationships are important sources of emotional, psychological, and physical well-being (Burman & Margolin, 1992; Wood, Rhodes, & Whelan, 1989). However, these associations have a dark side as well. For example, diaries kept by spouses indicate that intimates enact displeasurable instrumental and emotional behaviors toward one another on a daily basis (Wills, Weiss, & Patterson, 1974). In fact, even generally happy marriages are not immune from such problematic actions (Birchler, Weiss, & Vincent, 1975; Kirchler, 1988). Beyond experiencing mere irritations, intimate relationships are more likely to be physically and psychologically abusive than are less intimate associations (Larner & Thompson, 1982; Mason & Blankenship, 1987; Roscoe & Benaske, 1986; Stets & Pirog-Good, 1987, 1990). Indeed, a majority of individuals in abusive relationships report that aggression did not start until after they became seriously involved (Cate, Henton,

Koval, Christopher, & Lloyd, 1982; Gryl, Stith, & Bird, 1991; Henton, Cate, Koval, Lloyd, & Christopher, 1983).

The occurrence of negative intimate behavior can raise serious challenges for participants in interpersonal relationships. Not surprisingly, a spouse's displeasurable behavior is negatively related to daily marital satisfaction (Wills et al., 1974), particularly among couples who are chronically distressed (Jacobson, Follette, & McDonald, 1982; Jacobson, Waldron, & Moore, 1980). Similarly, the frequency with which a spouse is perceived to engage in provocative behavior adversely impacts a partner's marital satisfaction (Smolen, Spiegel, Bakker-Rabdau, Bakker, & Martin, 1985; Smolen, Spiegel, & Martin, 1986). Thus, negative behaviors both characterize intimate associations and are implicated in the erosion of satisfaction within those relationships.

In light of the prevalence and effect of negative behavior, scholars of interpersonal relationships should be motivated to identify how intimates maintain their relationships in the face of the inevitable hurtful and provocative behavior that occurs. Accordingly, this chapter reviews and critiques extant research focused on behaviors enacted in response to relational transgressions. Notably, most of the research in this area is not based on a "relational maintenance" perspective, nor is this label frequently found in the literature. Consequently, our synthesis views this scholarship from an alternative perspective. In doing so, we first explicate the concepts of relational conflict, transgression, and maintenance. Then, we discuss a variety of maintenance approaches for handling relational transgressions. Finally, several directions for future research are described.

Relational Conflict

Deutsch (1973) conceives of conflict as the existence of incompatible activity wherein the behaviors of one individual in a relationship prevent, obstruct, or make less likely or effective the behaviors of the other. Clearly, this definition is broadly cast, and indeed must be to capture the range of situations that people normally characterize as conflicts. Hence, this section explicates Deutsch's perspective to advance a definition of relational conflict.

Appropriately, Deutsch's definition does not identify any particular causes of incompatibility within interpersonal relationships. Passer, Kelley, and Michela (1978) found that the causes of a spouse's negative behavior are perceived to vary in the extent to which they (1) reflect a positive or negative attitude toward the partner, (2) are intentionally or unintentionally enacted, and (3) are due to the spouse's traits or to circumstances. Furthermore, Pinkley (1990) reports that accounts of everyday conflicts are perceived to vary on three dimensions: (1) whether the conflict is relational or task oriented, (2) the degree to which the conflict is focused on emotional or intellectual issues, and (3) the extent to which the conflict needs to be resolved through compromise or through competition. Thus, relational conflict is not restricted to conflicts arising from any particular source or conflicts associated with any particular issue or outcome.

This perspective on relational conflict also does not assume that conflict is inherently discussed by relational partners. Whereas some definitions of interpersonal conflict focus on the interactions through which partners negotiate goal incompatibility (e.g., Hocker & Wilmot, 1991), relational conflict can exist independent of such overt interaction. In fact, Roloff and Cloven (1990) found that dating partners do not express to each other roughly 40% of their relational grievances. Similarly, Baumeister, Stillwell, and Wotman (1990) discovered that 44% of victims of an anger-provoking incident reported that they withheld overt expression of their anger. Thus, the primary characteristic defining relational conflict is the occurrence of incompatible actions.

Although relational conflict is not limited to particular interpersonal contexts or causes, goal incompatibility has the potential for greater intensity as relational intimacy grows. Altman and Taylor (1973) speculate that intimate partners are more interdependent than nonintimates, which makes intimate conflict inevitable and often serious. Indeed, people report that their intimate relationships involve greater criticism and emotional conflict than is experienced in their less intimate associations (Argyle & Furnham, 1983). Given the association between conflict and dissatisfaction noted previously, this reasoning implies that intimate relationships are endangered entities.

However, one should not assume that all conflicts threaten the continuance of an intimate relationship. Coser (1956, pp. 73–74) argues that only conflicts over the fundamental basis of a relationship are sufficiently disruptive to endanger the association. He notes:

> Conflicts arising within the same consensual framework are likely to have a very different impact upon the relationship than those which put the basic consensus into question. Thus, within a marriage relation, a conflict on whether or not to have children involves the basic consensual agreement about the very purposes of the relationships. One may expect that this type of conflict will presumably have a more profound impact on the relationship than a conflict over particular plans to spend a vacation or to allocate the budget.

Although Coser's examples portray a somewhat archaic and restricted view of the purpose of marriage, his essential argument is compelling: Conflicts that call into question the fundamental understandings that guide a relationship are especially damaging. In our view, such incompatibilities constitute a relational transgression.

Relational Transgression

Our notion of *relational transgression* assumes that individuals have some conceptions about relational activities and purposes that embody or define their associations. The violation of these central views, then, calls into question the viability and desirability of staying in a given relationship. Hence, in our view, these violations constitute relational transgressions. To develop our perspective, this section discusses the various effects of such violations in close associations.

We recognize that relational understandings vary across individuals and cultures; however, researchers have identified a number of rules that illustrate how transgressions can cause the breakdown of a relationship. For example, many but not all married couples believe in a rule that specifies sexual monogamy (e.g., Blumstein & Schwartz, 1983). Not surprisingly, then, extramarital relations frequently appear in the accounts of why marriages ended in divorces (Kitson & Sussman, 1982; Spanier & Margolis, 1983). Moreover, Baxter (1986) analyzed the accounts of how 157 dating relationships ended and from them identified eight primary relational rules that were broken: (1) autonomy, (2) similarity display, (3) supportiveness, (4) openness, (5) loyalty/fidelity, (6) shared time, (7) equity, and (8) romance. Similarly, Argyle and Henderson (1984) interviewed 156 individuals about failed friendships and their analysis yielded nine violated rules: (1) not being jealous or critical of other relationships, (2) keeping confidences, (3) being tolerant of friends, (4) not criticizing the friend in public, (5) trusting and confiding, (6) volunteering help in time of need, (7) showing positive regard, (8) standing up for the friend in his/her absence, and (9) giving emotional support. Thus, the violation of central relational rules is implicated in the dissolution of intimate relationships.

Although relational transgressions appear to cause the breakup of relationships, it does not automatically follow that a single violation is sufficient to end a relationship. However, in some cases, an action so clearly violates a relational partner's personally important rule that it alone is sufficient to damage the relationship. For example, Davis and Todd (1985) found that 87% of a sample of individuals with former friends reported that a friendship was terminated because of a relational violation. Similarly, Knapp, Stafford, and Daly (1986) found that 20% of a sample of individuals who regretted having said something did so because their statement harmed their relationships.

In other instances, a disagreeable behavior must be repeated and/or occur in conjunction with other provocations before it is judged to be a relational transgression that threatens the association. Accordingly, Baxter (1984) found that the decision to exit from a dating relationship more frequently resulted from an incremental increase in relational problems, rather than from a single critical incident of major magnitude. Indeed, most individuals who are angry with someone report that the anger-provoking behaviors have been occurring for quite some time and are part of a pattern of multiple provocations (Baumeister et al., 1990). Hence, these findings suggest that intimates can tolerate a degree of conflict, and relationships become threatened only when some threshold of negative experience is surpassed.

The imperfect association between relational transgressions and breakdown could stem from the indefinite nature of relational conceptions. Given that relational rules are often stated at a high level of abstraction (e.g., intimates should be supportive), it is possible that under appropriate circumstances almost any conflict has the potential to be viewed as a relational transgression. Consistent with this view, individuals in chronically distressed marriages appear to be highly reactive to their spouse's negative behaviors (Jacobson et al., 1980), and perhaps are more likely to see any contrary action as being a relational transgression. Conversely, individuals may be able to reduce the degree to which a partner's behaviors violate fundamental relational rules. Hence, we believe that intimates often enact relational maintenance behaviors to limit the damage caused by either their own or their partner's behavior.

Relational Maintenance

From our perspective, *relational maintenance* involves the individual or joint approaches intimates take to limit the relational harm that may result from prior or future conflicts and transgressions. This definition has six important components.

First, relational maintenance may be enacted individually or jointly. This implies that intimates may act alone without letting their partners know that maintenance behavior is being enacted. Indeed, we speculate that intimates often try to cope with their partners' negative behavior prior to confrontation. For example, Lee (1984) found that some intimates delay confronting their partners with their complaints for extended periods even after they have

become dissatisfied with the relationship. Alternatively, relational maintenance may involve the joint action of partners that ensues when individuals
confront partners about transgressions.

Second, we mean relational maintenance "approaches" to encompass both
covert and overt maintenance behavior. Cloven and Roloff (1991) found that
the degree of intrapersonal mulling an individual did about a conflict, in
conjunction with the character of the interaction they had with their partner
about the issue, influenced their sense of the seriousness of the problem and
who was to blame. Hence, it is important that we focus on maintenance as it
occurs in both thought and talk.

Third, the goal of relational maintenance is to limit relational harm. Relational damage may take a variety of forms. In some cases, the partners try to
prevent their conflicts from affecting the quality of their relationship through
reduced levels of trust, love, or support. In the extreme, maintenance is
enacted to prevent the immediate dissolution of the association. Thus, relational maintenance approaches are intended to reduce a variety of potentially
negative effects associated with relational conflict.

Notably, relational maintenance is not focused on reducing the *personal*
distress that may be associated with a partner's negative behaviors. Although a
number of strategies to cope with both social and nonsocial sources of personal stress have been identified in prior research (Pearlin & Schooler, 1978),
our perspective emphasizes those approaches individuals take to maintain
their *relationships* in the face of possible transgressions. In fact, we recognize
that efforts to limit the negative relational ramifications of conflicts may
sometimes produce or exacerbate personal distress (cf. Gelles & Straus,
1988).

Fourth, we note that relational maintenance may be enacted proactively
and reactively. When individuals anticipate that their behaviors might be
interpreted as transgressions, they may try to reduce damages prior to their
partners' becoming aware of any conflicts. Conversely, once a conflict has
been perceived as a relational transgression, relational repair may be necessary and relational maintenance becomes focused on damage control.

Fifth, our definition of relational maintenance is exclusively focused on
limiting the damage produced by conflicts and transgressions. Indeed, this
aspect differentiates our perspective from other conceptions of relational
maintenance. For example, Dindia and Baxter (1987, p. 144) conceive of
relational maintenance as "an effort to continue the present state without
anything necessarily going wrong." Accordingly, they derived maintenance
strategies by asking individuals what they do to keep their relationship from
going downhill. Similarly, Stafford and Canary (1991) identified a variety of
strategies employed by individuals in romantic relationships to "maintain a

satisfactory relationship." Because the health of a relationship may be adversely affected by a variety of factors including conflict, our definition to some extent overlaps with this earlier work. In actuality, however, our approach may have greater commonality with Dindia and Baxter's notion of relational repair, which involves correcting something in the relationship that has gone awry.

Finally, we mean relational maintenance approaches to encompass clusters of behaviors that appear to serve the purpose of maintaining the relationship by accomplishing other ends. We chose to use the term "approach" rather than the more common label "strategy" to acknowledge that some of the maintenance behaviors may not be enacted with sufficient self-awareness so that individuals understand the dynamics of the particular approach. Hence, individuals may engage in behaviors that cause them to minimize the extent of their problems, but may not *choose* to enact such behaviors with the *explicit* goal of minimization. In our view, a definition of relational maintenance should encompass both forms of action.

In total, we advance a relatively broad conception of relational maintenance. In particular, our perspective includes individual or joint actions, covert and overt behaviors, proactive and reactive approaches, and explicitly or implicitly goal-directed action oriented toward limiting any form of relational damage associated with interpersonal conflict. However, thus far we have not addressed the core issue of what approaches intimates take when trying to maintain their violated relationships; therefore, the following section explores this question.

Relational Maintenance Approaches

As noted at the outset, research has not directly addressed the issue of how intimates try to prevent their conflicts from damaging their relationships. However, scholars have examined how individuals respond to disputes, and one can infer approaches to relational maintenance from these reports. Again, we note that maintenance approaches focus on preserving relationships, and may not otherwise benefit the individuals involved. Moreover, we do not intend to advocate any particular response to relational transgressions. Rather, this section discusses approaches implied in extant literature as instrumental in the maintenance of transgressed relationships. In particular, we describe five relational maintenance approaches: (1) retribution, (2) reformulation, (3) prevention, (4) minimization, and (5) relational justification.

Retribution

Felson (1984) defines retribution as the desire of an individual to see misbehavior punished. This desire may stem from either the loss of face that often is reported by the victims of relational inequities (Schafer, Keith, & Lorenz, 1984), or negative norms of reciprocity (e.g., "an eye for an eye," Foa & Foa, 1974). Not surprisingly, when individuals retaliate in a manner similar to that in which they were harmed, there is a reduction in hostility toward their transgressors (Donnenwerth & Foa, 1974).

Although retribution might be a motive more commonly expected after a relationship has been terminated, there is evidence that retribution occurs on a limited basis in ongoing intimate relations. For example, White (1980) found that some individuals who admitted trying to make their dating partners jealous did so out of a desire for revenge (10%) and punishment (1%). Similarly, Muehlenhard and Hollabaugh (1988) discovered that among females who denied their male dating partner's request for sex, 36% did so because they were angry with him. In addition, Bowman (1990) identified a set of behaviors including criticism, sarcasm, and revenge as one of five methods of coping with recurrent marital problems. Finally, Briere (1987) discovered that among a sample of college males, 75% indicated that they were at least somewhat likely to batter a wife if she had sex with another man, and 65% reported they were somewhat likely to batter a wife who told her friends that he was sexually pathetic. Thus, intimates are clearly willing to use retribution even within ongoing relationships.

Retribution may also affect the behavior of individuals who have transgressed. To avoid retribution, transgressors may express apologies, self-blame, or offers of compensation to their victims, particularly when their negative behaviors were accidental or due to their negligence (Gonzales, Manning, & Haugen, 1992). Presumably, such penitence restores a sense of justice to the relationship that would make revenge unnecessary and unjustified (O'Malley & Greenberg, 1983).

Despite this evidence, the effectiveness of retribution as a relational maintenance approach has not been addressed in prior work. Although speculative, we believe this approach could run the risk of conflict escalation, particularly when the transgressor believes the partner's retribution is excessive and itself warrants retribution. For example, Baumeister et al. (1990) found that individuals who have been confronted by another who is angry about their behavior tend to see the other's anger as both unjustified and an overreaction. Furthermore, the use of such conflictual coping behaviors has been associated with decreased relational satisfaction and perceptions of greater problem severity (Bowman, 1990). Hence, retribution is implicated as a relational maintenance approach, but one that could risk continued and/or escalated relational conflict.

Reformulation

Reformulation involves changing the nature of the relational understanding so that a given negative behavior no longer constitutes a transgression. This response does not prevent the behavior from occurring but simply redefines relational rules so that the behavior is less harmful or no longer violates the relational contract.

This approach is apparent in the behavior of individuals in sexually open relationships. In particular, Blumstein and Schwartz (1983) identified three sets of rules that couples develop to prevent extrarelational involvements from damaging their associations. One set of rules was aimed at preventing extrarelational activities from disrupting daily lives (e.g., don't be late to dinner, never spend money on other partners, practice safe sex). A second group was designed to keep affairs discrete (e.g., not letting significant others know about outside involvements). Finally, a third cluster of rules placed limits on emotional entanglements (e.g., never become involved with a mutual friend, never give out phone number, never see the same person twice). Thus, these couples designed relational rules such that extrarelational involvement in and of itself was not a relational transgression.

In a similar way, partners may formulate rules to limit the damage done during their arguments. Often people regret the direct attacks and criticisms they inflict on loved ones (Knapp et al., 1986). One response is to develop rules that keep arguments on an even keel. Accordingly, Jones and Gallois (1989) identified five clusters of conflict rules from the accounts of spouses: (1) be considerate, (2) be rational, (3) be specific, (4) try to resolve the dispute, and (5) keep the interaction positive. Again, these rules are designed to keep potentially negative behaviors from harming the relationship.

As with retribution, the effectiveness of reformulation as a relational maintenance approach is unclear, and we have reason to believe this approach could be problematic. In particular, reformulation does not stop a particular behavior (e.g., extrarelational affairs or arguing), but simply tries to eliminate its more objectionable features. For some, the behavior may be unacceptable regardless of modifications (e.g., extramarital affairs are viewed as inherently immoral). Moreover, new rules may be violated just as easily as the originals, especially given that the undesirable features of certain behaviors may be quite difficult to control. For example, arguments by their nature appear to be more negative and less supportive than other forms of communication (Resick et al., 1981); therefore, these behaviors may not be easily modified.

Thus, reformulation constitutes a second potentially ineffective relational maintenance approach.

Prevention

Prevention is a relational maintenance approach directed toward ensuring that there are no future occurrences of a transgression. Unlike reformulation, a prevention approach maintains that certain behaviors are illegitimate and attempts to eradicate such actions.

A variety of prevention strategies are indicated in extant research. For example, Gelles and Straus (1988) interviewed abused wives about the long-term strategies they employed to prevent their husbands' future violence. Regardless of the severity of the violence, the most frequent strategy was to avoid the husband or to avoid talking with him about certain topics (see also Cloven & Roloff, 1993). Women who used this strategy reported it as active and exhausting, as they tried to anticipate circumstances in which the husband might become violent. Other strategies included trying to talk the husband out of being aggressive, getting him to promise to stop, threatening to get a divorce, physically fighting back, hiding, threatening to call the police, and leaving the home for 2 or more days. Hence, these responses suggest that whereas some victims take the burden of prevention on themselves by trying to avoid behaviors that might provoke a negative response, others confront the transgressor or call on the assistance of others. In each case, the goal of the victim's action is to prevent future negative episodes.

As might be expected, prevention strategies vary considerably in effectiveness. After examining the costs and benefits of each strategy reported by the abused wives, Gelles and Straus (1988) concluded that the most effective prevention approach was to get the abusive husband to promise to stop being violent and to demand that he do so after the first incident. Delayed or covert reactions such as avoidance appeared to be far less effective. Similarly, a longitudinal study by Menaghan (1982) discovered that couples who initially attempted to cope with relational difficulties through negotiation reported fewer relational problems 4 years later. In comparison, less confrontational coping devices (e.g., ignoring problems or resigning oneself to them) increased marital distress, which in turn reduced the ability to control subsequent relational problems (Menaghan, 1982).

Because the work of both Gelles and Straus, and Menaghan is based on self-reports, we are reluctant to conclude that confrontation is always effective. However, preliminary evidence suggests confrontative preventive approaches may be superior to some forms of avoidance (Cloven & Roloff, 1991, in press). Indeed, regardless of whether such approaches are actually effective in reducing negative behaviors, it is clear that abused wives who stay with their husbands are more likely to do so because the husband promised to end the violence (Strube & Barbour, 1984).

Minimization

Minimization is an attempt to recast a conflict so that it is no longer a threat to the relationship. Whereas prevention is directed toward eliminating future conflicts and reformulation tries to eradicate their negative aspects, minimization does not alter the form of negative behaviors. Instead, the goal of minimization is to reduce the significance of a relational conflict within an association.

At least two forms of minimization seem to be employed in close relationships. First, the victim of a transgression may come to accept the blame for the problem, rather than attribute the relational conflict to the transgressor (e.g., Bowman, 1990). By doing so, an individual may be able to avoid seeing the transgressor and the relationship in a negative light. Consistent with this view, Andrews and Brewin (1990) found that abused wives who continued to live with their violent husbands blamed themselves more for the abuse than did abused wives who had left their husbands. Moreover, Herbert, Silver, and Ellard (1991) also found similar attributional patterns among abused wives. Neither the veracity of the attributions of the women sampled nor the direction of causal processes was addressed in these efforts; however, these findings imply that minimization may serve to keep an individual in a relationship.

A second form of minimization concerns perceptions of the frequency or severity of conflict. In particular, intimates may minimize relational conflicts by judging them to be relatively infrequent and not especially severe. For example, Bowman (1990) found that coping efforts in marital relationships included a group of behaviors involving denial or the suppression of negative feelings. In fact, although the use of such coping responses was negatively correlated with marital happiness, Bowman (1990) found that such minimization techniques were reported with greater frequency in marriages of longer durations. Moreover, Herbert et al. (1991) reported that abused wives who remained with their husbands were more likely than those who left their husbands to report that the abuse was not frequent or severe. Again, this evidence is merely correlational and based on self-reports; however, it does imply that relational partners may minimize their problems in a manner that allows the continuation of the relationships.

Notably, either of the minimization approaches to relational maintenance could be promoted by the transgressor, rather than by the victim. For example, transgressors may justify their behavior by downplaying negative effects, blaming the victim, stressing positive motives, or even fabricating supporting evidence (Gonzales et al., 1992). Thus, partners may "collude" to limit the potential damage created by relational conflict.

In evaluating minimization as a relational maintenance approach, one must keep in mind that the goals of these approaches is to limit the *relational* harm associated with negative behaviors. Hence, because the results previously described suggest that both forms of minimization are associated with maintained rather than dissolved relationships, minimization approaches appear to be somewhat effective. We recognize, however, that such strategies may result in ongoing commitment to a relationship that may be personally threatening. Moreover, because minimization does not result in cessation of the negative behaviors, the long term-effectiveness of this approach may be questionable.

Relational Justification

Relational justification, the fifth and final relational maintenance approach, is defined by a focus on the reasons for staying in the relationship. Thus, this approach ignores a transgression by shifting attention to motivations for remaining committed to the association. We believe justifications for continuing violated relationships could be threefold.

First, intimates may focus on beneficial aspects of the relationship. In fact, Bowman (1990) discovered that focusing on good memories, expressing positive affections, and initiating shared experiences comprised a prevalent strategy for coping with marital difficulties. Furthermore, Herbert et al. (1991) found that abused wives who stayed with their husbands were more likely to view their marriage as being better than most, and less likely to see their husbands' positive behavior as manipulative when compared to women who had separated from abusive husbands. Similarly, studies of abused wives have found that some women stay with their husbands because of love (Strube & Barbour, 1983, 1984), and 26% to 29% of dating abuse victims interpret violent behaviors as a sign of love (Cate et al., 1982; Henton et al., 1983). Moreover, 85% of a sample of dating college students reported that relationships either stayed the same or improved as a result of physical violence (Gryl et al., 1991). Hence, individuals appear to emphasize either rewards in a relationship or the rewarding aspects of negative action to justify maintaining a relationship.

A second focus of relational justification approaches to maintenance may emphasize the perceived obligations within a relationship. For example, a study of unhappily married couples who had been together 15 years or more revealed that the primary reasons for keeping such marriages intact included beliefs that marriage is a long-term commitment, marriage is sacred, and enduring marriages are central to a stable society (Lauer & Lauer, 1987). Not surprisingly, 47% of these couples reported they stayed together because of their children (see also Heaton & Albrecht, 1991). These responses suggest that some people may endure unhappy relations not because of the benefits to themselves, but because of the obligations they feel toward others (see also Attridge, this volume).

Finally, intimates may justify relational maintenance through a focus on the absence of alternatives. Strube and Barbour (1984) found that abused wives were more likely to remain with their husbands if the wife was unemployed, feared economic hardship from separation, and felt that she had nowhere else to go. In fact, relational alternatives have been found to play a central role in an individual's decisions about how to respond to a variety of relational dissatisfactions (Cloven & Roloff, 1993; Roloff & Cloven, 1990; Rusbult, 1987; Rusbult, Johnson, & Morrow, 1986; Rusbult, Verette, Whitney, Slovik, & Lipkus, 1991; Rusbult, Zembrodt, & Gunn, 1982). Apparently, in some situations, the individual feels entrapped in the relationship and may become resigned to accommodate negative behaviors.

Once again, little research has examined the effectiveness of relational justification as a maintenance approach. Focusing on positive aspects of relationships has been associated with lower levels of relational distress, greater satisfaction, decreased problem severity, and/or fewer later problems (Bowman, 1990; Menaghan, 1982, 1983); however, the role of the remaining justifications for staying in violated relationships has not been directly examined. As with some of the other relational maintenance approaches, justification does not attempt to eradicate the negative behaviors producing conflict. Thus, although this approach may promote the continuation of some relationships, positive long-term and personal outcomes could be limited.

To summarize, intimates take a variety of approaches to maintaining their relationships when faced with relational conflicts. Indeed, during the course of a relationship, individuals may enact multiple maintenance approaches until they either find an effective approach or combination of approaches, or give up on the relationship altogether. Consistent with this view, Strube and Barbour (1984) found that abused wives who left their husbands reported having first tried a variety of coping devices. Thus, people may use a variety of relational maintenance approaches, alone or in combination, and discontinue their associations only if these attempts fail to reconcile the relationships and their inherent conflicts.

Directions for Research

The relative lack of research directly addressing relational transgression and maintenance leaves open a wide variety of research needs. In particular, we see at least four primary directions for further study: (1) verifying the maintenance approaches, (2) addressing unit of analysis issues, (3) identifying determinants of approaches, and (4) evaluating the effectiveness of the different approaches. This section describes each of these directions in greater detail.

Verification of Relational Maintenance Approaches

Clearly, researchers need to verify the existence of the relational maintenance approaches we advance and to identify others not anticipated. Although we relied on the accounts of respondents in other studies, our secondary analysis may be incomplete. Moreover, this literature lacks a comprehensive empirical examination of the approaches individuals use to maintain associations in the face of relational transgressions. Thus, such investigations are warranted.

However, we caution that researchers must be mindful of two problems that have plagued similar attempts in other research areas. First, we must recognize the influence of context on both the particular approaches that might be adopted and their behavioral manifestations. For example, our review noted evidence that individuals use reformulation when dealing with extrarelational sexual involvements; however, we found no evidence of this approach among victims of abuse. Indeed, it is difficult to imagine how individuals might create rules that would make physical aggression less damaging. Thus, if the goal is to establish general relational maintenance approaches, researchers will need to explore a wide variety of transgressive situations.

Second, researchers need to remain aware that the establishment of valid measures of relational maintenance approaches does not substitute for the development of theoretical frameworks for explaining and predicting their use and effects. Too often, methodological and psychometric zeal diverts attention from the construction of theoretical perspectives and results in disjointed research findings. Therefore we advocate the verification of approaches to maintaining violated relationships within a theoretical perspective incorporating the conditions promoting these responses and the associated outcomes.

Unit of Analysis

In our discussion of relational maintenance approaches, we intentionally left ambiguous the unit of analysis. By doing so, we hoped to avoid prematurely truncating the range of relevant levels at which maintenance behavior could be examined. In fact, we believe that research employing a variety of units of analysis could be enlightening.

For example, researchers might focus on the maintenance approaches taken by either an individual or by the dyad forming the relationship. On the one hand, examining individual actions could provide insight into both the overt and covert approaches that people employ when partners transgress. Alternatively, focusing on the dyad incorporates the approaches taken by both partners. Indeed, more importantly, a dyadic analysis would emphasize the way relational maintenance approaches are derived and modified as partners interact with one another. Hence, whereas the former perspective highlights the responses of one individual, the latter addresses the degree to which the maintenance strategies of one partner are stimulated, reinforced, and perhaps altered by those of the other.

In addition, a theoretical framework for explaining relational maintenance approaches and outcomes would benefit from investigations of maintenance approaches at both micro and macro levels of analysis. In fact, although we described specific behaviors that might reflect broader approaches (e.g., thinking about relational obligations represents a general approach of relational justification), we anticipate some ambiguity in examining the correspondence between micro-level behaviors and macro approaches. For example, Felson (1984) noted that coercive behavior may reflect a desire for retribution and/or a desire to deter future misbehavior (in our terms, prevention). Although this possibility complicates research, the fact that a single maintenance behavior may be motivated by multiple purposes or serve several functions is in itself an important idea that warrants research.

Determinants of Approaches

To predict and explain the use of various maintenance approaches within violated relationships, research efforts should focus on identifying determinants of approaches within relationships. Certainly, extant research has revealed associations between relational and personal variables and how people respond to interpersonal problems (e.g., Bowman, 1990; Cloven & Roloff, 1993; Roloff & Cloven, 1990; Rusbult et al., 1986; Rusbult et al., 1982); however, this research has not focused expressly on the selection of methods to maintain relationships in the face of relational transgressions. Moreover, research that clarifies causal relations and explicates *how* or *why* social and personal factors promote particular maintenance approaches is wanting.

We should note that our conception of relational maintenance taps a process different from the conflict behaviors that may be enacted during the "heat of the moment;" therefore, our perspective implies unique determinants. For example, Gelles and Straus (1988) interviewed abused wives about how they reacted during the most recent violent encounter. Those responses included crying, yelling, running to another room, hitting back, running from the house, calling a friend or a relative, and calling the police. These behaviors understandably reflect escape and defensive action, rather than maintenance. However, as we previously noted, these same women reported somewhat different responses when queried about the long-term strategies they employed to try to end the violence. Answers to the latter seem to reflect behaviors aimed at limiting the damage that aggression might do to the relationship and also seemed to reflect a degree of planning. Hence, relational maintenance may be something individuals choose to do after reflecting about the transgression in a less arousing environment.

The implied role of reflection in relational maintenance responses suggests that the deliberative environment may be critical to understanding the type of maintenance approach individuals adopt in violated associations. In fact, our earlier work found that mulling about relational problems in social isolation was associated with defining a conflict as more serious and attributing greater blame for the dispute to the partner relative to judgments when mulling occurred in conjunction with social contact (Cloven & Roloff, 1991). Moreover, these findings imply that isolated individuals may choose to seek retribution, whereas those in contact with others may choose alternative maintenance approaches. Although speculative, this example suggests that a focus on the cognitive and social processes that affect how individuals make sense of their disputes may be a valuable framework through which to explain how individuals act to maintain violated relationships (Cloven & Roloff, in press).

In addition, research focused on the determinants of relational maintenance approaches should not overlook the role of sociological variables in shaping these behaviors. Given that preferences for conflict strategies are influenced by an individual's cultural background (Cahn, 1985), we expect culture to play a role in the selection of relational maintenance approaches. Furthermore, future research should investigate the possibility that males and females maintain violated relationships through different approaches. In fact, the bulk of the research previously discussed on how people cope with violence in intimate associations focused exclusively on the actions or perceptions of abused women (e.g., Gelles & Straus, 1988). Males, however, are also the recipients of violence in personal relationships and may respond uniquely to such relational transgressions (e.g., Gryl et al., 1991).

Approach Effectiveness

Finally, our discussion of relational maintenance approaches noted the paucity of research speaking to the effectiveness of various techniques. Thus, discovering the extent to which different approaches actually serve to maintain violated relationships is needed to understand how individuals manage relational transgressions in ongoing associations. However, we recognize that the issue of what constitutes an effective relational maintenance strategy is a difficult one.

On the one hand, we noted earlier that the primary goal of relational maintenance is to reduce the *relational* damage arising from conflict. Hence, effective maintenance could be defined by any of the following: ensuring that a partner does not become alienated from the relationship, persuading oneself to remain within the association, and maintaining consistent levels of satisfaction within a relationship. Thus, to the extent the relational partners view their relationship as interdependent, stable, committed, and/or satisfying, we might conclude that the approach was effective.

From another perspective, however, this view is problematic. Should we define as successful relational maintenance approaches that allow individuals to remain within an ongoing abusive or exploitative relationship? Indeed, individuals who successfully maintain their own or their partner's commitment to an association may, in effect, be promoting the continuation of a personally harmful and threatening interpersonal association. Therefore, we caution researchers to note that relational maintenance possesses a positive connotation which may be undeserved given the nature of some associations.

To summarize, we direct future research efforts to investigate a variety of issues toward clarifying how individuals maintain violated interpersonal associations. First, the domain of maintenance approaches should be empirically investigated and validated across a variety of relational transgression types. In addition, we call for research at individual and dyadic, and micro and macro levels. Third, investigations of the determinants of maintenance approaches are warranted, and we recommend a focus on the process by which individuals make sense of transgressions within close relationships. Finally, the effectiveness of maintenance behaviors should be evaluated, but we note that definitions of effective relational maintenance should not be confounded with the desirability of these outcomes.

Conclusion

Overall, we believe that the study of relational maintenance is a critical area. Given the increasing stresses placed on intimates, the likelihood of conflict and transgressions seems assured. Although relational transgressions have the potential to end relationships, people can manage to continue associations despite such violations. Of interest, then, are the approaches individuals use to maintain interpersonal associations in the face of violations to fundamental or defining aspects of their relationships. We know that relational transgression occur with unfortunate frequency; however, at this point, we have limited knowledge as to how individuals might reduce the damage of these stresses. Thus, our goal in this chapter has been to explicate a variety of relational maintenance approaches to provide a framework for further study on how people maintain violated interpersonal associations.

References

Altman, I., & Taylor, D. A. (1973). *Social penetration: The development of interpersonal relationships.* New York: Holt, Rinehart, & Winston.

Andrews, B., & Brewin, C. R. (1990). Attributions of blame for marital violence: A study of antecedents and consequences. *Journal of Marriage and the Family, 52,* 757–767.

Argyle, M., & Furnham, A. (1983). Sources of satisfaction and conflict in long-term relationships. *Journal of Marriage and the Family, 45,* 481–493.

Argyle, M., & Henderson, M. (1984). The rules of friendship. *Journal of Social and Personal Relationships, 1,* 211–237.

Baumeister, R. F., Stillwell, A., & Wotman, S. R. (1990). Victim and perpetrator accounts of interpersonal conflict: Autobiographical narratives about anger. *Journal of Personality and Social Psychology, 59,* 994–1005.

Baxter, L. A. (1984). Trajectories of relationship disengagement. *Journal of Social and Personal Relationships, 1,* 29–48.

Baxter, L. A. (1986). Gender differences in the heterosexual relationship rules embedded in break-up accounts. *Journal of Social and Personal Relationships, 3,* 189–306.

Birchler, G. R., Weiss, R. L., & Vincent, J. P. (1975). Multimethod analysis of social reinforcement exchange between maritally distressed and nondistressed spouse and stranger dyads. *Journal of Personality and Social Psychology, 31,* 349–360.

Blumstein, P., & Schwartz, P. (1983). *American couples: Money, work, sex.* New York: Morrow.

Bowman, M. L. (1990). Coping efforts and marital satisfaction: Measuring marital coping and its correlates. *Journal of Marriage and the Family, 52,* 463–474.

Briere, J. (1987). Predicting self-reported likelihood of battering: Attitudes and childhood experience. *Journal of Research in Personality, 21,* 61–69.

Burman, B., & Margolin, G. (1992). Analysis of the association between marital relationships and health problems: An interactional perspective. *Psychological Bulletin, 112,* 39–63.

Cahn, D. (1985). Communication competence in the resolution of intercultural conflict. *World Communication, 14,* 85–94.

Cate, R., Henton, J. M., Koval, J., Christopher, F. S., & Lloyd, S. (1982). Premarital abuse: A social psychological perspective. *Journal of Family Issues, 3,* 79–90.

Cloven, D. H., & Roloff, M. E. (1991). Sense-making activities and interpersonal conflict: Communicative cures for the mulling blues. *Western Journal of Speech Communication, 55,* 134–158.

Cloven, D. H., & Roloff, M. E. (in press). Sense-making activities and interpersonal conflict: II. The effects of communicative intention on internal dialogue. *Western Journal of Speech Communication.*

Cloven, D. H., & Roloff, M. E. (1993). The chilling effect of aggressive potential on the expression of complaints in intimate relationships, *Communication Monographs, 60,* 199–219.

Coser, L. (1956). *The functions of social conflict.* New York: The Free Press.

Davis, K. E., & Todd, M. J. (1985). Assessing friendship: Prototypes, paradigm cases and relationship description. In S. Duck & D. Perlman (Eds.), *Understanding personal relationships: An interdisciplinary approach* (pp. 17–38). Beverly Hills, CA: Sage.

Deutsch, M. (1973). *The resolution of conflict: Constructive and destructive processes.* New Haven, CT: Yale University Press.

Dindia, K., & Baxter, L. A. (1987). Strategies for maintaining and repairing marital relationships. *Journal of Social and Personal Relationships, 4,* 143–158.

Donnenwerth, G. V., & Foa, U. G. (1974). Effect of resource class retaliation to injustice in interpersonal exchange. *Journal of Personality and Social Psychology, 29,* 785–793.

Felson, R. B. (1984). Patterns of aggressive social interaction. In A. Mummendey (Ed.), *Social psychology of aggression: From individual behavior to social interaction* (pp. 107–126). New York: Springer-Verlag.

Foa, U. G., & Foa, E. B. (1974). *Societal structures of the mind.* Springfield, IL: Charles C. Thomas.

Gelles, R. J., & Straus, M. A. (1988). *Intimate violence.* New York: Simon and Schuster.

Gonzales, M. H., Manning, D. J., & Haugen, J. A. (1992). Explaining our sins: Factors influencing offender accounts and anticipated victim responses. *Journal of Personality and Social Psychology, 62,* 958–971.

Gryl, F. E., Stith, S. M., & Bird, G. W. (1991). Close dating relationships among college students: Differences by use of violence and by gender. *Journal of Social and Personal Relationships, 8,* 243–264.

Heaton, T. B., & Albrecht, S. L. (1991) Stable unhappy marriages. *Journal of Marriage and the Family, 53,* 747–758.

Henton, J., Cate, R., Koval, J., Lloyd, S., & Christopher, S. (1983). Romance and violence in dating relationships. *Journal of Family Issues, 4,* 467–482.

Herbert, T. B., Silver, R. C., & Ellard, J. H. (1991). Coping with an abusive relationship: I. How and why do women stay? *Journal of Marriage and the Family, 53,* 311–325.

Hocker, J. L., & Wilmot, W. W. (1991). *Interpersonal Conflict* (3rd ed.). Dubuque, IA: Wm. C. Brown.

Jacobson, N. S., Follette, W. C., & McDonald, D. W. (1982). Reactivity to positive and negative behavior in distressed and nondistressed married couples. *Journal of Consulting and Clinical Psychology, 50,* 706–714.

Jacobson, N. S., Waldron, H., & Moore, D. (1980). Toward a behavioral profile of marital distress. *Journal of Consulting and Clinical Psychology, 48,* 696–703.

Jones, E., & Gallois, C. (1989). Spouses' impressions of rules for communication in public and private marital conflicts. *Journal of Marriage and the Family, 51,* 957–967.

Kirchler, E. (1988). Marital happiness and interaction in everyday surroundings: A time-sample diary approach for couples. *Journal of Social and Personal Relationships, 5,* 375–382.

Kitson, G., & Sussman, M. (1982). Marital complaints, demographic characteristics, and symptoms of mental distress in divorce. *Journal of Marriage and the Family, 44,* 87–101.

Knapp, M. L., Stafford, L., & Daly, J. A. (1986). Regrettable messages: Things people wish they hadn't said. *Journal of Communication, 36,* 40–58.

Larner, M. R., & Thompson, J. (1982). Abuse and aggression in courting couples. *Deviant Behavior, 3,* 229–244.

Lauer, R. H., & Lauer, J. C. (1987). Factors in long-term marriages. *Journal of Family Issues, 7,* 382–390.

Lee, L. (1984). Sequences in separation: A framework for investigating endings of the personal (romantic) relationship. *Journal of Social and Personal Relationships, 1,* 49–73.

Mason, A., & Blankenship, V. (1987). Power and affiliation motivation, stress, and abuse in intimate relationships. *Journal of Personality and Social Psychology, 52,* 203–210.

Menaghan, E. (1982). Measuring coping effectiveness: A panel analysis of marital problems and coping efforts. *Journal of Health and Social Behavior, 23,* 220–234.

Menaghan, E. (1983). Coping with parental problems: Panel assessments of effectiveness. *Journal of Marriage and the Family, 4,* 483–506.

Muehlenhard, C. L., & Hollabaugh, L. C. (1988). Do women sometimes say no when they mean yes? The prevalence and correlates of women's token resistance to sex. *Journal of Personality and Social Psychology, 54,* 872–879.

O'Malley, M. N., & Greenberg, J. (1983). Sex differences in restoring justice: The down payment effect. *Journal of Research in Personality, 17,* 174–185.

Passer, M. W., Kelley, H. H., & Michela, J. L. (1978). Multidimensional scaling of the causes for negative interpersonal behavior. *Journal of Personality and Social Psychology, 36,* 951–962.

Pearlin, L. I., & Schooler, C. (1978). The structure of coping. *Journal of Health and Social Behavior, 19,* 2–21.

Pinkley, R. L. (1990). Dimensions of conflict frame: Disputant interpretations of conflict. *Journal of Applied Psychology, 75,* 117–126.

Resick, P. A., Barr, P. K., Sweet, J. J., Kieffer, D. M., Ruby, N. L., & Spiegel, D. K. (1981). Perceived and actual discriminators of conflict from accord in marital communication. *The American Journal of Family Therapy, 9,* 58–68.

Roloff, M. E., & Cloven, D. H. (1990). The chilling effect in interpersonal relationships: The reluctance to speak one's mind. In D. D. Cahn (Ed.), *Intimates in conflict: A communication perspective* (pp. 49–76). Hillsdale, NJ: Lawrence Erlbaum.

Roscoe, B., & Benaske, N. (1986). Courtship violence experienced by abused wives: Similarities in patterns of abuse. *Family Relations, 34,* 419–424.

Rusbult, C. E. (1987). Responses to dissatisfaction in close relationships: The exit–voice–loyalty–neglect model. In D. Perlman & S. Duck (Eds.), *Intimate relationships: Development, dynamics, and deterioration* (pp. 209–237). Beverly Hills, CA: Sage.

Rusbult, C. E., Johnson, D. J., & Morrow, G. D. (1986). Determinants and consequences of exit, voice, loyalty, and neglect: Responses to dissatisfaction in adult romantic involvements. *Human Relations, 39,* 45–63.

Rusbult, C. E., Verette, J., Whitney, G. A., Slovik, L. F., & Lipkus, I. (1991). Accommodation processes in close relationships: Theory and preliminary empirical evidence. *Journal of Personality and Social Psychology, 60,* 53–78.

Rusbult, C. E., Zembrodt, I. M., & Gunn, L. K. (1982). Exit, voice, loyalty, and neglect: Responses to dissatisfaction in romantic involvements. *Journal of Personality and Social Psychology, 43,* 1230–1242.

Schafer, R. B., Keith, P. M., & Lorenz, F. O. (1984). Equity/inequity and self-concept: An interactionist analysis. *Social Psychology Quarterly, 47,* 42–49.

Smolen, R. C., Spiegel, D. A., Bakker-Rabdau, M. K., Bakker, C. B., & Martin, C. (1985). A situational analysis of the relationship between spouse-specific assertiveness and marital adjustment. *Journal of Psychopathology and Behavioral Assessment, 7,* 397–410.

Smolen, R. C., Spiegel, D. A., & Martin, C. J. (1986). Patterns of marital interaction associated with marital dissatisfaction and depression. *Journal of Behavioral Therapy and Experimental Psychiatry, 17,* 261–266.

Spanier, G. B., & Margolis, R. L. (1983). Marital separation and extramarital sexual behavior. *The Journal of Sex Research, 19,* 23–48.

Stafford, L., & Canary, D. J. (1991). Maintenance strategies and romantic relationship type, gender and relational characteristics. *Journal of Social and Personal Relationships, 8,* 217–242.

Stets, J. E., & Pirog-Good, M. A. (1987). Violence in dating relationships. *Social Psychology Quarterly, 50,* 237–246.

Stets, J. E., & Pirog-Good, M. A. (1990). Interpersonal control and courtship aggression. *Journal of Social and Personal Relationships, 7,* 371–394.

Strube, M. J., & Barbour, L. S. (1983). The decision to leave an abusive relationship: Economic dependence and psychological commitment. *Journal of Marriage and the Family, 45*, 785–844.

Strube, M. J., & Barbour, L. S. (1984). Factors related to the decision to leave an abusive relationship. *Journal of Marriage and the Family, 46*, 837–844.

White, G. L. (1980). Inducing jealousy: A power perspective. *Personality and Social Psychology Bulletin, 6*, 222–227.

Wills, T. A., Weiss, R. L., & Patterson, G. R. (1974). A behavioral analysis of the determinants of marital satisfaction. *Journal of Consulting and Clinical Psychology, 42*, 802–811.

Wood, W., Rhodes, N., & Whelan, M. (1989). Sex differences in positive well-being: A consideration of emotional style and marital status. *Psychological Bulletin, 106*, 249–264.

Steady as (S)he Goes

Relational Maintenance as a Shared Meaning System

Steve Duck

Departments of Communication Studies and Psychology
University of Iowa
Iowa City, Iowa

The sociology of knowledge must not only be concerned with the great universes of meaning that history offers up for our inspection but with the many little workshops in which living individuals keep hammering away at the construction and maintenance of these universes.

(Berger & Kellner, 1964, p. 24)

Introduction

Relationship maintenance refers generally to the vast unstudied void in relational research—that huge area where relationships continue to exist between the point of their initial development (which has been intensively studied) and their possible decline (which has also been studied but somewhat less intensively). For most people in most relationships, this period of continuous existence *is* the relationship, as they experience it (Duck, 1988). Yet we researchers began to focus on it only relatively recently (Ayres, 1983; Dindia & Baxter, 1987; Shea & Pearson, 1986; Stafford & Canary, 1991). The research which has been done has focused mostly on strategies for the active

Communication and Relational Maintenance

and conscious sustaining of relationships and thus implicitly assumes that people think about it, plan it, do it, and do it repeatedly—or else their relationships would not work (see, however, Dainton & Stafford, 1993). It is as if the underlying research model is of a relational automobile that is never able to go anywhere without a feverish intellectual mechanic working continually on parts under the hood even as the vehicle speeds down the freeway.

By contrast, this chapter emphasizes the space between the car's annual services: the structures, routines, and automatic, self-adjusting activities that occur all the time without anyone's intervention except for the occasional strategic tune-up. In short, I wish to argue that relational maintenance contains two elements, not one: the first is strategic planning for the continuance of the relationship; and the second is the breezy allowance of the relationship to continue by means of the everyday interactions and conversations that make the relationship what it is.

This approach is in contrast, but not in opposition, to the sort of psychological and communicative emphasis that has focused on the careful assessment of a person's thoughts about continuing a relationship. Thus, even when not focused exclusively on relationship maintenance, various discussions of relationships can have implications for maintenance processes. If, for example, one writes about the activities relevant to marital stability (e.g., Acitelli, 1992), one is, in a sense, saying something about relationship maintenance even though it is obliquely referenced. Also if one writes about the balancing of costs and benefits that people consider in order to sustain an acceptable reward–cost ratio, and which prevent them from leaving a relationship (e.g., Rusbult, 1983), then again one is implicitly writing about activities relevant to relational maintenance. If one writes about the barriers that would need to be overcome in order to get out of a relationship (see Attridge, this volume; Levinger, 1976), or the relative consideration of alternatives before one would think of leaving (Thibaut & Kelley, 1959), then one is also talking about relational maintenance.

Earlier and cruder views of relationships focused only on the costs and rewards of the person reviewing the relationship (Homans, 1961). If the person's checks and balances checked and balanced, then the person would happily stay in place and all would be well. Thibaut and Kelley's (1959) model based on the comparison of one's own input–outcome equation against a Comparison Level for Alternatives (CL_{alt}) and an absolute comparison level (CL) is also a variation on these themes that contributes much to current thinking about relational maintenance.

Some theorists (e.g., Hatfield [Walster], Walster & Berscheid, 1978) have argued that people assess their inputs and outcomes in relationships relative to one another and to their partner's patterns of inputs and outcomes. A state of rough equivalence of the two, relative to the partner's input–outcome ratio, is termed *equity* and is one of three types of fairness measures that people perceive and use to evaluate their relationships (La Gaipa, 1977). When fairness is maintained in a way that is felt by the person to be suitable to the circumstances, the person's desire to continue the relationship is also sustained. La Gaipa (1977) distinguished two other types of Fairness: one is *equality*, where people are satisfied enough to stay in relationships where each of them receives the same outcome regardless of inputs, the other is *Marxist justice*, where maintenance is achieved when the person with means provides for the person with needs, rather than everyone getting the same outcome or being rewarded in terms of effort. Unfortunately, researchers have done relatively little to discover the circumstances or the principles through which couples decide which pattern of fairness should be applied in particular circumstances within their relationship.

Even using explicit social exchange approaches or other approaches, there are two implicit models for thinking about relational maintenance, each containing different unexpressed "theorettes" about the nature of relational maintenance (Duck, 1992). One model suggests that relationships are naturally somehow held together unless something pulls them apart; the other suggests that they will naturally fall apart unless partners do something to keep them together. Although I still believe that these models do underlie much of the thinking about the topic, I have come to feel, since first noting the distinction (Duck, 1988), that relationship maintenance is probably a mixture of both, but that there is more that unconsciously keeps them together than we have typically supposed.

The approach developed here, therefore, is not, as I noted, in opposition to an exchange view of relationships. I assume that some sort of careful accounting of relational commodities is indeed undertaken in relationships from time to time. It seems likely to be very important, particularly at the points where partners are considering change in a relationship or want (to continue the metaphor) to take stock of it. Disputes about relationships are a well-known feature of human life and very often are quite obviously either explicit or implicit inventory-taking exercises.

However, relationships are not made up only of significant cost–reward tabulations, nor of dramatic stock-takings, nor even of excitement, drama, or pyrotechnical conflicts. Much of the time they just "are." As Berger and Kellner (1964) pointed out, the routine behaviors of life are often those that bind and cement social structures or social relationships together. We do not wake up each morning and think carefully and strategically before kissing our partner in case he or she does not deserve it on the relationship stock exchange (even though stock markets themselves go up and down rather unpredictably most days). Neither do we arrange to meet friends for lunch only after we have calculated our cost–benefit ratio for that relationship. Rather, such relationships tend to be taken for granted and continued *because* they exist, not in order to *make* them exist. It is true that in the long haul, partners do probably check out the winners and losers. Yet also in the long haul, the monumentally normal experience will be that partners stay in their relationships "because the relationships are there." They continue because the two partners are in them, or rather, because the routine behaviors of life, especially day-to-day conversations, structure and sustain the relationship in various subtle ways that we shall explore here.

This chapter develops and explores this radical view. It is radical, however, only if one starts from the perspective of a field of research that has typically not attended adequately to the daily conduct of relational life (Duck, 1986, 1992). It will not be seen as radical by persons (including reflective research scientists) who are actually conducting those lives, all of whom will take it for granted as they chat away with their friends, lovers, and spouses in the talk of everyday life. That talk, I shall argue, is the essence of relational maintenance for three important reasons. First, talk provides a "rhetorical vision" or persuasive image of what the relationship is and will be. Second, talk provides relational partners with the method for sharing one another's worlds of experience. Third, to follow Berger and Kellner (1964), talk serves to sustain the reality of the world by continually hardening or stabilizing the "commonly objectivated reality" that a relationship represents to the partners.

An Analogy: "Maintaining" Conferences and Maintaining Relationships

Let me draw an analogy from relationships to conferences in order to help argue these points. The things said about conferences can be translated into things said about relationships quite directly, but the contrast in our assumptions about each of them is quite instructive. We normally do not think of *conferences* needing to be "maintained," on the one hand, yet we do tend to think that friendships need to be. Nevertheless both are voluntarily entered, have a discernible structure, endure over time, and have purposes that can be considered in exchange terms. In addition, both involve and have their existence in many ways through talk, and both are reported to others in summary ways that obscure important components of their real nature. So what differences and similarities are there in the ways in which conferences and relationships begin and continue? Why, then, do we feel that we need to explain *maintenance* in one and not the other?

The mere creation of an opportunity for a conference is not all that there is to it. One can construct the shell, as it were, but the interesting part is how it hatches. Having organized several International Conferences on Personal Relationships, I know that even if you announce one, much could go wrong in its unfolding. Its day-to-day conduct matters quite as much as the simple "track" that it appears to be set on. Difficulties such as unavailability of rooms or nonappearance of key speakers can be reduced by careful strategic planning, obviously, but the availability of rooms and the keynote speakers do not in themselves guarantee success of the conference. Success is guaranteed by the way the individual delegates interact and stimulate one another. People go to conferences for good scholarly discourse, but also for collegial and intellectual sociality. Conference attenders do talk about the "important" things that we are supposed to discuss. In reality, though, conference sites are usually chosen and advertised in ways that give us a clue about human behavior: they are usually in nice places, advertised as having great social events, zoos or shopping malls, bars, restaurants, and "atmosphere." For all the serious purposes and intellectual heat that is often observed at conferences, it is usually not long before the wine appears and the conversation naturally turns to gossip and the important trivialities of regular conference life. A full conference experience is not limited to those things that we report on when we return home to the department.

The analogy, of course, is that relationships also have serious purposes and significant occurrences within them, but that this is not all that they have. Also, relational researchers ask subjects to explain their relationships in the researchers' chosen terms on questionnaire reports, which the subjects duly do, just as conference delegates report to colleagues using respectable formal terms or answering the questions as asked on the report form. But neither conference delegates nor research subjects describing their relationships make such reports to one another during the real experiences described on those forms. Subjects' answers to research questions are, after all, like conference delegates' "official" reports, informative only to the extent that the researchers' questions about the topic are really important reflections of the processes under investigation. They are not all that is relevant to the processes being explored.

Conferences may well be initially structured by some exterior force, but once the opportunity is born, people enter the process by registering for them and arriving for them in different degrees of preparedness. Then it all "just happens" through the medium of everyday talk and in the inertia of the processes. Because people are in the same place and because the day proceeds without anyone's intervention, conferences continue from start to finish. In such a view, maintenance of conferences requires no constant effort by organizing forces. The conference just is, and the whole social proceeding carries on unaided until we reach the final paper and the fat lady sings. This view suggests that conferences [and relationships] actually proceed, once started, by reason of the simple advance of *time*.

Finally, conferences are *varied* experiences, not just a flat or steadily increasing line on the graph of satisfaction. It just is not true, however we characterize the conference to others, that it was experienced all the way through as equally enjoyable, stimulating, or whatever, at each and every moment. Some papers are good and some not; some parties work and some do not; some interactions are stimulating and others are not; but we do not get up and leave as soon as we have had one negative experience. When we report to other people about the conference, however, we are very likely to encapsulate such variability into a single thematic description—perhaps overlaid with some cautionary preliminary statement about "variability" that is sure to be ignored or else translated to mean that the *whole thing* was "mixed."

Likewise in relationships, people *can* focus on only significant things, people *can* use talk strategically, and they obviously do (e.g., Baxter & Dindia, 1990; Dindia & Baxter, 1987), so it is important that we understand the processes going on there. But that is not all that people use talk for. People also report single-minded summary experiences, but that is not what they had. So it is also important that we research and understand not only that people summarize their experiences, and so leave out some of the detail, but also what happens psychologically when they do that. What they leave out is often a description of how they experience relationships or conferences moment by moment, which raises the question of how people get from the full experience to the brief overview and what the psychological and relational processes are that are involved in doing so. However, we must not forget that this encapsulation is what occurs and that much important and time-consuming triviality can be omitted when encapsulated in a single summary. Yet that does not mean that triviality has had no cumulative effects. In most cases the importance of individual interactions lies in their simple and spontaneous occurrence, in the fact that the delegates arrange to meet one another—without permission and without checking with the motivational organizers each time to see if it is (1) advantageous in terms of exchanged resources, or (2) is significant, or (3) is going anywhere.

Back to Relationships

The preceding analogy about conferences alerts us to several factors in the ordinary conduct of daily life (even in special settings) that are as relevant in personal relationships. To focus on these factors, however, is to shift attention away from some of the ways in which relationships are most typically represented in current research.

In my recent work (Duck, 1990, 1991), I have been stressing not exchange variables but the relational importance of the "effort after meaning" that Bartlett (1932) detected in subjects remembering stories: a tendency to struggle to find a pattern or a frame or a coherence in what had been heard, even when it was heard in bits and pieces. Bartlett observed that rememberers (1) made errors of recall that helped the various parts hang together into something meaningful, (2) tended to forget things that did not fit, and (3) made up "missing links" that produced a sensible report—even when the original material did not make sense. I believe that the same process is relevant in interpreting the maintenance of relationships. Individuals in all their lively interaction seek to impose order and meaning on the flow of experience, whether those individuals are examined in dyadic personal relationships, in large conferences or at work, or just as human beings facing life. The specific instances of exchange variables, self-disclosure, and strategy that have been studied to explain relational maintenance are, in this view, important Big Instances of the effort after meaning, but are not the whole process. Of course we try to understand a self-disclosure, comprehend a strategy, or put meaning to exchange outcomes, but we do not switch on "meaning" only when such things occur. We look for meaning all the time, constantly making sense of what we see, even if it appears to be trivial. As Berger and Kellner (1964) noted, trivial rituals of conversation actually serve to create and sustain reality for married couples. I am going further and saying that people do it for all relationships, by creating meaning. Meaning sustains relationships.

Relationships, like conferences, keep going because they are filled with juicy meaning for the partners. *Period.* This juicy meaning is created in talk and the mere occurrence of talk in everyday relationships not only satisfies the partners that the relationship exists and is important *irrespective of the content of the talk*, it also reifies, sustains, and produces the relationship (Duck & Pond, 1989). Duck, Rutt, Hurst, and Strejc (1991) have shown that the mere occurrence of conversations is more important than the topics discussed, or whether the conversation was with a friend, best friend, or family. Subjects indicated that the perpetuation of the relationship through talk was more important than any self-disclosing or other "significant" content of the talk. The perpetuation is both the purpose and the result of such talk.

In the context of relationship maintenance, this reminds me of Herzberg's (1966) comments on motivations in organizations: that there exist two sorts of factors relevant to motivation. On the one hand there are so-called "hygienic factors" from the absence or inadequacy of which dissatisfaction arises. According to Herzberg (1966), their simple presence does not increase satisfaction; indeed, workers will always want "better" or "more" of them. Rather, it is the absence of hygienic factors that reduces satisfaction. Examples would be status, company policy, good relationships with other workers, and salary. On the other hand, there are factors that increase motivation directly, such as the degree of interestingness of the work, feelings of significance about one's contribution, and feelings of personal growth; however, the effects of these factors are predicated on the fact that some acceptable level of the hygienic factors is present first. So I think it is with relational maintenance: some factors, like easy regular interaction, talk, and chatter, are hygienic and some, like conscious strategies, are deliberately maintaining. However, you cannot have the second without the first.

Talk Is the Essence of Relational Maintenance

Talk is the essence of relational maintenance not only because it achieves the discussion and assessment of relational exchanges or provides some of the topics for it, but also because it serves to do something that communication scholars have long attributed to political speeches and other forms of public address. Like these other declarations (but on a much less noble scale), everyday talk presents a *rhetorical vision* and hence projects a continued future for the relationship.

A rhetorical vision is easily understood as an image or impression of some topic, particularly one that creates an expectation for the future form of an institution or relationship. In this case, one of the functions and consequences of everyday talk is to present to the two partners an image or impression of the relationship itself and how it may continue. This may be done by the relatively crude and direct means of open statements about the relationship (e.g., "I love you," "Let's bury the hatchet," "Let's be friends"). Yet this rhetorical vision is more likely and more frequently accomplished by both the style of the performance (see Baxter, 1992, on play in relationships) and the mere occurrence of the talk (Duck et al., 1991). Just as partners indicate their degree of love by their nonverbal communication (see Rubin, 1974), so they can indicate to self and others something about the friendliness or lovingness of their relationship by a variety of conversational devices such as the immediacy of language (Mehrabian, 1971), accommodation to the listener (Giles, 1989), the development of relational personal idioms (Bell, Buerkel-Rothfuss, & Gore, 1987; Hopper, Knapp, & Scott, 1981), the use of playful banter (Baxter, 1992) and teasing (Shapiro, Baumeister, & Kessler, 1991), or simply by the sheer enjoyment of their interactions together (Burleson, Samter, & Lucchetti, in press). In short, a multitude of everyday communicative interactive behaviors define and redefine the relationship.

This chapter develops the view that talk maintains relationships by presenting symbolic evidence to the partners that the two of them share an appreciation of the relationship and that they also happen to approach important experiences in similar ways. The apparently idle chatter of partners serves to demonstrate a "symbolic union" between their two independent ways of looking at life; that is to say, it shows a shared, similar, and connected way of conceiving of the relationship, each other, and the forms of connectedness between them. Thus talk functions communicatively to endorse their views and sustain them in their relationship in an implicit, subtle way that does not always need strategic activity.

Shared Meaning as Relationship Maintenance and Vice Versa

Duck and Pond (1989) proposed that people do many things when they talk. Sometimes they perform instrumental tasks, like requesting a favor from someone else or asking them on a date. Talk can also be used to indicate the status of the relationship, whether by a direct statement ("I love you") or by the use of intimate and immediate language, pet names, or distant formal modes of address. Talk also serves as a medium that creates, embodies, or "essentializes" the relationship; that is to say, it becomes the relationship and is the essence of the relationship. Thus the occurrence of everyday talk is essential in the long-term existence of typical relationships.

The preceding points have intriguing implications for the present discussion. When one starts to look at the functions of everyday talk (Nofsinger, 1990) and to strip it away from the special circumstances of the lab, transplanting it back to real-life contexts, one begins to see just how silly and trivial most of it seems to be. Whereas lab work focuses on serious stuff like intelligent, planned talk (Berger, 1987), or strategic message selection (Cody & McLaughlin, 1985), or persuasive discourse (Tracy, Craig, Smith, & Spisak, 1984), if you just hang out and listen to what is said by people in the daily concourse of existence, it is pretty banal. However, that does not mean that it is unimportant or that the other important things do not occur or have significance in the full picture. It merely indicates that investigators have so far focused only on some of the picture, or acted as if, as it were, all that makes humans stay alive is the heart, rather than the liver, lymph nodes, epithelial cells, and the communal interaction of all the other bits (however humble).

What is it that people are achieving by holding silly and insignificant conversations about trivial topics, telling one another jokes, discussing the clothing or demeanor of passersby, complaining about other people, speculating about other people's relationships, suggesting where to go for lunch, teasing one another, arguing and debating, or cajoling others? People are achieving two results. First, as *individuals*, they are "giving off" meaning: they are manifesting their attitudes on a whole variety of things; showing their priorities, indicating their ways of looking at the world, declaring their vision of things, symbolizing their affection for one another, embodying their relationship, conveying the manner in which they understand the world, denoting their perspectives on things, representing their universes of comprehension. Second, as *partners*, they are colluding with the other partner in the embodiment of the relationship (Berger & Kellner, 1964).

That is what *they* are doing, but what are their partners doing? Their partners are doing precisely the same thing back to them, and the reason that communication works is precisely because the two persons know one another sufficiently well to understand what the other person is communicating both as an individual and as a partner. Whether it is the two strangers talking the talk of the truly superficial interaction, or the two lovers talking the talk of affectionate superficial interaction, the thing that keeps the two people in the kind of relationship that they have is the extent to which they each comprehend the other person as an individual and as a partner. People can play a role in social processes with someone else only to the extent that they comprehend the other's frames of reference, meaning, and talk. It is that extent of comprehension that effectively determines (in the sense of limits) the boundaries of the relationship they each have with the other, as Kelly (1955) first pointed out.

Thus, in the seemingly trivial talk that bombards us daily, people are signifying the essence of their relationships with each other and doing so because they share enough understanding of one another to make this mutual interpretation possible. Everyday talk continues relationships because it continues to embody partners' understanding or shared meaning, and it continues to represent their relationship to one another in ways that each accepts and is comfortable with, or which "ratify" the relationship.

Some of these propositions were examined by Duck et al. (1991). In three separate studies, we explored the patterns of daily communication that subjects reported in everyday interaction with six types of possible partners (strangers, acquaintances, friends, best friends, lovers, and family). These studies, taken as a whole, showed that there are consistent differences between the everyday talk that characterizes different types of relationships, which confirms the preceding points about the enactment of relationships' essential character in talk.

Duck et al. also discovered that the differences between relationships were not necessarily those intuitively proposed by previous scholars. For example, talk with lovers was generally regarded as being of *lesser* quality than talk with friends, and talk with a best friend was rated as of the highest quality. It thus appears that talk operationalizes intimacy on a day-to-day basis in ways that are different from those proposed by scholars who suppose a graduation of intimacy from strangers through friends to lovers. Talk with lovers tended to be characterized by lower quality that could not be attributed to consistently greater conflict, but was instead due to greater variability in the quality of conversation. Evidently, lovers maintain their relationships with greater difficulty and at greater cost than friends do. Given that in Duck et al. (1991) the relationships with lovers all were cross-sex relationships, whereas those with friends tended to be same-sex ones, it is likely that the maintenance of lover relationships through talk simply involves a mixture of greater differences in conversational style, a need to organize roles in the relationship in ways that may be difficult to negotiate, and the discussion of a different range of issues (such as sexual satisfaction) that do not arise with simple friendship. Monsour (1992) similarly has shown that the meaning of intimacy differs for female and male subjects and that in cross-sex friendship there are differences in managing the distance between friends on sexual and emotional expressive elements of intimacy that are not present in same-sex friendships.

These findings thus indicate that everyday talk manifests differences in the meanings and understandings that are shared in different sorts of relationships. They also show that the maintenance of relationships involves some relatively simple social routines having to do with everyday conversations. In short, people are organizing and giving meaning to relationships by dealing with the variabilities that confront them across time in dealing with their partners, both as individuals and as partners in relationship to self. It is also worth noting that maintenance of some sorts of relationships appears to be different from maintenance of other sorts of relationships, a point about which research in this field may need to pay closer attention.

People also organize and give meaning to relationships, and to the variabilities of their experience, through the organization of memory and the systematizing effects the mind produces in its reduction of a hundred little details to one overall summary statement. The principles here are complex and interdependent, but they bear importantly on the maintenance of relationships because they are the psychological processes by which a sense of continuity in a relationship is retained. Edwards and Middleton (1988) have already demonstrated the role of conjoint remembering on the development of a child's sense of place in the family history. Duck and Miell (1986) have shown how a secure sense of steadiness in relationships is made by development of conjoint memories of the origin of the relationship. We found that histories of the origin of relationships changed over time, partly, we suspected, as a productive part of the process of forming a relationship and a sense of belonging, rather than simply as the *cause* of it. Yet, Duck and Miell failed to carry this analysis as far as I now think it can be taken—to the full range of experiences of a relationship across time. The partners in relationships are notoriously able to create shared memories of one another and of their relationship (Berger & Kellner, 1964), often to the point where one will "correct" the other about an event in the other's past before they even met! Such memories and steadiness are likewise embodied and celebrated in the conversations of everyday life (Duck et al., 1991), some of which have to do with reminiscing, or the recall of particularly important relational experiences (Baxter, 1988). Honeycutt (1993) has shown how such memory processes are tied to personal and cultural scripts for relational growth and decline, and do not happen on their own as the simple recounting of experience. Andersen (1993) also relates such activity to cultural and other schemata that allow people to create meaning for relational events by connecting them to other patterns. Such patterns are, of course, preexisting ways of organizing meaning in relationships that transcend individual relational exchanges and serve to provide implicit relational continuities.

On each occasion of everyday talk, one unseen consequence is the partial or even total confirmation of the fact that the partners agree on other aspects of the world (Duck & Pond, 1989; Duck, in press). The everyday conversations of life confirm the fact that the partners share the attachment of meaning to, and evaluation of, certain aspects of the world. The occurrence of everyday conversation simply presents (and continues over time to present) partners with increasing numbers of chances to discover and to verify similarities of evaluation that they share with one another.

This is not very interesting taken out of context, but is significant when one remembers the obvious fact that people in relationships and interaction do not necessarily agree initially about the events and experiences that they share and report. In fact, different people almost always have different accounts of the "same events." Previous researchers (Christensen, Sullaway & King, 1983) have taken differences in perspective to be a methodological annoyance based on simple human error or inaccuracy. Yet a much more exciting theoretical position is that the ubiquity of such differences is meaningful and important to people (Duck & Sants, 1983). Recently, Duck, Pond, and Leatham (in press) have shown that there are meaningful and systematic differences in the perceptions of people in the selfsame interaction witnessing exactly the same communicative interchange. For example, lonely people rated their own relationships more negatively after viewing them on a videotape than did any other viewers, and "observers" rated the relational interactions lower in quality than the participants themselves did. In everyday life, when partners realize through their conversations that at some important level they are seeing things in general agreement, or that they share priorities and values, the relationship sustains itself from that realization.

This latter point reemphasizes the notion that relationships are unfinished business, as is life itself (Billig, 1987). Recognition of this fact orients people toward the future (Duck, 1990; Kelly, 1969). In other words, no matter what the history of a relationship (whether it be friends or family), there is no certainty that it will continue forever exactly as it has. No matrix of exchange, no union of symbols, no initial degrees of similarity or patterns of interdependence can guarantee that a relationship will *never* change in the future. Thus, I assume that even trivial references to the stability of a relationship, such as are provided by recognition of shared meanings, are helpful in sustaining continuity. We have all recognized this on some human level, but perhaps too readily focus our research on events such as critical turning points where we researchers can then come in and apply our craft to something important and dramatic (e.g., Surra, 1987).

However, I believe that we should explore relationships and relational life also from the point of view of their routine, daily, and trivial processes. This means on the one hand that we should recognize the fundamental role of perpetual change in human experience and the importance to people of stabilizing it so that they can attach meaning to it. Thus, relational maintenance occurs through stabilization of tensions between conflicting forces rather than by setting something on a permanent course. Relationship maintenance is, like "the poor" in the Bible, always with us. It is perpetual, routinely executed, and carried out unconsciously as well as consciously.

Conclusion

Thus, as I reach the point where as an author I am obliged to say "More research needs to be done," I can be quite specific about the directions in which I believe that work should take us. We need to spend more time looking at everyday behaviors, especially as they embody a relationship, and deal with the ways in which diurnal triviality cements relationships—not just looking at the difficult negotiative issues that partners in relationships face from time to time. We should be seeking out the boring stabilities that are created by the sharing of meaning in conversations. This will, I believe, focus us on the variability of experience across time in relationships and on the ways in which people experience it, and not just on the ways in which they smooth it out (though we should try to understand that, too). We should also seek to understand the different ways in which different sorts of relationships are maintained, before we too readily conclude that "relationship maintenance" is always one sort of process for all relationships.

I believe that we shall learn something deep about relationships (and conferences) when we stop focusing on The Significant and focus on the fact that
in the trivial realities that we all inhabit, there are many unseen and unex-
plored forces that keep things in animated suspension like the circus ball
dancing on the air jets. Exchange and a lot of other things can help turn up
the pressure of those air jets, but the jets themselves would not be necessary
without the all-embracing and ever-present gravitational forces that no one
can see. Basically, the ever-present tiny things are what sustain relationships.
These tiny things happen in the context of some big things, like the passage
of time, but cataclysm is not the major element of maintained lives. The
major element is routine daily talk in routine daily lives.

References

Acitelli, L. K. (1992). Gender differences in relationship awareness and marital satisfaction
    among young married couples. *Personality and Social Psychology Bulletin, 18,* 102–110.
Andersen, P. (1993). Cognitive schemata in personal relationships. In S. W. Duck (Ed.), *Under-
    standing relationship processes 1: Individuals in relationships.* 1–22. Newbury Park, CA: Sage.
Ayres, J. (1983). Strategies to maintain relationships: Their identification and perceived usages.
    Communication Quarterly, 31, 62–67.
Bartlett, F. (1932). *Remembering.* Cambridge, UK: Cambridge University Press.
Baxter, L. A. (1988). A dialectical perspective on communication strategies in relationship devel-
    opment. In S. W. Duck, D. F. Hay, S. E. Hobfoll, W. Ickes, & B. Montgomery (Eds.),
    Handbook of personal relationships (pp. 257–273). Chichester: Wiley.
Baxter, L. A. (1992). Forms and functions of intimate play in personal relationships. *Human
    Communication Research, 18,* 336–363.
Baxter, L. A., & Dindia, K. (1990). Marital partners' perceptions of marital maintenance strate-
    gies. *Journal of Social and Personal Relationships, 7,* 187–208.
Bell, R. A., Buerkel-Rothfuss, N., & Gore, K. (1987). "Did you bring the yarmulke for the
    Cabbage Patch Kid?" The idiomatic communication of young lovers. *Human Communication
    Research, 14,* 47–67.
Berger, C. R. (1987). Planning and scheming: Strategies for initiating relationships. In R. Bur-
    nett, P. McGhee, & D. Clarke (Eds.), *Accounting for relationships* (pp. 158–174). London:
    Methuen.
Berger, P., & Kellner, H. (1974). Marriage and the construction of reality: An exercise in the
    microsociology of knowledge. *Diogenes, 46,* 1–24.
Billig, M. (1987). *Arguing and thinking: A rhetorical approach to social psychology.* Cambridge, UK:
    Cambridge University Press.
Burleson, B., Samter, W., & Lucchetti, A. E. (in press). Similarity in communication values as a
    predictor of friendship choices: Studies of friends and best friends. *Southern Communication
    Journal.*
Christensen, A., Sullaway, M., & King, C. (1983). Systematic error in behavioral reports of
    dyadic interaction: Egocentric bias and content effects. *Behavioral Assessment, 5,* 129–142.
Cody, M. J., & McLaughlin, M. L. (1985). The situation as a construct in communication
    research. In M. L. Knapp & G. R. Miller (Eds.), *Handbook of interpersonal communication* (pp.
    263–312). Beverly Hills, CA: Sage.
Dainton, M., & Stafford, L. (1993). Routine maintenance behaviors: A comparison of relation-

ship type, partner similarity and sex differences. *Journal of Social and Personal Relationships, 10,* 255–271.

Dindia, K., & Baxter, L. A. (1987). Strategies for maintaining and repairing marital relationships. *Journal of Social and Personal Relationships, 4,* 143–158.

Duck, S. W. (1986). *Human relationships* London: Sage.

Duck, S. W. (1988). *Relating to others.* Monterey, CA: Brooks/Cole.

Duck, S. W. (1990). Relationships as unfinished business: Out of the frying pan and into the 1990s. *Journal of Social and Personal Relationships, 7,* 3–28.

Duck, S. W. (1991, May). *New lamps for old: A new theory of relationships and a fresh look at some old research.* Paper presented to the third conference of the International Network on Personal Relationships, Normal IL.

Duck, S. W. (1992). *Human relationships* (2nd ed.). London: Sage.

Duck, S. W. (in press). *Meaningful relationships: Talking, sense, and relating.* Newbury Park, CA: Sage.

Duck, S. W., & Miell, D. E. (1986). Charting the development of personal relationships. In R. Gilmour & S. W. Duck (Eds.), *Emerging field of personal relationships* (pp. 133–144). Hillsdale, NJ: Lawrence Erlbaum.

Duck, S. W., & Pond, K. (1989). Friends, Romans, countrymen, lend me your retrospective data: Rhetoric and reality in personal relationships. In C. Hendrick (Ed.), *Review of social psychology and personality: Vol. 10: Close relationships* (pp. 3–27). Newbury Park, CA: Sage.

Duck, S. W., Pond, K., & Leatham, G. B. (1991, May). *Remembering as a context for being in relationships: Different perspectives on the same interaction.* Paper presented to the third conference of the International Network on Personal Relationships, Normal, IL.

Duck, S. W., Pond, K., & Leatham, G. B. (in press). Loneliness and the evaluation of relational events. *Journal of Social and Personal Relationships.*

Duck, S. W., Rutt, D. J., Hurst, M. H., & Strejc, H. (1991). Some evident truths about everyday conversation: All communications are not created equal. *Human Communication Research, 18,* 228–267.

Duck, S. W., & Sants, H. K. A. (1983). On the origin of the specious: Are personal relationships really interpersonal states? *Journal of Social and Clinical Psychology, 1,* 27–41.

Edwards, D., & Middleton, D. (1988). Conversational remembering and family relationships: How children learn to remember. *Journal of Social and Personal Relationships, 5,* 3–25.

Giles, H. (1989, May). *Gosh, you don't look it: Intergenerational communication in relationships.* Paper presented to the Iowa Conference on Personal Relationships, Iowa City, IA.

Hatfield [Walster], E., Walster, G. W., & Berscheid, E. (1978). *Equity Theory and Research.* Boston: Allyn & Bacon.

Herzberg, F. (1966). *Work and the nature of man.* Cleveland, OH: World.

Homans, G. C. (1961). *Social behavior: Its elementary forms.* New York: Harcourt, Brace, and World.

Honeycutt, J. M. (1993). Memory structures for the rise and fall of personal relationships. In S. W. Duck (Ed.), *Understanding relationship processes 1: Individuals in relationships.* 60–86. Newbury Park, CA: Sage.

Hopper, R., Knapp, M. L., & Scott, L. (1981). Couples' personal idioms: Exploring intimate talk. *Journal of Communication, 31,* 23–33.

Kelly, G. A. (1955). *The psychology of personal constructs.* New York: Norton.

Kelly, G. A. (1969). Ontological acceleration. In B. Maher (Ed.), *Clinical psychology and personality: The collected papers of George Kelly* (pp. 7–45). New York: Wiley.

La Gaipa, J. J. (1977). Interpersonal attraction and social exchange. In S. W. Duck (Ed.), *Theory and practice in interpersonal attraction* (pp. 129–164). London: Academic Press.

Levinger, G. (1976). A social psychological perspective on marital dissolution. *Journal of Social Issues*, *31*, 21–47.

Mehrabian, A. (1971). *Silent messages*. New York: Fumbleton Press.

Monsour, M. (1992). Meanings of intimacy in cross-sex and same-sex friendships. *Journal of Social and Personal Relationships*, *9*, 277–296.

Nofsinger, R. (1990). *Everyday conversation*. Newbury Park, CA: Sage.

Rubin, Z. (1974). From liking to loving: Patterns of attraction in dating relationships. In T. L. Huston (Ed.), *Foundations of interpersonal attraction* (pp. 233–260). New York: Academic Press.

Rusbult, C. E. (1983). A longitudinal test of the investment model: The development (and deterioration) of satisfaction and commitment in heterosexual involvements. *Journal of Personality and Social Psychology*, *45*, 101–117.

Shapiro, J. P., Baumeister, R. F., & Kessler, J. V. (1991). A three component model of children's teasing: Aggression, humor and ambiguity. *Journal of Social and Clinical Psychology*, *10*, 459–472.

Shea, B. C., & Pearson, J. (1986). The effects of relationship type, partner intent, and gender on the selection of relationship maintenance strategies. *Communication Monographs*, *53*, 352–364.

Stafford, L., & Canary, D. J. (1991). Maintenance strategies and romantic relationship type, gender, and relational characteristics. *Journal of Social and Personal Relationships*, *8*, 217–42.

Surra, C. A. (1987). Reasons for changes in commitment: Variations by courtship style. *Journal of Social and Personal Relationships*, *4*, 17–33.

Thibaut, J. W., & Kelley, H. H. (1959). *The Social Psychology of Groups*. New York: Wiley.

Tracy, K., Craig, R. T., Smith, M., & Spisak, F. (1984). The discourse of requests: Assessment of a compliance gaining approach. *Human Communication Research*, *10*, 513–538.

A Social Skills Approach to Relationship Maintenance

How Individual Differences in Communication Skills Affect the Achievement of Relationship Functions

Brant R. Burleson

Department of Communication
Purdue University
West Lafayette, Indiana

Wendy Samter

Department of Communication
University of Delaware
Newark, Delaware

Introduction

This chapter develops a social skills approach to the study of relationship maintenance. Our framework is an outgrowth of what has been termed a *functional analysis* of interpersonal relationships, a position emphasizing what relationships do for those involved in them. Bochner (1984) characterizes the functional perspective as a general approach for analyzing interpersonal relationships, one that assumes there are

> a common set of functional requirements for comprehensive dyads such as friendships and marriages; that these functional requirements impose certain communicative demands on

Communication and Relational Maintenance

> enduring twosomes; that these demands are sometimes contradictory, resulting in dyadic
> stress; and that this tension is accommodated by varying communicative and perceptual
> mechanisms that, though not always successful, are targeted at combating distress, dishar-
> mony, or disunion. I propose that a functional perspective can account for much of the
> communicative activity and difficulty that is experienced in enduring relationships. (p. 557)

A functional approach thus stresses the things that certain relationships typically *do* for people and, consequently, the things that people come to look to
those relationships *for.* Further, the functional perspective focuses on communication as the means through which people both pursue and service
relevant relationship functions.

Extending Bochner's functional approach, the current chapter suggests
that maintaining satisfying interpersonal relationships is an ability—an ability at which individuals may be differentially skilled. More specifically, we
believe one important way in which people maintain relationships is through
the enactment of various communication skills that contribute to the achievement of the functions that define those relationships. As with most forms of
skilled behavior, however, it is likely that individuals differ with respect to the
communication skills that contribute to the maintenance of significant relationships. Thus, we examine whether there are measurable individual differences in the ability to maintain desirable personal relationships; we further
seek to specify the cognitive and behavioral skills that lead some persons to be
more effective than others at maintaining personal relationships.

To date, most studies examining relationship maintenance from a social
skills vantage point have operated from what might be termed a "main effects" model. That is, much existing work on the contributions of social skills
to relationship maintenance rests on the assumption that individual differences in social skills exert a *main* or *direct effect* on the maintenance of intimate relationships such as friendship and marriage. Thus, the core hypothesis put forth in such studies has been that individuals with comparatively
developed social skills will be more effective at maintaining desirable social
relationships. Although some research supports the main effects model, other
recent studies provide more limited support for this model.

In this chapter we propose an elaboration of the social skills model that
considers how the cognitive representations individuals hold for certain relationships influence the kinds of skills needed to maintain those relationships.
More specifically, we propose a "skill similarity" model which suggests that
similarity in the nature and level of partners' social skills may be more important to relationship maintenance than the absolute level of skill sophistication
of the partners. The skill similarity model also emphasizes that relationship
maintenance is a dyadic process: Relationship maintenance may be less a
matter of what one individual does for (or to) another, and more a matter of
what partners do *with* each other. The skill similarity model thus posits that

the maintenance-enhancing effects of individuals' communication skills are moderated by the skill levels of their partners. The final section of the chapter reviews several recent studies supporting the skill similarity model.

A central issue in any social skills approach to relationship maintenance has to do with identifying the particular skills facilitating the continuation of a healthy relationship. We suggest that the cognitive and behavioral skills contributing to the maintenance of personal relationships can be identified by carrying out detailed functional analyses of those relationships. Different relationships serve distinct functions in people's lives; for example, the functions served by the marital relationship are distinct from those served by close friendships. Communication skills that foster the maintenance of any given relationship, then, are those which enable individuals to accomplish the functions associated with that particular relationship. In what follows, we present a set of theoretical questions to guide analyses of relationship maintenance—questions that may aid researchers in identifying important relationships, the functions individuals associate with these relationships, and the skills partners must possess in order to accomplish relevant relational functions. To situate our social skills approach to relationship maintenance, we begin the chapter with a brief review of existing work on relationship maintenance. Much of what we currently know about relationship maintenance is based on research assuming that people consciously and strategically seek to maintain relationships with significant others through intentional actions designed to address perceived relationship exigencies (broadly defined).

Approaches to the Study of Relationship Maintenance

Prevailing Approaches to the Study of Relationship Maintenance

In comparison to work on relationship escalation and deterioration, work on relationship maintenance is in its early stages of development (see Duck, 1986; Stafford & Canary, 1991). Perhaps it is not surprising, then, that several different conceptualizations of relationship maintenance can be identified in the literature. For example, some researchers (e.g., Dindia, 1989; Baxter & Dindia, 1990) define maintenance in "preventative" terms, as behaviors actors employ to ensure or "uphold" satisfaction in their relationships. Other researchers such as Stafford and Canary (1991) view maintenance as proactive efforts directed at preserving a particular relationship definition. Ayres (1983) and Shea and Pearson (1986) conceptualize maintenance in terms of the strategies individuals use to keep relationships stable when faced with a partner's desire to increase or decrease levels of intimacy.

Still others (e.g., Duck, 1988) have suggested that relationship maintenance can involve specific acts undertaken to repair a damaged or distressed relationship.

Maintenance as a Response to a Relational Exigence

Although there are clear differences in how researchers define relationship maintenance, there is remarkable similarity in the methods used by many researchers to assess relationship maintenance. Typically, researchers have elicited persons' maintenance strategies by asking them to either (1) construct messages, that is provide open-ended descriptions of the strategies they think they use (or might use) to maintain a particular relationship, or (2) select messages, that is rate a set of maintenance strategies supplied by the researcher for frequency or likelihood of use (for a general discussion of the advantages and limitations of message construction *versus* message selection methods, see Burleson et al., 1988). Researchers using these methods appear to assume that relationship maintenance is a relatively conscious process in which persons intentionally enact behaviors strategically designed to achieve some "maintenance" goal (see Duck, 1988, this volume). Further, most research has assumed that maintenance behaviors are enacted when an individual encounters some *relational exigence*, a desired goal state that may be marked by some urgency. Thus, from this view, maintenance behaviors are strategic efforts intended to manage or overcome some relational exigence. In research stemming from this relational exigence approach, people have been asked to report specific things they might say or do (or have done) to achieve a desired level of intimacy, to keep relationships stable, to ensure satisfaction, or to repair a breech of relationship rules.

In studies equating maintenance with intimacy control and stability, for example, participants have been instructed to imagine an exigence wherein one party wants to move the relationship toward greater or lesser levels of intimacy while the other wishes to keep intimacy at its current level; subjects are then asked to rate how likely they would be to use various strategies designed to "keep the relationship stable." Findings indicate that common responses to this sort of exigence include direct inquiries about relational goals, statements reminding partners of earlier relationship definitions, or the avoidance of particular topics of talk (Ayres, 1983). In contrast, other research shows that when the exigence is one of preserving a particular relationship definition, maintenance efforts are directed toward conveying positive feelings and assurances (see Stafford & Canary, 1991). Finally, when asked what strategies they would use to maintain a relationship in the face of a partner's breech of relational rules, participants report that talking about the problem, acquiescing, or giving an ultimatum are among the more common strategies they would employ (Dindia & Baxter, 1987; Duck, 1985).

Although the handling of exigencies certainly constitutes an important part of relationship maintenance, strategic actions directed specifically at some "maintenance exigence" are not the only behaviors that function to sustain relationships. As Duck (1988) and others (e.g., Hays, 1989) have recently argued, a broad array of behaviors that partners enact may contribute to the maintenance of a relationship.

Maintenance as the Enactment of Behavioral Routines and Rituals

Duck (1988) suggests an alternative approach to relationship maintenance where virtually every action—especially mundane, routine actions—are the vehicles by which relationships are maintained. As he argues:

> The maintenance of relationships is accomplished by a complex combination of individual strategic inputs, mundane routines, social pressures, ritual actions that celebrate the relationship, personal attention to partner's needs, adherence to relational rules, and social skills, among other things. Relationships are sustained not merely by people's feelings for one another but also by people's routines, their trivial interconnectedness and presence in one another's spheres of life, by their strategic behavior intended to sustain the relationships and also by the actions and communications of other friends, mutual acquaintances, or colleagues. (p. 100)

Duck suggests that in a very real sense relationships are maintained by existing—by being enacted. Thus, *all* behavior in a relationship serves to maintain that relationship. However, Duck further suggests that because certain behavioral routines or rituals (which may be highly idiosyncratic to a particular couple) acquire significant symbolic value for relationship partners, the enactment of those routines or rituals may serve especially important maintenance functions.

Consistent with his view that virtually all behavior serves to maintain a relationship, Duck advocates increased study of everyday relational behaviors, and especially the daily routines and rituals enacted by partners. The aim of such research (e.g., Duck, Rutt, Hurst, & Strejc, 1991) is to illuminate how a variety of mundane events serve to stabilize and sustain relationships.

An Alternative Approach to Relationship Maintenance: The Social Skills Perspective

In the approach to the study of relationship maintenance developed here, we feature the role that nonstrategically enacted routines serve in binding people together. We argue that different relationships perform specific functions for the partners in those relationships, and, in order for these relationships to serve their characteristic functions, partners must control appropriate social skills through which these functions can be realized. For us, then, relationships are maintained through the routine enactment of skills that enable partners to accomplish the functions associated with various relationship types. In other words, *relationship maintenance occurs whenever persons enact behaviors that service the particular tasks or functions defining a particular relationship.*

People may be more or less skilled in addressing the tasks or functions that define a relationship, and thus relationships may be more or less well maintained. Relationship maintenance may be viewed as a normative and continuous construct—a relationship may be more or less effectively maintained. Well-maintained relationships are those in which people smoothly accomplish the tasks and functions that define that relationship. Less well-maintained relationships are those characterized by some inadequacies in the extent to which necessary tasks and functions are achieved. Poorly maintained relationships are marked by serious inadequacies in the achievement of relationship functions. "Failed relationships" may be viewed as those where the achievement of relationship functions was so lacking that one or both parties exited from the relationship.

Our approach to relationship maintenance differs from those just described in three significant ways. First, we believe that relationships are maintained through the enactment of many different behaviors, not just those undertaken with a conscious intention to maintain, stabilize, or restore a relationship. Theorists representing perspectives as diverse as constructivism (Clark & Delia, 1979), speech act theory (Searle, 1969), and systems theory (Watzlawick, Beavin, & Jackson, 1967) have emphasized that virtually all interactional behaviors communicate "relational messages," and thus may be viewed as defining or maintaining the relationship. However, the relational messages inherent in the vast majority of interactional behaviors are implicit. Indeed, behaviors undertaken with the specific intention of defining, negotiating, and/or maintaining the relationship may be comparatively rare, especially in long-lasting or well-developed relationships. Certainly, circumstances do occur where partners consciously and strategically enact behaviors designed to maintain a relationship; studies such as those reported by Dindia and Baxter (1987) and Stafford and Canary (1991) provide ample evidence of this. Like Duck, though, we see relationships being maintained through the enactment of a broad array of behavioral routines characteristic to particular relationships—routines unconnected to any conscious effort to "maintain" the relationship. Unlike Duck, however, we argue that individuals may be more or less skilled in how they carry out the routine forms of communication characterizing their relationships, and that these differences in skill levels have significant consequences for how well the relationship is maintained.

More specifically, we believe people hold tacit definitions of relationships

—and of the functions they serve—and that these beliefs guide behavior at a global level. To use Duck's terms, skills may be "strategic inputs" from individuals; but they are strategic in the sense of contributing to the accomplishment of particular functions or tasks that define a given relationship, not in the sense of indexing differences in some limited, finite set of strategic behaviors that maintain all relationships. For example, most young adults see close friends as their primary source of emotional support; during times of distress, they expect their friends to function as providers of support (i.e., to comfort, advise, listen, soothe, etc.). When called on to fill this function, friends do so not because they perceive their support-giving efforts as strategic, conscious attempts to "maintain" the relationship, but rather because they recognize at some tacit level that the provision of emotional support is a common element of close friendship (i.e., "That's what friends do for one another"). Thus, from our perspective, a tacit understanding of what friends "do for one another" drives the enactment of various behaviors, and these behaviors, in turn, have the effect of sustaining the relationship. In other words, our analysis focuses on skills and behaviors that are not strategically intended by individuals to maintain their relationships, but that nevertheless function to do so.

A second way in which our approach to relationship maintenance differs from others is in furnishing a framework for identifying the forms of behavior centrally contributing to specific relationships. Most studies of relationship maintenance (including those that would follow from Duck's arguments) provide little theoretical basis for understanding the specific routines that must be enacted effectively on a regular basis if a relationship is to be sustained. Although some scholars believe all behaviors in a relationship may make some contribution to its maintenance, certain types of behavior (or behaviors addressing some issues) are likely to be more important than others with respect to maintaining the relationship. Existing approaches to relationship maintenance do not provide a principled basis for identifying, *a priori*, the specific behaviors likely to have the greatest impact on relationship maintenance. The following approach to relationship maintenance provides a principled basis for identifying the types of behavior in specific relationships likely to have special significance in maintaining those relationships.

Relationships are differentially functional; that is, people expect different types of relationships to provide them with different things, to accomplish for them distinct pragmatic, social, and emotional goals. The functions individuals associate with marriage, for instance, are likely to differ from those they associate with close friendship. This suggests that the routines and tasks partners must enact to accomplish the functions associated with marriage will differ from the routines and tasks individuals must enact to accomplish the functions associated with close friendship. Examining the functions different relationships serve for people thus should provide a theoretical basis for identifying the routine behaviors serving to sustain different relationships.

A third way in which our approach to relationship maintenance is distinct lies in its focus on individual differences. Neither the relational exigence approach nor Duck's approach provides an analysis of systematic individual differences in the ability to maintain particular types of relationships. Yet, some individuals are more effective than others at maintaining certain types of relationships. For example, extensive research indicates that some children effectively maintain peer friendships, and do so consistently from one year to the next, whereas other children have serious difficulties in sustaining any significant peer relationships (see Coie, Dodge, & Kupersmidt, 1990). Similarly, research indicates that some young adults are able to sustain mutually satisfying dating relationships with relatively few problems, whereas others have significant difficulties in initiating and maintaining such relationships (see Curran, Wallander, & Farrell, 1985).

We assume that individuals differ in their control of skills needed to accomplish the tasks associated with the functions defining a particular relationship. That is, our analysis suggests the successful maintenance of any given relationship depends, in part, on the skillfulness individuals exhibit in the communicative activities that enable them to achieve important relational functions. Understanding that individuals differ with respect to relationally relevant communication skills thus provides a theoretical basis for explaining why some people are more successful or effective than others at maintaining relationships.

In sum, we suggest that a relationship is maintained when it more or less fulfills the functions with which participants associate it. For relationships to be maintained, then, partners must control the social and communication skills needed to realize relevant functions. The following section further elaborates the social skills approach, identifying critical theoretical and methodological concerns addressed within this approach.

Issues Framing a Social Skills
Analysis of Relationship Maintenance

Our analysis of relationship maintenance is framed by three theoretical questions concerning (1) the kinds of relationships that are important in people's lives, (2) the functions individuals associate with these relationships, and (3) the skills partners must control to realize the relevant functions. Each question, in turn, raises methodological issues concerning how researchers can identify important relationships, understand the functions they serve, and target the skills necessary for the effective maintenance of those relationships. In what follows, we briefly discuss each theoretical question and the attendant methodological issues it suggests. We then illustrate our analysis by presenting in some detail a social skills approach to the maintenance of a particular relationship, that of friendship.

What Relationships Are Significant in People's Lives?

People maintain a variety of relationships on a day-to-day basis, some of which are subjectively significant (e.g., relationships with spouses, friends, romantic partners, and family members) and some of which are less significant, at least personally (e.g., relationships with co-workers, acquaintances, local merchants, neighbors, and service professionals). Determining the types of relationships that populate life at a given time, and the social and personal significance of these relationships, requires consideration of multiple dimensions of human experience. In particular, efforts to identify significant forms of human relationship must be informed by an understanding of biology, sociology, and psychology.

Some relationships inhere in human biology. Humans are intrinsically social creatures; they survive and prosper as members of groups and communities. Thus, a fundamental relationship for virtually all people is that of group or team member. Other biological facts have important relationship implications: reproduction of the human species is a social process; the human newborn is relatively helpless for the first dozen years of life; and human beings further lack the instincts necessary to ensure survival. In a very real sense, children must be taught what it means to "be human" and how to survive as a human (Berger & Luckmann, 1967). These circumstances mean that the parenting relationship is a biological necessity. Further, varied forms of the marital relationship may be seen as a biologically based support system for the parenting relationship.

A vast number of relationships are the product of particular cultural formations. The types of relationships in which an individual may engage are largely determined by the role structure of a social system. For example, certain relationship possibilities inhere in tribal societies, whereas vastly different relationship possibilities inhere in advanced industrial societies. The historical legacy and traditions of a society further shape the contours of relationship possibility: The nature and character of potential relationships in modern Japan differ significantly from those in modern America, even though both are advanced industrial societies.

Other human relationships may be grounded primarily in the psychological needs of individuals. Most people have needs for affiliation, confirmation, and acceptance that can be fully met only in voluntary relationships such as friendship. Personal desires for esteem, validation, or power may motivate individuals to pursue relationships in social hierarchies such as gangs. Other personal desires, such as those for security, attachment, and love, provide powerful psychological incentives to pursue biologically necessary familial relationships.

In sum, our analysis of relationship maintenance begins with asking, What kinds of relationships are particularly important in people's lives? Generating answers to this question rests on sociological and psychological analysis of relationships. Relationships are sociologically significant when they fulfill some kind of necessary institutional function. Relationships are psychologically significant when they fulfill some sort of important personal or emotional need that if left unmet will impede an individual's optimal functioning.

What Functions Are Served by Particular Relationships?

Once a significant relationship is isolated on the basis of the sociological and psychological needs it meets, the specific functions individuals associate with that relationship can be identified. Thus, the second set of questions in our three-part analysis of relationship maintenance asks, What are the functions particular relationships serve in people's lives and how are they determined?

As noted earlier, we believe relationships are differentially functional. By asking individuals how they think about and what they want from a particular relationship, researchers can acquire a sense of how people define that relationship, what they expect partners to do in that relationship, and what pragmatic, social, and emotional goals are associated with it. Thus, one way to ascertain the functions associated with a particular relationship is to examine people's conceptions of and expectations for that relationship. This has been a particularly popular method for studying the friendship relation in recent years (e.g., Damon, 1977; Rawlins & Holl, 1987; Selman, 1980; Youniss, 1980).

The functions individuals associate with particular relationships suggest a set of tasks around which those relationships are organized. In other words, the functions people expect specific relationships to fulfill imply a set of tasks either that they want accomplished or that must be accomplished if the relationship is to continue (see McFall, 1982; Renshaw & Asher, 1982).

Sometimes the expectations people voice for a relationship directly imply tasks integral to the process of maintaining a relationship. For example, the expectation that "friends will pick you up when you are feeling down," directly implies the tasks of providing comfort, reassurance, and support. Occasionally, the expectations voiced by naive actors may provide a fairly exhaustive catalogue of the functions served by a relationship. Often, however, direct inquiries about relationship conceptions and expectations must be supplemented by what Burleson (1991) has called a "logical analysis" of relationship characteristics and properties. Such logical analyses aim to reveal features, challenges, and demands of particular relationships that are rarely made explicit in the relationship descriptions directly articulated by naive actors. Rawlins' (1989, 1992) work on the dialectical tensions inherent in the friendship relation is an example of such a logical analysis. Thus, logical analyses of relationship types can suggest a somewhat different set of tasks partners face (i.e., the successful management of dialectical tensions inherent to the relationship) than what is suggested by a straightforward empirical survey of actors' conceptions.

What Skills Are Needed to Accomplish the Functions Associated with a Particular Relationship?

The third question in our analysis of relationship maintenance asks, What are the skills individuals must possess to achieve the functions associated with a given relationship? The tasks around which particular relationships are organized provide information about the duties of and demands on partners in those relationships. These tasks, in turn, suggest something about the particular skills and behaviors partners need to enact if the relationship is to be maintained. An understanding of the tasks partners must accomplish— and the attendant duties these tasks obligate partners to perform—provides the foundation for identifying skills necessary to sustain relationships. The skills individuals must possess for a relationship to be maintained, then, are those which enable them to fulfill specific obligations suggested by the tasks around which the relationship is organized.

The social skills approach to relationship maintenance is therefore framed by a set of theoretical questions that seek to (1) identify relationships that serve important needs for the individual and society, (2) isolate the functions and tasks around which these relationships are organized, and (3) target the forms of communication which, if enacted skillfully, enable individuals to accomplish the relational duties such tasks obligate them to perform. We believe these theoretical questions can be used to understand how communication skills contribute to the maintenance of any important relationship. In the next section, we demonstrate how these questions inform our analysis of the role communication skills play in the maintenance of one particular relationship: the close friendship.

An Example of the Social Skills Approach
to Relationship Maintenance: The Case of Close Friendship

The commitments and potential contributions of the social skills approach to relationship maintenance are best illustrated by presenting an extended example. We have chosen to illustrate our approach with close friendship because this relationship occupies a central place in most contemporary cultures and, in recent years, has been the target of extensive research.

The Sociological and Psychological Significance of Friendship

Friendship is an important relationship for both institutional (sociological) and personal (psychological) reasons. Sociologically, friendship is a context in which socializing impulses may be productively channeled; Simmel (1908/ 1950) identifies friendship as an important outlet for the impetus to "sociate." Early in life, friendship serves as a "laboratory" in which children acquire and practice numerous social skills (see the reviews by Burleson, 1986; Ginsberg, Gottman, & Parker, 1986). Individuals experiencing dysfunctions in friendship early in life may have continuing personal and social difficulties later on (e.g., Cowen, Pederson, Babigian, Izzo, & Trost, 1973; Roff, Sells, & Golden, 1972). Throughout life, friendships provide tangible, informational, emotional, and other forms of support. In some communities, such as certain groups of the aged, friends provide the care, companionship, and material support traditionally given by the family (e.g., Heinemann, 1985; Shea, Thompson, & Blieszner, 1988). But friendships do more than support individuals; they also serve as a means through which larger social entities may achieve important goals. For example, Lincoln and Miller (1979) studied friendships in the work environment and concluded that the friendship networks they observed served as "systems for making decisions, mobilizing resources, concealing or transmitting information, and performing other functions closely allied with work behavior and interaction" (p. 197). Across the life course, then, friendships provide important contexts for socialization and important vehicles for the achievement of personal, communal, and institutional purposes.

Friendships also serve important psychological needs for the individual (e.g., Duck, 1986; Hays, 1988; Rawlins, 1992). Across the life span, friends are key sources from which people gain a sense of psychological connectedness, inclusion, and affiliation. In comparison to individuals with close friends, those without close friends tend to be dissatisfied with themselves, their relationships, and, ultimately, their lives. Research indicates, for example, that people who lack significant ties to friends are lonely (e.g., Jones & Moore, 1989; Peplau & Perlman, 1982), prone to depression, anxiety, and fatigue (e.g., Cobb, 1976; Hojat, 1982; Jones, Freemon, & Goswick, 1981), feel they have little control over social situations (e.g., Jones et al., 1981; Moore & Sermat, 1974), and have low levels of self-esteem (e.g., Cutrona, 1982; Hojat, 1982; Horowitz & French, 1979).

In fact, studies suggest that at several life stages friends are the most important source from which people derive a sense of "belonging" and that this sense of belonging has several pragmatic benefits. For example, in a study of college students, Cutrona (1982) found that satisfaction with current friendships was a better predictor of loneliness during freshman year than was satisfaction with family or romantic relationships. Her results also indicated that students who overcame loneliness by the end of freshman year did so because they developed new friendships, not because they initiated romances or maintained close ties with family members. Other work has shown that in comparison to family members, friends play a greater role in supporting a person's sense of self esteem and usefulness during old age (Blau, 1973), helping widowed individuals overcome grief (Arling, 1976), and providing social and emotional support during recovery from physical illness (Croog, Lipson, & Levine, 1972).

People's Conceptions of and Expectations for Friendship: What They Say about the Functions of Friendship and the Skills Needed for Their Accomplishment

During the last 15 years, researchers have intensively examined people's conceptions of and expectations for the friend relationship (e.g., Damon, 1977; La Gapia, 1981; Selman, 1980; Smollar & Youniss, 1982; see the reviews by Serafica, 1982; Tesch, 1983). These empirical investigations have been directed at showing how ordinary people conceptualize friendship, their expectations for friends, the duties and obligations seen as inhering in the friend relationship, appropriate activities and conversational topics for friends, and so forth (see also Rawlins, this volume).

Very diverse methods and subject samples have been used in these studies. Despite such diversity, the results of this research paint a remarkably consistent picture of how adults in contemporary American society think about friends and what they expect from them. From adolescence onward, most people see friendship in terms of deep psychological characteristics. That is, friends are described in terms of trustworthiness, loyalty, commitment, affection, acceptance, and support. The latter two qualities appear to be particularly important in people's conceptions of friendship: a central component of friendship is defined by expectations that friends provide validation and acceptance, and also varied forms of support during times of need or emotional distress. Acceptance and support thus appear to lie near the heart of what most people mean by friendship.

The core significance of acceptance and support are nicely illustrated in a recent study by Secklin (1991), who analyzed interviews with 44 pairs of young-adult best friends. For the most part, these pairs characterized the essence of friendship as "being there" for each other. According to Secklin, "being there" meant the willingness to "do just about anything" or "whatever it takes to support" a friend through the hassles of everyday life or through more difficult emotional crises. Being there represented the tacit understanding that one was never alone, that there was always someone who accepted you and to whom you could turn. Several other researchers report that when asked to define friendship, both young and older adults commonly respond by saying "friends are people with whom one can discuss personal matters" (Phillips & Metzger, 1976), "friends are people you can talk to and trust," "friends call on one another for help" (Crawford, 1977), and that "people want their friends to "be there" to talk to and to help or to celebrate" (Rawlins, 1992, p. 201).

These expectations are reflected in the activities of friends. Work by Kon (1981) and Adelman, Parks, and Albrecht (1987) suggests that young adults not only expect friends to function as their primary sources of acceptance and emotional support, but actually turn to friends for help in difficult times. Other studies indicate that much of the time friends spend together revolves around disclosure of private facts and feelings (Morton, 1978) and talk focusing on doubts and fears, relationships, and social and emotional problems (e.g., Aries, 1976; Aries & Johnson, 1983).

Studies of friendship conceptions and expectations suggest, then, that a central task facing young adult friends is the provision of emotional acceptance and support. To maintain a close friendship, partners are thus obligated to provide comfort, help solve problems, work through uncertainties, celebrate victories, offer encouragement, validate motivations, and so on. Communication skills enabling individuals to fulfill these obligations—that is, to accomplish the task of providing acceptance and emotional support—are thus essential to friendship maintenance.

Ego support and comforting are two forms of communication that focus on the provision of emotional acceptance and support. Ego support is defined as the general ability to make others feel good about themselves (Burleson & Samter, 1990; Samter & Burleson, 1990a). Two forms of ego support skill have been identified: one that focuses on encouraging another to undertake a difficult or challenging task (called *encouraging* ego support), and one that focuses on celebrating another's personal success (called *celebratory* ego support). Skillful or sophisticated ego support messages signal an understanding and acceptance of who the other is and what he or she wants to do. Because friends are expected to validate and support each other's personhood and goals, we believe skillful communication aimed at making others feel good about themselves is integral to the maintenance of close friendships.

Comforting skill has been defined as the ability to alleviate another's emotional distress (Burleson, 1984). Because friends often look to one another as chief sources of emotional support, the ability to provide comfort in a sensitive and effective manner should be important to the process of maintaining close friendship. In sum, communication skills such as providing ego support and emotional comfort appear vital to the maintenance of friendships because these skills are the vehicles through which core tasks inherent in the friend relationship get addressed.

Logical Analyses of the "Dialectics" of Friendship:
What They Say about the Functions and Tasks of Friendship
and the Skills Needed for Their Accomplishment

The relevance of ego support and comforting skills to the maintenance of friendships is directly suggested by empirical investigations of friendship conceptions and expectations. However, Rawlins' (1989, 1992) logical analysis of the "dialectics" of friendship reveals several significant tensions inherent in this social relationship. These tensions make the outbreak of interpersonal disputes possible at any time and, therefore, suggest that conflict management skill may also play an important role in the successful maintenance of close friendship.

Of course, it is not novel to suggest that conflict is a common, even inevitable, feature of close relationships such as friendship (see Fitzpatrick & Winke, 1979; Hocker & Wilmot, 1991; Sillars, 1980; Sillars & Weisberg, 1987). However, most analyses of conflict in close relationships have viewed it as stemming from factors such as (1) competition over scare resources ("I want to do this and you want to do that"), (2) failure to live up to the obligations of the relationship ("you done me wrong"), or (3) differences in attitudes or values ("we just disagree"). There is no question that these are potent and continuing sources of conflict in close relationships. However, Rawlins' dialectical analysis of friendship shows that there are different, even deeper sources of conflict between friends, sources built into the very structure of the friend relationship (see Rawlins, this volume).

Rawlins identifies four dialectical principles that characterize the interactions of friends. The dialectic of *affection and instrumentality* arises from the circumstance that although true friendships are ideally based on mutual affection, friends often prove useful to one another. Yet, those who seek instrumental support run the risk of being viewed as "using" their friends. The dialectic of *judgment and acceptance* arises from the circumstance that although friends are expected to accept one another "warts and all," real friends are also expected to be trusted sources of feedback which, of course, implies critical evaluation. Paradoxically, too much acceptance of a friend may suggest a *laissez faire* lack of caring, whereas too much judgment may convey a lack of understanding, solidarity, and support. The dialectic of *expressiveness and protectiveness* arises from the circumstance that although friends should be free to communicate openly, saying anything to each other, such open communication often reveals areas of personal vulnerability and implies critical evaluation. Open, unrestrained communication about a friend's qualities or behaviors may lead to embarrassment or hurt. Finally, the dialectic of *independence/dependence* arises because friends expect from each other the freedom to pursue life interests without interference, but simultaneously maintain the privilege of calling on one another in times of need: friends should not *impede* each other, but neither should they *impose* on one another.

These dialectics both organize and compose "ongoing challenges and antagonistic choices in the practical management of communication sustaining friendships" (Rawlins, 1989, p. 170). Further, each dialectic expresses a fundamental, unresolvable contradiction lying at the core of friendship. Rawlins emphasizes that conflicts can arise not only from the contradictions inherent in each of the dialectics, but also from how friends seek to manage and balance dialectical tensions. Moreover, any balance friends happen to strike between the dialectical contradictions is temporary; there can be no permanent resolution to these fundamental tensions. In sum, Rawlins' work shows that conflict is an intrinsic part of friendship. In a very real sense, friends are perpetually on the edge of conflict.

Because conflict is built into the very structure of friendship, conflict management is an ongoing task in which friends must engage. Rawlins' work clearly shows that the sources of conflict do not decrease as a friendship deepens; if anything, the contradictions faced by friends become more complicated and demanding as intimacy increases. Thus, the ability to manage conflict in sensitive and nonthreatening ways should be vital to the maintenance of close friendship.

Summary
Analyses of people's conceptions of and expectations for the friendship relation indicate that two important duties of friends include providing emotional acceptance and social support. This suggests that communication directed at validating another's successes (celebrating ego support skill), encouraging another to undertake a challenging task (encouraging ego support skill), and alleviating another's emotional distress (comforting skill) should be important communicative vehicles for the maintenance of friendships. Rawlins' logical analyses of the dialectical tensions inherent in friendships suggest that conflict is an inevitable part of close friendship. Because friends must somehow manage disputes arising from these, sophisticated conflict management skills should contribute to effective friendship maintenance as well.

Research assessing people's evaluations of ego support, comforting, and conflict management skills further suggests their relevance to the maintenance of friendships. Samter and Burleson (1990b) found that individuals' ratings of the importance of ego support and comforting skills in the friend relationship were positively associated with a measure of peer acceptance and negatively associated with self-reports of loneliness. Further, these researchers found that self-reported loneliness was negatively associated with individuals' ratings of the importance of conflict management skill. In sum, there are both theoretical and empirical reasons for viewing ego support, comforting, and conflict management skills as significant predictors of friendship maintenance. The next section of this chapter reviews empirical research directly assessing the contributions of comforting, ego support, and conflict management skills to the maintenance of friendships.

Skills for Maintaining Friendships: Two Models for Interpreting the Impact of Individual Differences in Communication Skills

---

To this point, our analysis implies the hypothesis that persons with relatively advanced ego support, comforting, and conflict management skills should be more successful than less skilled persons at maintaining friendships. This hypothesis expresses what we term the *main effects model:* the notion that the individuals' skills exert a direct effect on how well relationships such as friendship are maintained.

There is, however, an alternative to the main effects model that is still generally consistent with our functional analysis of interpersonal relationships. This alternative, which we term the *skill similarity model*, examines the skills of both parties in a relationship and suggests that *similarities in levels of partners' skills* will be more predictive of relationship satisfaction and maintenance than the absolute level of skillfulness exhibited by the parties. This portion of the chapter evaluates both of these models in light of the data currently available.

The Main Effects Model

Studies assessing the main effects of individual differences in communication skills on the maintenance of friendships have often proceeded in the following manner. First, a social group with relatively definite boundaries is identified (e.g., a classroom of elementary school children, a housing unit such as a college fraternity, a project team in a work environment). Such groups are contexts from which individuals typically draw friends; moreover, "social success" in such groups is often viewed in terms of developing and maintaining friendships with group members. Research assessing the main effects models would have each individual in the group complete a battery of tests assessing relevant social skills, including measures of targeted communication skills (e.g., comforting skill, conflict management ability). Sociometric methods are used to assess the quantity and quality of the social relationships each member of the group shares with other members. For example, patterns of friendship are often determined through "peer nomination" procedures, and patterns of liking can be assessed through "peer rating" procedures. Sociometric information is especially useful for generating indices of peer acceptance, peer popularity, and related constructs (for a review of sociometric methods, see Ladd & Asher, 1985). To assess the main effects of individual differences in communication skills on friendships, researchers typically correlate individuals' scores on the communication skill assessments with indices generated from the sociometric measures.

Research stemming from the main effects model has met with only limited success in showing that persons with advanced communication skills are better able to form and maintain friendships. Studies (e.g., Yeates, Schultz, & Selman, 1991; see the review by Burleson, 1986) have consistently found that children with poor conflict management skills are less liked by and less popular with their peers. The relevance of conflict management skill to the maintenance of adult friendships is less clearly established, however, and the "main effects" of ego support and comforting skills on ongoing friendships have not been established for either children or adults.

For example, Burleson et al. (1986) had a sample of first- and third-grade children complete a series of tasks assessing their comforting, referential, persuasive, and listener-adapted communication skills. Sociometric nominations were used to identify groups of accepted and rejected children. Children rejected by their peers had less developed comforting and referential communication skills than those accepted by peers. Burleson and Waltman (1987) attempted to extend these results by assessing how the communication skills of fifth and sixth graders influenced their acceptance by classmates. These researchers obtained measures of children's comforting, conflict management, and persuasion skills; however, individual differences in these skills were not related to any measure of the children's popularity with or acceptance by peers.

In a study designed to provide a rigorous test of the main effects model, Samter and Burleson (1990a) investigated the influence of individual differences in comforting, ego support, and conflict management skills on the degree of peer acceptance enjoyed by college students living in fraternities and sororities. These researchers had each person living in a fraternity or sorority house complete a battery of communication skill assessments. The participants also completed sociometric nominations and ratings for their house members; these latter data were used to generate multiple indices of peer acceptance. Individual differences in communication skills were found to be only infrequently and weakly associated with the peer acceptance indices; rejection by peers was negatively associated with individuals' comforting skills and conflict management skills ($r = -.12$, $p < .05$, for both skills). None of the communication skills were positively associated with any of the peer acceptance indices. In sum, there is only weak and inconsistent evidence supporting the notion that individual differences in certain communication skills exert a main effect on the maintenance of friendships.

There are several reasons why efforts testing the main effects model may have met with limited success. First, it is possible that a flawed or incomplete analysis of the functions served by friendship may have resulted in important communication skills being ignored. Several recent studies (e.g., Duck et al., 1991; Hays, 1989; Rawlins, 1992) emphasize that friendship is rooted in the sharing of fun and playful activities as much as it is in the sharing of intimacies and the provision of support. Indeed, "having fun" may be the most frequent function served by many friendships. This suggests communication skills such as conversational ability, narrative ability, and related verbal abilities that contribute to "having a good time" serve an important, and perhaps critical, role in the maintenance of friendships. Certainly, future tests of the main effects model should include measures of such skills.

Second, the procedures employed in these studies provided assessments of how accepted or well liked an individual was within a certain peer group, not how well individuals maintained specific, reciprocated friendships. Some researchers (e.g., Bukowski & Hoza, 1989) emphasize that there are important differences in constructs such as "friendship," "popularity," "acceptance," and so on. Thus, the sociometric assessments of popularity and peer acceptance obtained in these studies may not be appropriate indicators of friendship maintenance. A related problem stems from the subject samples employed in the studies: participants were limited to indicating friends they had only in the closed social systems examined (i.e., the classroom or the fraternity house). It is possible that most of the relationships in these social systems constitute relatively casual "friendly relations" (Kurth, 1970) rather than deep friendships.

There are, then, several theoretical and methodological problems in existing research that may explain why these studies provide little support for a main effects model. However, it is also possible that the main effects model is just *wrong*. The main effects model focuses exclusively on how characteristics of the individual contributes to the maintenance of a dyadic relationship. The model does not provide for how characteristics of partners contribute to maintaining the relationship. This may be an inherent flaw in the main effects model; efforts directed at accounting for the maintenance of a relationship may need to focus on qualities of the dyad rather than characteristics of individuals. For example, it seems possible that the maintenance-enhancing effects of individuals' communication skills may be moderated by the skill levels of their partners.

The Skill Similarity Model

The notion that similar individuals will be more attracted to each other than dissimilar others is a mainstay of modern social psychology, with much research (e.g., Byrne, 1971) having focused on how similarities in attitudes and other cognitive variables promote attraction. The most probative versions of the similarity/attraction hypothesis are those coupled with "filter" theories of relationship development (e.g., Duck, 1977; Kerckhoff & Davis, 1962). The fundamental idea underlying filter theories is that people expect and receive different things from particular relationships at various points in the history of those relationships. Consequently, potential partners are "filtered" or "screened" for how well they serve the functions appropriate to a given level of relationship development. Those who adequately fulfill the expectations of a relationship at a given point in development remain available for further relationship development.

Filter theories emphasize that the functions of relationships change as those relationships and the people in them develop. That is, neither people nor relationships are static, both change and develop over time. Thus, understanding the functions served by relationships at given points in time requires the articulation of "doubly developmental" models of relationships. One sense in which relationships develop is that every relationship has a history. Any relationship, including close friendship, will have passed through a series of phases in getting to its current state. Several researchers have charted the phases of friendship development from initial acquaintanceship to intimate friendship (e.g., Hays, 1988; Levinger, 1974). Such developmental models of close friendship not only provide a description of the sequence in which the relationship comes to be, they also provide—at least implicitly—a typology of friendship categories (e.g., acquaintanceship, casual friends, good friends, close friends, and best friends).

The distinctions naive actors make when talking about different phases or categories of friendship development reveal underlying differences in how the relationship is conceptualized and in the expectations held for relationship partners. This point is nicely illustrated by Kurth (1970), who found that people associated different functions with what she termed "friendly relations" and close friendships. Whereas cordiality and politeness characterized the conceptions people held about friendly relations, commitment, sacrifice, and intimacy were seen as the defining features of close friendships. Thus, the tasks, duties, and skills contributing to the maintenance of friendly relations probably differ significantly from the tasks, duties, and skills contributing to the maintenance of close friendships.

Just as close friendship may be said to develop over time, people's conceptions of and expectations for friendship also develop over the course of the life cycle. Considerable research (e.g., Berndt, 1986; Damon, 1977; Tesch, 1983) shows that how people think about close friendship, what they do with their intimate friends, and the meaning of concepts directly implicated in the friendship bond (e.g., intimacy, loyalty, commitment, and trust) change dramatically over the course of childhood, adolescence, and into adulthood. Whereas children typically view close friends as playmates, adults typically view close friends as confidants. Again, because conceptions of close friendship change (in this case because of psychological development), tasks that must be accomplished to maintain this social relationship are likely to vary over time as well. By extension, skills enabling individuals to perform the duties suggested by such tasks will differ for children and adults.

Appreciation of the ontogenetic changes occurring in friendship conceptions, expectations, and activities provides a fresh perspective on the similarity/attraction thesis. Specifically, we have proposed that similarity in underlying cognitive representations of relationships, similarity in expectations for relationship partners, and similarity in levels of the social skills used to address relationship tasks may be especially conducive to relationship development and maintenance (Burleson & Denton, 1992; Burleson & Lucchetti, 1990, 1991; Burleson & Samter, 1992; Burleson, Samter, & Lucchetti, 1992). Unlike most social psychology research that focuses on how similarity in general attitudes and values contributes to attraction, we suggest that similarity in the social skills that facilitate enjoyable, rewarding interactions should be particularly important determinants of relationship growth and maintenance. Moreover, our reanalysis of the similarity/attraction thesis provides a framework for explaining how individual, as well as developmental, differences in social cognition and social skills contribute to the development and maintenance of relationships. Within any age group some individuals have comparatively advanced relationship conceptions, cognitive structures, and social skills while others have less mature modes of thinking and behaving. Consequently, even among people of the same age, compatibility may be greater among those with similar levels of social–cognitive and behavioral development. In other words, individual differences in levels of social–cognitive abilities and communication skills should predict interpersonal attraction and relationship maintenance. People are likely to find interaction with others having similar skill levels more enjoyable and, hence, should be more likely to develop and successfully maintain relationships with them.

Several recent studies support the notion that similarities in relationship conceptions and communication skills contribute to relationship maintenance. One line of research has focused on how similarity in people's conceptions of the functions served by a relationship promotes maintenance of that relationship. Burleson et al. (1992) argue that individuals' evaluations of the importance of different communication skills in a relationship provides one index of how that relationship is conceptualized. Two samples of subjects, pairs of "best friends" and pairs of less well-acquainted "just friends," rated the importance of eight different communication skills in the friend relationship. Burleson et al. found that friends' evaluations of several communication skills were significantly correlated, and that pairs of friends had significantly more similar evaluations of communication skills than randomly generated nominal pairs. Moreover, the degree of similarity in friends' evaluations of communication skills generally did not change as a function of length of relationship, suggesting that these similarities were not the outcome of a maintained relationship, but rather contributed to relationship growth and maintenance.

Interestingly, Burleson, Birch, and Kunkel (1993) found that the degree of similarity in the communication skill evaluations of dating couples was associated with the couple's commitment to and satisfaction with the relationship. In couples expressing low levels of satisfaction with the relationship there was little similarity in skill evaluations, whereas among couples expressing a high level of satisfaction with the relationship there was substantial similarity in partners' skill evaluations. These latter findings suggest that although similarities in skill evaluations may not attract dating partners to one another initially, they do contribute to the development of a satisfying relationship that partners feel committed to maintain. In sum, research on the communication skill evaluations of friends and dating couples suggests that those having similar evaluations of skills—and thus similar conceptions of the functions of the relationship—are more likely to form enduring, mutually satisfying relationships.

Several other studies have provided direct assessments of the claim that similarities in social skills contribute to the development and maintenance of friendships and other close relationships. Burleson and Lucchetti (1991) obtained assessments of four different social-cognitive abilities and five different communication skills from classes of elementary school children. Sociometric methods were used by these researchers to identify both those peers to whom children were attracted and those with whom they formed reciprocated friendships. These researchers found significant, moderate associations between the children's own skill levels and the skill levels of those to whom they were attracted (i.e., those they said they liked). Moreover, the skill levels of pairs of reciprocal friends were significantly correlated, indicating that friend pairs exhibited similar social–cognitive and communicative abilities. Thus, these results suggest that cognitively and behaviorally mature children cultivate each other as friends, whereas those with lesser degrees of maturity gravitate toward one another.

Similar procedures were employed by Burleson and Samter (1992) in reanalyzing the data these researchers had collected from fraternity and sorority residents (see the previous discussion of Samter & Burleson, 1990a). The sociometric nomination data obtained from participants was analyzed to identify both those persons to whom individuals were attracted and those with whom they formed reciprocated friendships. Individuals' scores on six social skills ("interpersonal cognitive complexity"—a measure of social–cognitive ability—and five communication skills, including measures of comforting, ego support, and conflict management ability) were then correlated with (1) the averaged skill levels of those to whom they were attracted, and (2) the skill levels of those with whom they had formed reciprocated friendships. Individuals were both attracted to and maintained reciprocated friendships with those having levels of social skills similar to their own. In particular, there were significant similarities in friends' levels of comforting and conflict management skills. Thus, data that had provided only weak support for the "main effects" model furnished considerably more support for the skill similarity model.

Finally, Burleson and Denton (1992) examined similarities in the communication skills of married couples. Although this study obviously did not deal with same-sex friends, it nonetheless constitutes an assessment of the skills similarity model. Measures of interpersonal cognitive complexity and three general communication skills (accuracy at perceiving another's intentions, accuracy at predicting the emotional impact of one's messages, and effectiveness at achieving intended communication outcomes) were obtained from 60 married couples. The levels of the spouses' social skills were significantly correlated; spouses had significantly more similar levels of social skills than randomly generated nominal pairs. Further, there was a trend for relatively happy couples to exhibit greater similarity in skill levels than less happy couples. Finally, Burleson and Denton found that couples where spouses had similarly low levels of skills were no less satisfied with their partner or marriage than couples where spouses had similarly high levels of skills. Thus, these results suggest that skill similarity may be a more important predictor of relationship satisfaction than the absolute level of skillfulness exhibited by partners.

Conclusion

We have outlined an approach to the study of relationship maintenance built on an analysis of the functions served by various relationships. From the functional perspective, a relationship is maintained when persons enact behaviors that service the tasks and functions that define a particular relationship. In particular, we have suggested that because communication skills contribute to the achievement of relationship functions, individual differences in communication skills play an important role in the maintenance of relationships such as friendship.

Our analysis of the functions served by close friendship suggested that skills such as ego support, comforting, and conflict management should facilitate the maintenance of friendships. However, empirical tests of both the "main effects" and "skill similarity" models indicate that although these skills are relevant to the maintenance of friendship, similarity in levels of partners' skills makes a stronger contribution to relationship maintenance than the absolute level of partners skills.

Although the skill similarity model has received greater empirical support than the main effects model, the former model is counter-intuitive in one important respect. Theorists and educators have almost always assumed that good (i.e., highly developed) social perception and communication skills will facilitate the development and maintenance of successful, satisfying interpersonal relationships. Thus, it seems quite reasonable that highly skilled individuals would enjoy interacting with each other more than with less skilled individuals. But why should low-skilled individuals maintain friendships with other low-skilled individuals rather than with highly skilled persons, especially when in the case of friendship, the skills in focus include such basic matters as ego support, comforting, and conflict management? There are at least two possible answers to this question.

First, it is possible that the less skilled may not actually enjoy interacting with similarly skilled individuals, but end up maintaining friendships with such persons because they are the interactional partners left available. That is, if highly skilled individuals generally select as friends other highly skilled individuals and reject the less skilled, there may be few highly skilled persons available to form friendships with the less skilled, and fewer still who are willing to maintain enduring friendships with the low skilled. Research on the friendship networks of socially rejected children (Kupersmidt, Coie, & Dodge, 1990) and lonely college students (Samter, 1992) provides support for this hypothesis: Socially rejected children and lonely college students appear to become friends with one another because they are the only ones who will *have* each other as friends. If this account has merit, then low-skilled friendship pairs should be less satisfied with their relationship and partners than high-skilled friendship pairs. This hypothesis should be evaluated in future research.

A second possibility—one supported by Burleson and Denton's (1992) examination of married couples—is that less skilled individuals genuinely enjoy interacting with those having similar skill levels more than with highly skilled persons. Several recent critiques (e.g., Bochner, 1981; Parks, 1981; Sillars & Weisberg, 1987) suggest that the tendency by communication researchers to assume the desirability of accurate and sensitive communication reflects an "ideology of intimacy." There may be substantial segments of the population for whom achieving accurate and sensitive understandings through verbal interaction just is not that important. Further, the highly skilled individual's concern with validating the other's view of self and the world, with exploring the feelings and motivations of the other, with working out disagreements by developing greater mutual understanding, with soothing upset and distress by helping the other articulate and elaborate his or her feelings, and so forth, may be seen as obsessive, boring, and intrusive by "less skilled" individuals. Consistent with this view, persons with "less developed" social–cognitive abilities have been found to view nonaffectively oriented communication skills (e.g., narrative ability) as more important in friendships, view affectively oriented skills (e.g., comforting and ego support) as less important, and converse about external events and activities more than personal feelings and aspirations when self-disclosing (e.g., Burleson & Samter, 1990; Delia, Clark, & Switzer, 1979). Future research should further examine how much low- and high-skilled individuals enjoy maintaining relationships with partners of similar and dissimilar skill levels.

More generally, we believe the functional perspective outlined here can provide a useful framework for examining how a broad array of relationships are maintained. Certainly, relationships are maintained by many behaviors other than those consciously intended by partners to stabilize, maintain, or repair the relationship. The routines and rituals of daily life serve to bind people together in powerful ways. However, it is likely that some forms of everyday behavior are more important than others in keeping particular relationships going. The functional perspective approaches the study of relationship maintenance by asking what relationships *do* for those involved in them, and in so doing encourages researchers to identify and scrutinize the communicative behaviors that make distinct ways of relating possible.

References

Adelman, M. B., Parks, M. R., & Albrecht, T. L. (1987). Supporting friends in need. In T. L. Albrecht, M. B. Adelman & Associates (Eds.), *Communicating social support* (pp. 105–125). Beverly Hills, CA: Sage.

Aries, A. (1976). Interactional patterns and themes of male, female, and mixed groups. *Small Group Behavior, 7,* 7–18.

Aries, A., & Johnson, F. L. (1983). Close friendship in adulthood: Conversational content between same-sex friends. *Sex Roles, 9,* 1183–1196.

Arling, G. (1976). The elderly widow and her family, neighbors, and friends. *Journal of Marriage and the Family, 38,* 757–768.

Ayres, J. (1983). Strategies to maintain relationships: Their identification and perceived usage. *Communication Quarterly, 31,* 62–67.

Baxter, L. A., & Dindia, K. (1990). Marital partners' perceptions of marital maintenance strategies. *Journal of Social and Personal Relationships, 7,* 187–208.

Berger, P. L., & Luckmann, T. (1967). *The social construction of reality: A treatise in the sociology of knowledge.* New York: Anchor Books.

Berndt, T. J. (1986). Children's comments about their friendships. In M. Perlmutter (Ed.), *The Minnesota Symposium on Child Psychology: Vol. 18. Cognitive perspectives on children's social and behavioral development* (pp. 189–212). Minneapolis: University of Minnesota Press.

Blau, Z. (1973). *Old age in a changing society.* New York: New Viewpoints.

Bochner, A. P. (1981). On the efficacy of openness in close relationships. In M. Burgoon (Ed.), *Communication yearbook 5* (pp. 109–124). New Brunswick, NJ: Transaction Press.

Bochner, A. P. (1984). The functions of human communication in interpersonal bonding. In C. C. Arnold & J. W. Bowers (Eds.), *Handbook of rhetorical and communication theory* (pp. 544–621). Boston: Allyn and Bacon.

Bukowski, W. M., & Hoza, B. (1989). Popularity and friendship: Issues in theory, measurement, and outcome. In T. J. Berndt & G. W. Ladd (Eds.), *Peer relationships in child development* (pp. 15–45). New York: Wiley.

Burleson, B. R. (1984). Comforting communication. In H. E. Sypher & J. L. Applegate (Eds.), *Communication by children and adults: Social cognitive and strategic processes* (pp. 63–104). Beverly Hills, CA: Sage.

Burleson, B. R. (1986). Communication skills and childhood peer relationships: An overview. In M. L. McLaughlin (Ed.), *Communication yearbook 9* (pp. 143–180). Beverly Hills, CA: Sage.

Burleson, B. R. (1991, November). *Communication skills that promote the maintenance of friendships: Contributions of comforting and conflict management.* Paper presented at the Speech Communication Association convention, Atlanta, GA.

Burleson, B. R., Applegate, J. L., Burke, J. A., Clark, R. A., Delia, J. G., & Kline, S. L. (1986). Communicative correlates of peer acceptance in childhood. *Communication Education, 35,* 349–361.

Burleson, B. R., Birch, J., & Kunkel, A. W. (1993). Similarities in the cognitions of romantic partners. Unpublished data, Department of Communication, Purdue University, W. Lafayette, IN.

Burleson, B. R., & Denton, W. H. (1992). A new look at similarity and attraction in marriage: Similarities in social-cognitive and communication skills as predictors of attraction and satisfaction. *Communication Monographs, 59,* 268–287.

Burleson, B. R., & Lucchetti, A. E. (1990, July). *Similarity–attraction revisited: Similarity in communication skills and values as predictors of friendship choices in two age groups.* Paper presented at the Fifth International Conference on Personal Relationships, Oxford University, Oxford.

Burleson, B. R., & Lucchetti, A. E. (1991, November). *Friendship and similarity in levels of social-*

cognitive and communicative functioning: Social skill bases of interpersonal attraction in childhood. Paper presented at the Speech Communication Association convention, Atlanta, GA.

Burleson, B. R., & Samter, W. (1990). Effects of cognitive complexity on the perceived importance of communication skills in friends. *Communication Research, 17,* 165–182.

Burleson, B. R., & Samter, W. (1992, November). *Attraction and friendship as a function of similarity in social-cognitive and communication abilities: Social skill bases of relationship development among young adults.* Paper presented at the Speech Communication Association convention, Chicago.

Burleson, B. R., Samter, W., & Lucchetti, A. E. (1992). Similarity in communication values as a predictor of friendship choices: Studies of friends and best friends. *Southern Communication Journal, 57,* 260–276.

Burleson, B. R., & Waltman, P. A. (1987). Popular, rejected, and supportive preadolescents: Social-cognitive and communicative characteristics. In M. L. McLaughlin (Ed.), *Communication yearbook 10* (pp. 533–552). Newbury Park, CA: Sage.

Burleson, B. R., Wilson, S. R., Waltman, M. S., Goering, E. M., Ely, T. S., & Whaley, B. R. (1988). Item-desirability effects in compliance-gaining research: Seven studies documenting artifacts in the selection procedure. *Human Communication Research 14,* 429–486.

Byrne, D. (1971). *The attraction paradigm.* New York: Academic Press.

Clark, R. A., & Delia, J. G. (1979). Topoi and rhetorical competence. *Quarterly Journal of Speech, 65,* 187–206.

Cobb, S. (1976). Social support as a moderator of life stress. *Psychosomatic Medicine, 38,* 300–314.

Coie, J. D., Dodge, K. A., & Kupersmidt, J. B. (1990). Peer group behavior and social status. In S. R. Asher & J. D. Coie (Eds.), *Peer rejection in childhood* (pp. 17–59). Cambridge: Cambridge University Press.

Cowen, E. L., Pederson, A., Babigian, H., Izzo, L. D., & Trost, M. A. (1973). Long-term follow-up of early detected vulnerable children. *Journal of Consulting and Clinical Psychology, 41,* 438–446.

Crawford, M. (1977). What is a friend? *New Sociology, 20,* 116–117.

Croog, S. H., Lipson, A., & Levine, S. (1972). Help partners in severe illness: The roles of kin network, non-family resources, and institutions. *Journal of Marriage and the Family, 32,* 32–41.

Curran, J. P., Wallander, J. L., & Farrell, A. D. (1985). Heterosexual skills training. In L. L'Abate & M. A. Milan (Eds.), *Handbook of social skills training and research* (pp. 136–169). New York: Wiley.

Cutrona, C. E. (1982). Transitions to college: Loneliness and the process of social adjustment. In L. A. Peplau & D. Perlman (Eds.), *Loneliness: A sourcebook of current theory, research, and therapy* (pp. 291–309). New York: Wiley Interscience.

Damon, W. (1977). *The social world of the child.* San Francisco: Jossey-Bass.

Delia, J. G., Clark, R. A., & Switzer, D. E. (1979). The content of informal conversations as a function of interactants' interpersonal cognitive complexity. *Communication Monographs, 46,* 274–281.

Dindia, K. (1989, May). *Toward the development of a measure of marital maintenance strategies.* Paper presented at the annual conference of the International Communication Association, San Francisco.

Dindia, K., & Baxter, L. A. (1987). Strategies for maintaining and repairing marital relationships. *Journal of Social and Personal Relationships, 4,* 143–158.

Duck, S. W. (1977). *The study of attraction.* Farnborough, England: Saxon House.

Duck, S. W. (1985). Social and personal relationships. In M. L. Knapp & G. R. Miller (Eds.), *Handbook of interpersonal communication* (pp. 655–686). Beverly Hills, CA: Sage.

Duck, S. W. (1986). *Human relationships: An introduction to social psychology.* Beverly Hills, CA: Sage.

Duck, S. W. (1988). *Relating to others*. Chicago: Dorsey Press.

Duck, S. W., Rutt, K. J., Hurst, M. H., & Strejc, H. (1991). Some evident truths about everyday conversation: All communications are not created equal. *Human Communication Research, 18*, 228–267.

Fitzpatrick, M. A., & Winke, J. (1979). You always hurt the one you love: Strategies and tactics in interpersonal conflict. *Communication Quarterly, 27*, 3–11.

Ginsberg, D., Gottman, J. M., & Parker, J. G. (1986). The importance of friendship. In J. M. Gottman & J. G. Parker (Eds.), *Conversations of friends: Speculations on affective development* (pp. 3–50). Cambridge: Cambridge University Press.

Hays, R. B. (1988). Friendship. In S. Duck (Ed.), *Handbook of personal relationships* (pp. 391–408). London: Wiley.

Hays, R. B. (1989). Day-to-day friendships. *Journal of Social and Personal Relationships, 6*, 21–38.

Heinemann, G. D. (1985). Interdependence in informal support systems: The case of elderly, urban widows. In W. A. Peterson & J. Quadagno (Eds.), *Social bonds in later life: Aging and interdependence* (pp. 165–186). Beverly Hills, CA: Sage.

Hocker, J. L., & Wilmot, W. W. (1991). *Interpersonal conflict* (3rd ed.). Dubuque, IA: Wm. C. Brown.

Hojat, M. (1982). Loneliness as a function of selected personality variables. *Journal of Clinical Psychology, 38*, 136–141.

Horowitz, L. M., & French, R. de S. (1979). Interpersonal problems of people who describe themselves as lonely. *Journal of Consulting and Clinical Psychology, 47*, 762–764.

Jones, W. H., Freemon, J. E., & Goswick, R. A. (1981). The persistence of loneliness: Self and other determinants. *Journal of Personality, 49*, 26–48.

Jones, W. H., & Moore, T. L. (1989). Loneliness and social support. In M. Hojat & R. Crandall (Eds.), *Loneliness: Theory, research, and applications* (pp. 145–156). Newbury Park, CA: Sage.

Kerckhoff, A. C., & Davis, K. E. (1962). Value consensus and need complementarity in mate selection. *American Sociological Review, 27*, 295–303.

Kon, I. S. (1981). Adolescent friendship: Some unanswered questions for future research. In S. Duck & R. Gilmour (Eds.), *Personal relationships: Vol. 2. Developing personal relationships* (pp. 187–204). New York: Academic Press.

Kupersmidt, J. B., Cole, J. D., & Dodge, K. A. (1990). The role of poor peer relationships in the development of disorder. In S. R. Asher & J. D. Coie (Eds.), *Peer rejection in childhood* (pp. 274–307). Cambridge: Cambridge University Press.

Kurth, S. B. (1970). Friendships and friendly relations. In G. J. McCall, M. M. McCall, N. K. Denzin, G. D. Suttles, & S. B. Kurth (Eds.), *Social relationships* (pp. 136–170). Chicago: Aldine de Gruyter.

Ladd, G. L., & Asher, S. R. (1985). Social skill training and children's peer relations. In L. L'Abate & M. Milan (Eds.), *Handbook of social skills training* (pp. 219–244). New York: Wiley.

La Gaipa, J. J. (1981). Children's friendships. In S. Duck & R. Gilmour (Eds.), *Personal relationships, 2: Developing personal relationships* (pp. 161–186). New York: Academic Press.

Levinger, G. (1974). A three-level approach to attraction: Toward an understanding of pair relatedness. In T. L. Huston (Ed.), *Foundations of interpersonal attraction* (pp. 100–120). New York: Academic Press.

Lincoln, J. R., & Miller, J. (1979). Work friendships and ties in organizations: A comparative analysis of relational networks. *Administrative Science Quarterly, 24*, 181–199.

McFall, R. M. (1982). A review and reformulation of the concept of social skills. *Behavioral Assessment, 4*, 1–33.

Moore, J. A., & Sermat, V. (1974). Relationship between loneliness and interpersonal relationships. *Canadian Counselor, 8*, 84–89.

Morton, T. L. (1978). Intimacy and reciprocity of exchange: A comparison of spouses and strangers. *Journal of Personality and Social Psychology, 36,* 72–83.

Parks, M. R. (1981). Ideology of interpersonal communication: Off the couch and into the world. In M. Burgoon (Ed.), *Communication yearbook 5* (pp. 79–108). New Brunswick, NJ: Transaction Press.

Peplau, L. A., & Perlman, D. (Eds.). (1982). *Loneliness: A sourcebook of current theory, research, and therapy.* New York: Wiley Interscience.

Phillips, G. M., & Metzger, N. J. (1976). *Intimate communication.* Boston: Allyn and Bacon.

Rawlins, W. A. (1989). A dialectical analysis of the intentions, functions, and strategic challenges of communication in young adult friendships. In J. A. Anderson (Ed.), *Communication yearbook 12* (pp. 157–189). Newbury Park, CA: Sage.

Rawlins, W. K. (1992). *Friendship matters: Communication, dialectics, and the life course.* New York: Aldine de Gruyter.

Rawlins, W. K., & Holl, M. (1987). The communicative achievement of friendship during adolescence: Predicaments of trust and violation. *Western Journal of Speech Communication, 51,* 345–363.

Renshaw, P. D., & Asher, S. R. (1982). Social competence and peer status: The distinction between goals and strategies. In K. H. Rubin & H. S. Ross (Eds.), *Peer relationships and social skills in childhood* (pp. 375–395). New York: Springer-Verlag.

Roff, M., Sells, S. B., & Golden, M. M. (1972). *Social adjustment and personality development in children.* Minneapolis: University of Minnesota Press.

Samter, W. (1992). Communicative characteristics of the lonely person's friendship circle. *Communication Research, 19,* 212–239.

Samter, W., & Burleson, B. R. (1990a, June). *The role of affectively oriented communication skills in the friendships of young adults: A sociometric study.* Paper presented at the International Communication Association convention, Dublin.

Samter, W., & Burleson, B. R. (1990b). Evaluations of communication skills as predictors of peer acceptance in a group living situation. *Communication Studies, 41,* 311–326.

Searle, J. (1969). *Speech acts: An essay in the philosophy of language.* Cambridge: Cambridge University Press.

Secklin, P. (1991, November). *Being there: A qualitative study of young adults' descriptions of friendship.* Paper presented at the Speech Communication Association convention, Atlanta, GA.

Selman, R. L. (1980). *The growth of interpersonal understanding: Developmental and clinical analyses.* New York: Academic Press.

Serafica, F. C. (1982). Conceptions of friendship and interaction between friends: An organismic-developmental perspective. In F. C. Serafica (Ed.), *Social-cognitive development in context* (pp. 100–132). New York: Guilford.

Shea, B. C., & Pearson, J. C. (1986). The effects of relationship type, partner intent, and gender on the selection of relationship maintenance strategies. *Communication Monographs, 53,* 352–364.

Shea, L., Thompson, L., & Blieszner, R. (1988). Resources in older adults' old and new friendships. *Journal of Social and Personal Relationships, 5,* 83–96.

Sillars, A. L. (1980). Attributions and communication in roommate conflicts. *Communication Monographs, 47,* 180–200.

Sillars, A. L., & Weisberg, J. (1987). Conflict as a social skill. In M. E. Roloff & G. R. Miller (Eds.), *Interpersonal processes: New directions in communication research* (pp. 140–171). Newbury Park, CA: Sage.

Simmel, G. (1908/1950). [*The sociology of Georg Simmel*]. K. Wolff (Ed. and Trans.). Glencoe, IL: Free Press.

Smollar, J., & Youniss, J. (1982). Social development through friendship. In K. H. Rubin & H. S. Ross (Eds.), *Peer relationships and social skills in childhood* (pp. 279–298). New York: Springer-Verlag.

Stafford, L., & Canary, D. J. (1991). Maintenance strategies and romantic relationship type, gender, and relational characteristics. *Journal of Social and Personal Relationships, 8,* 217–242.

Tesch, S. A. (1983). Review of friendship development across the life span. *Human Development, 26,* 266–276.

Watzlawick, P., Beavin, J. H., & Jackson, D. D. (1967). *Pragmatics of human communication.* New York: Norton.

Yeates, K. O., Schultz, L. H., & Selman, R. L. (1991). The development of interpersonal negotiation strategies in thought and action: A social-cognitive link to behavioral adjustment and social status. *Merrill-Palmer Quarterly, 37,* 369–406.

Youniss, J. (1980). *Parents and peers in social development: A Sullivan-Piaget perspective.* Chicago: University of Chicago Press.

A Multiphasic View of Relationship Maintenance Strategies

Kathryn Dindia
Department of Communication
University of Wisconsin, Milwaukee
Milwaukee, Wisconsin,

Introduction

Research on relationship development strategies has tended to be phase bound. That is, relationship development strategies have been studied within the boundaries of a particular stage of relationship development. "Relationship development" refers to all phases and/or stages of relationships including relationship de-escalation and termination. For example, there are typologies of relationship initiation strategies (e.g., Baxter & Philpott, 1982), relationship escalation strategies (e.g., Tolhuizen, 1989, 1992), relationship maintenance strategies (e.g., Dindia & Baxter, 1987; Stafford & Canary, 1991), and relationship termination strategies (e.g., Baxter, 1984, 1985).

The purpose of this chapter is to discuss the generalizability of relationship development strategies across stages of relationship development, in particular, relationship maintenance. I will argue that relationship development strategies are multiphasic. Uniphasic strategies are strategies that are specific to a particular stage of relationship development. Multiphasic strategies are strategies that are applicable to a number of stages of relationship development. Thus, I will argue that strategies used to initiate and escalate relation-

Communication and Relational Maintenance

ships are also used to maintain relationships and these are the opposite of strategies to de-escalate and terminate a relationship. In addition, I will propose a typology of relationship development strategies that is applicable to all stages of relationship development, including relationship maintenance.

Such a typology has important theoretical implications for personal relationships. Two criteria frequently mentioned for evaluating theories are generality and parsimony (Reynolds, 1971). A typology of relationship development strategies that generalizes to all stages of relationship development is better, if adequate, than separate typologies of relationship initiation, escalation, maintenance, de-escalation, and termination strategies. In addition, a typology of relationship development strategies that is generalizable to all stages of relationship development would have important implications for relationship maintenance. A multiphasic approach to relationship maintenance is important for understanding the similarities and differences between relationship maintenance and other stages of relationship development as well as the similarities and differences between relationship maintenance strategies and other relationship development strategies.

Review of Literature

Several researchers have discussed the multiphasic nature of relationship maintenance strategies. For instance, Duck (1988, p. 100) claims that "some means for developing relationships are also means for maintaining them," and Buley (1977, p. 143) asserts, "If you know the behaviors required to strengthen a relationship, these are the same behaviors required to keep it strong." I will, in the following section, review several theoretical perspectives which have implications for the argument that relationship development strategies, in particular, relationship maintenance strategies, are multiphasic.

Theoretical Perspectives on Relationship Development

Morton and Douglas (1981) reviewed three theoretical approaches from the fields of sociology, communication, and social psychology to the study of relationship development in order to identify the central dimensions and characteristics of relationship development. Two major dimensions of change appeared in the process of relationship development: familiarity with or personal knowledge of the other person, and attraction and connectedness. "Intimacy is generally construed as high familiarity, and knowledge of private, highly unique and personalistic information about the other" (Morton &

Douglas, 1981, p. 9). *Connectedness* refers to the causal interconnections between individuals. Connections become more frequent, more diversified, and stronger as a relationship escalates. In other words, relationship escalation is marked by an increased frequency in the participants' interaction, a diversification of their shared activities, and a strengthening of the ability to influence one another (Levinger, 1983).

Other researchers of personal relationships have posited other fundamental dimensions of relationship development (e.g., Burgoon & Hale, 1987). Regardless of what one considers the basic dimensions of relationship development to be, the important point is that these characteristics of relationships are thought to change systematically as relationships develop (i.e., "grow" as a relationship grows and "decline" as a relationship declines). Thus, Morton and Douglas state, "development [escalation] involves quantitative increases in intimacy and attraction, as well as attendant qualitative changes in these dimensions" (1981, p. 3).

From this perspective on relationship development, it can be argued that the initiating stage of relationship development is the phase in which these underlying dimensions of relationship development (e.g., familiarity, attraction, connection) first come into existence. Relationship escalation is the stage in which these characteristics grow. Relationship maintenance refers to the period in which advanced levels of these characteristics are sustained. Relationship de-escalation is the phase in which these characteristics decline. Finally, relationship termination occurs when these characteristics come to an end.[1]

Strategies are plans, methods, or a series of maneuvers or stratagems for obtaining a specific goal or result. Relationship development strategies are strategies to initiate, escalate, maintain, de-escalate, or terminate relationships. Thus, according to this perspective, relationship development strategies are similar across stages of relationships because they are designed to influence the underlying dimensions of relationship development. Relationship initiation strategies are strategies to bring into existence important characteristics of relationship development, such as familiarity, attraction, and connectedness. Relationship escalation strategies are strategies to increase these characteristics. Relationship maintenance strategies are intended to sustain advanced levels of these characteristics. Relationship de-escalation strategies are strategies to decrease these characteristics. Relationship termination strategies are designed to put an end to these characteristics. Using the example of self-disclosure, to initiate a relationship, an individual begins to self-disclose; to escalate a relationship, an individual increases the breadth and depth of self-disclosure; to maintain a relationship, an individual sustains

[1]See Baxter (1985) for argument that familiarity does not decrease as a relationship dissolves.

the breadth and depth of self-disclosure; to de-escalate a relationship, an individual decreases the breadth and depth of self-disclosure; and to terminate a relationship, an individual stops self-disclosing. Thus, according to this perspective, relationship development strategies, including relationship maintenance strategies, are multiphasic.

An alternative perspective on relationship development posits a set of external forces that act either to hold a relationship together (centripetal forces) or to pull it apart (centrifugal forces). Lewin (1951) labeled these forces *driving forces* and *restraining forces.* Levinger (1965, 1976) called them *attractions* and *barriers.* Davis (1973) referred to them as *social forces.*

According to this perspective, relationship development strategies can focus on any of the forces that affect a relationship. For example, Levinger (1979) indicates that a traditional strategy for maintaining marriage was to keep up the barriers preventing divorce and to remove all realistic alternatives; whereas, a contemporary maintenance strategy is to revive or raise the couple's mutual feelings of attraction. Similarly, Davis (1973) observed that "individuals who want to engage in an intimate relation must generate certain social forces to fasten themselves together" (p. xxiii). Alternatively, individuals who want to terminate a relationship must generate social forces that pull them apart and/or deactivate the forces holding them together.

According to this perspective, relationship development strategies would also be multiphasic. Relationship initiation strategies are designed to activate the forces holding a relationship together. Relationship escalation strategies are intended to increase the forces holding a relationship together. Relationship maintenance strategies are used to maintain the forces holding the relationship together (and to hold at abeyance all of the forces that pull a relationship apart). Relationship de-escalation and termination strategies are strategies to deactivate the forces holding a relationship together and to activate the forces pulling it apart.

Byrne and Murnen (1988) disagree with the preceding perspectives. They argue that "relationship maintenance involves something beyond the mere repetition of those variables that initiated attraction in the first place and something besides the mere absence of the variables that are associated with relationship failure" (p. 294). At the same time, they propose that the "*constructs* identified as crucial to attraction are also crucial to maintaining or failing to maintain a relationship" (p. 294). According to Byrne and Murnen, attraction is an important aspect of relationships, but what causes attraction in initial stages of relationship development may not be the same as what maintains attraction in a long-term relationship. Byrne and Murnen use the example of physical attractiveness, which is an important cause of initial attraction but may have nothing to do with maintaining attraction. Similarly, Byrne and Murnen state that arguments and negative behaviors characterize deteriorating relationships but that the absence of these variables may not maintain relationships.

Byrne and Murnen posit an affective model of attraction in which the ratio of positive to negative feelings in a relationship determines attraction. These authors propose three major constructs crucial to maintaining attraction: similarity, habituation (i.e., familiarity can breed contempt and boredom), and evaluation (i.e., the ratio of positive to negative interactions). These three factors are important to relationship maintenance because they affect levels of attraction between partners: more specifically, the ratio of positive to negative feelings in a relationship. However, these three factors may not be crucial to attraction in other stages of relationships. For example, habituation is likely to influence attraction only in the maintenance stage of relationships.

Thus, Byrne and Murnen posit that attraction is the underlying dimension of relationships or the force that holds a relationship together. Byrne and Murnen argue that what causes attraction may differ at different stages of relationship development; however, they also argue that the underlying basis for attraction, the ratio of positive to negative feelings in a relationship, is crucial to attraction across stages of relationships. According to this perspective, relationship development strategies are those that influence the ratio of positive to negative feelings in a relationship. However, strategies that influence the ratio of positive to negative feelings in a relationship would not necessarily be the same across stages of relationship development.

Empirical Research on Relationship Development Strategies

Most research on relationship development strategies is phase bound. That is, in general, relationship development strategies have been studied as they pertain to a particular stage of relationship development. As a consequence, there exists a number of typologies of relationship development strategies. Specifically, there are separate typologies of relationship initiation, escalation, maintenance, and termination strategies. The following discussion reviews the research on these typologies.

Typologies of Relationship Initiation Strategies

Baxter and Philpott (1982) examined ingratiation tactics (strategies a person uses to enhance another person's liking for him or her) used to initiate a relationship. Six ingratiation tactics were examined: other enhancement (cues that demonstrate high regard for the other), similarity (demonstration of commonality with the other), self-presentation (presentation of a unique and favorable image of oneself), favor-rendering (doing favors or giving rewards), information acquisition (solicit information about the other), and inclusion (activities that bring the other person into one's presence). The results of their research indicated that all six strategies were reported to initiate relationships.

Similar to Baxter and Philpott, Bell and Daly (1984) examined affinity-seeking strategies, the communication strategies people use to get others to like and feel positive toward them. Bell and Daly developed a typology of 25 strategies that people can say or do to get others to like them. They found that people who were thought to use many affinity-seeking strategies were judged to be attractive and likable. They also found that three basic dimensions underlie the affinity-seeking strategies: active–passive, aggressive–unaggressive, and self-oriented/other-oriented. Finally, the strategies fell into seven clusters in this three-dimensional space. The first cluster was labeled *control and visibility* and included the following strategies: personal autonomy, reward association, assume control, dynamism, present interesting self, and physical attractiveness. The second cluster was labeled *mutual trust* and included two strategies, trustworthiness and openness. The third cluster was labeled *politeness* and included two strategies, conversational rule-keeping and concede control. The fourth cluster involved strategies that communicate *concern and caring* (self-concept confirmation, elicit other's disclosures, listening, supportiveness, sensitivity, and altruism). The fifth cluster was labeled *other involvement* and included three strategies: facilitate enjoyment, inclusion of other, nonverbal immediacy. The sixth cluster was labeled *self involvement* and included two strategies: self-inclusion and influence perceptions of closeness. The seventh cluster was labeled *commonalities* and included three strategies: similarities, assuming equality, and comfortable self. (See Bell and Daly (1984) for conceptual definitions and examples for each strategy.)

Typologies of Relationship Escalation Strategies

Tolhuizen (1989, 1992) devised a typology of communication strategies for intensifying dating relationships. Sixteen strategies were inductively derived from written accounts of participants' attempts to intensify dating relationships. The 16 strategies were increased contact, relationship negotiation, social support and assistance (asking for advice or assistance from social network members), increase rewards, direct definitional bid (making a direct request for a closer relationship), tokens of affection, personal communication (using self-disclosure and supportiveness), idiomatic speech, verbal expressions of affection, suggestive actions (using hints, flirting, and other tactics characterized by subterfuge or deception), nonverbal expressions of affection, social enmeshment, accept definitional bid (agreeing to a direct request for a closer relationship), personal appearance, sexual intimacy, and behavioral adaptation (acts designed to impress partners or lead them to form a more favorable impression).

Tolhuizen (1989) asked participants to describe the things they said and did to change their most recent serious dating relationship from one of casual dating to one of serious and exclusive dating. Tolhuizen (1992) asked participants to indicate how many times they had used each of the intensification strategies in the last two weeks in a current dating relationship. The most frequently reported strategies in both studies were increased contact (reported by 39% of the participants in the 1989 study and an average of 3.04 increased contact strategies was reported in the 1992 study), personal communication (15%, $M = 2.79$), increase rewards (18%, $M = 2.70$), and verbal expressions of affection (14%, $M = 2.62$). Participants tended to report using more than one strategy and some strategies tended to be reported in combination (Tolhuizen, 1989). For example, increased contact and increase rewards were frequently reported together. Also, the use of intensification strategies increased linearly over relationship escalation (Tolhuizen, 1992).

Multivariate analysis (Tolhuizen, 1989) revealed that intimate versus nonintimate, and dominant versus submissive were underlying dimensions of the typology. The strategies grouped together into four clusters. The first cluster was labeled *social rewards and attraction*, and included tokens of affection, increase rewards, behavioral adaptation, personal appearance, and social enmeshment. The second cluster was labeled *implicitly expressed intimacy*, and included suggestive actions, nonverbal expressions of affection, and sexual intimacy. The third cluster was labeled *passive and indirect*, and included accept definition bid and social support and assistance. The fourth cluster was labeled *verbal directness and intimacy*, and included relationship negotiation, direct definitional bid, personalized communication, verbal expressions of affection and increased contact.

Typologies of Relationship Maintenance Strategies

Four typologies of relationship maintenance strategies have recently emerged in the literature (Ayres, 1983; Bell, Daly, & Gonzales, 1987; Dindia & Baxter, 1987; Stafford & Canary, 1991). Typically, relationship maintenance researchers are concerned with strategies for keeping a relationship at an advanced level of intimacy, thus preventing it from de-escalating and terminating. However, in developing the first of these typologies, Ayres (1983) was concerned with keeping the relationship the way it was regardless of the level of intimacy, thus preventing the relationship from escalating or de-escalating.

In Ayres' study, males and females were given a scenario and asked the likelihood of their using 38 strategies to maintain the hypothetical relationship. A factor analysis of the 38 strategies suggested three factors or sets of strategies used to maintain relationships. The first factor, Avoidance Strategies, included ignoring things the other person might do to change a relationship and avoiding doing things that might alter the relationship trajectory. The second factor, Balance Strategies, involved keeping the number of favors and emotional support levels constant or balanced. The third factor, Directness Strategies, involved directly telling the other person that the relationship should remain unchanged.

Whether one partner was trying to prevent the relationship from escalating or de-escalating affected the use of avoidance, balance, and directness strategies. Participants who wanted to maintain the level of the relationship but who were told that their partner wanted to escalate the relationship were most likely to report avoidance strategies. Participants who were told that their partner wanted to de-escalate the relationship were more likely to report balance strategies than those who were told that their partner wanted to escalate the relationship. Participants who were told that their partner wanted to escalate or de-escalate the relationship reported more directness strategies than participants who were told that their partner wanted to maintain the level of the relationship. Shea and Pearson (1986), in an extension of Ayres' research, found three factors that resembled, but were not identical to, Ayres' factors. In addition, they found that only partner intent affected balance strategies.

Bell et al. (1987) examined affinity-maintenance strategies used in marital relationships. The researchers developed a typology of affinity-maintenance strategies by asking subjects to describe, in writing, the things they said and did in their marriages which they thought maintained liking and solidarity. The subjects' responses were content analyzed and used to develop a typology that consisted of 27 strategies. The strategies were altruism, concede control, conversation rule-keeping, dynamism, elicit other's disclosures, equality, facility enjoyment, faithfulness, honesty, inclusion of other, influence perceptions of closeness, listening, openness, optimism, physical affection, physical attractiveness, present interesting self, reliability, reward association, self-concept confirmation, self-improvement, self-inclusion, sensitivity, shared spirituality, supportiveness, third party relations, and verbal affection. Conceptual definitions and examples for each strategy can be found in Bell et al. (1987). Wives' perceptions of husbands' maintenance strategies were moderately related to wives' marital satisfaction.

In a third line of research a typology of marital maintenance and repair strategies was generated using deductive and inductive methods (Dindia & Baxter, 1987). Davis' (1973) research on maintaining relationships was used as the deductive basis for the development of this typology. The strategy types discussed by Davis were supplemented with additional types that the authors inductively derived by reanalyzing the 652 strategies found in an earlier study of married couples (Dindia & Emery, 1982). The resulting typology consisted of 49 categories that were clustered into 11 superordinate types: changing the external environment, communication, metacommunication, avoid metacommunication, antisocial strategies (e.g., costs), prosocial strategies (e.g., rewards), ceremonies (e.g., celebrations, rituals), antirituals/spontaneity, togetherness, seeking/allowing autonomy, and seeking outside help. Conceptual definitions for each superordinate and subordinate category can be found in Dindia and Baxter (1987).

This typology of marital maintenance and repair strategies was used to categorize the marital maintenance and repair strategies reported by 50 couples ($N = 100$ spouses) (Dindia & Baxter, 1987). Strategies were categorized into the 11 superordinate categories. Respondents most frequently reported the use of prosocial, ceremonial, communication, and togetherness strategies. Changing the external environment, avoid metacommunication, antisocial strategies, and seeking/allowing autonomy were seldom reported.

A second study was conducted to assess the representational validity of this typology (Baxter & Dindia, 1990). Spouses sorted the 50 strategy types into categories. Results indicated that husbands and wives sorted the maintenance strategies similarly. Three underlying dimensions were found for the strategies: constructive/destructive communication styles, ambivalence-based versus satiation-based conditional use, and proactivity/passivity. The first dimension refers to whether the strategies are perceived as negative, destructive, and damaging to the relationship versus positive and constructive. The second dimension refers to strategies that are likely to be used only periodically or occasionally. Ambivalence-based conditional strategies are strategies characterized by widely disparate perceptions as to their constructive or destructive nature, or strategies that could be constructive but not without risk or effort. By contrast, satiation-based conditional strategies are positive strategies whose effectiveness depends on only periodic or sparing use, such as surprises, celebrations, and gifts. The third dimension refers to whether strategies are proactive or passive strategies. Six clusters of strategies were situated in the three-dimensional space: last resort, satiation, inward withdrawal, problem avoidance, destructive, and constructive. The findings differed substantially from the a priori classification employed by Dindia and Baxter (1987).

Stafford and Canary (1991) derived five relational maintenance strategies through factor analysis: positivity (being positive and cheerful), openness (self-disclosure and open discussion about the relationship), assurances (stressing commitment, showing love, and demonstrating faithfulness), network (spending time with common friends and affiliations), and sharing tasks (sharing with household tasks). Results indicated that relationship type moderately affected perceptions of partner maintenance strategies. Specifically, engaged and seriously dating individuals perceived greater partner positivity and openness than married or dating persons. Married, engaged, and seriously dating participants saw more use of assurances and sharing tasks than did those who had just begun dating. Married persons reported greatest perceptions of partner use of social networks to maintain relationships.

Typologies of Relationship Repair Strategies

To my knowledge, there are no separate typologies of relationship repair strategies. Both Davis (1973) and Dindia and Baxter (1987) defined relational maintenance to include both strategies to maintain the relationship (preventive maintenance) and strategies to repair the relationship (corrective maintenance). Thus, Dindia and Baxter's (1987) typology of relational maintenance strategies is also a typology of relational repair strategies. Dindia and Baxter found that not all strategies used to maintain a relationship were also used to repair a relationship. Specifically, metacommunication occurred more frequently when the goal was repairing the relationship than when the goal was maintaining the relationship. Introducing variety, novelty, and spontaneity into the relationship occurred more frequently when the goal was maintaining the relationship than when the goal was repairing the relationship. In addition, more strategies were reported for maintenance than repair indicating that individuals' repertoires of strategies for maintaining their relationship is larger than their repertoire of strategies for repairing their relationship.

Typologies of Relationship Termination Strategies

Baxter and Philpott (1982) examined strategies for terminating relationships. Baxter and Philpott examined six tactics to terminate a relationship: other negation (cues which demonstrate that the other is not liked), difference (demonstrating that one does not have things in common with the other), self-presentation (presentation of one's negative attributes), cost-rendering (ceasing favors and increasing costs to the other), disinterest (ceasing to acquire additional information about the other), and exclusion (avoiding having the other in one's presence). The results of the study indicated that individuals primarily use exclusion and other negation to terminate a relationship.

Baxter conducted several other studies examining strategies to terminate relationships. In factor analyzing strategies from hypothetical relationship terminations Baxter (1982) found four types of relational termination strategies: withdrawal/avoidance strategies, manipulatory strategies, positive tone strategies, and open confrontation strategies. In examining retrospective reports of termination strategies (Baxter, 1984, 1985) found eight termination strategies. They were withdrawal (avoidance behaviors in which intimacy and/or frequency of contact with a partner is reduced), pseudode-escalation (a declaration to the other party that the disengager desires a transformed relationship of reduced closeness when, in fact, the desire is to end the relationship), cost escalation (behavior that increases the partner's relational costs), fait accompli (an explicit declaration to the other party that the relationship is over, with no opportunity for discussion or compromise), state-of-the-relationship talk (an explicit statement of dissatisfaction and desire to exit in the context of a bilateral discussion of the relationship's problems), fading away (an implicit understanding that the relationship has ended), attributional conflict (a conflict, not over whether or not to exit, but on why the exit is necessary), and negotiated farewell (explicit communication between the parties which formally ends the relationship and which is free of hostility and argument).

Baxter (1984, 1985) noted that two underlying dimensions, directness and other-orientation, underlie these strategies. Direct strategies explicitly state a desire to exit the relationship, whereas indirect strategies try to accomplish the breakup without an explicit statement of the goal. Other-orientation refers to the degree to which the disengager attempts to avoid hurting the other party in the breakup. Indirect, unilateral strategies to exit a relationship included withdrawal, pseudo-deescalation, and cost escalation. Indirect, bilateral strategies included fading away and pseudo-deescalation. Pseudo-deescalation is similar to that discussed in the previous sentence, but the deception is mutual. Direct, unilateral strategies included fait accompli and state-of-the-relationship talk. Direct, bilateral strategies included attributional conflict and negotiated farewell. Baxter found that termination strategies are more likely to be indirect (primarily withdrawal) than direct.

Among other things, Baxter's typology is the first to explicitly include the variable of unilateral versus bilateral relational termination. Previous typologies of relational development strategies were exclusively of individual, rather than joint, strategies.

Cody (1982) asked students to recall a heterosexual relationship in which they had taken the initiative in terminating. Termination strategies formed five groupings: positive tone (i.e., end relationship on positive note), negative identify management (e.g., "I think you should start dating other people"), justification (i.e., legitimate reasons for breakup), behavioral de-escalation (i.e., withdrawal), and de-escalation (e.g., suggest a trial separation). The results of the study were that more intimate relationships were more likely to involve justification, de-escalation, and positive tone. Less intimate relationships were more likely to involve behavioral de-escalation.

Multiphasic Research
on Relationship Development Strategies

Very little research has examined relationship development strategies across stages of relationships. However, a few studies have examined the multiphasic nature of relationship development strategies. To provide empirical support for the argument that relational development strategies are multiphasic, these studies will be reviewed.

Baxter and Philpott (1982) argued that ingratiation tactics used to initiate relationships could be reversed to constitute a set of tactics to terminate a relationship. Six tactics and their opposites were examined for their role in initiating and terminating relationships. Respectively, they were other enhancement and other negation, similarity and difference, self-presentation (of positive attributes) versus self-presentation (of negative attributes), favor-rendering and cost-rendering, information acquisition and disinterest, and inclusion and exclusion. All six initiation strategies were reported to initiate relationships. Primarily exclusion and other negation were reported to terminate relationships. Thus, inclusion (activities that bring the two persons into contact) is used to initiate relationships; its opposite, exclusion (avoiding contact with the other), is used to terminate relationships. Similarly, other enhancement (cues that demonstrate liking for the other person) is used to initiate relationships; its opposite, other negation (cues which demonstrate that the other is not liked) is used to terminate relationships.

Bell and Daly (1984) and Bell, et al. (1987) developed typologies of affinity-seeking strategies and affinity-maintenance strategies, respectively. Most of the strategies for facilitating liking among nonintimates were the same as the strategies for maintaining liking among intimates. In particular, the following strategies were reported both to facilitate and maintain liking: altruism, assume equality, concede control, conversational rule-keeping, dynamism, elicit other's disclosures, facilitate enjoyment, inclusion of other, influence perceptions of closeness, listening, openness, optimism, physical attractiveness, present interesting self, reward association, self-concept confirmation, self-inclusion, sensitivity, and supportiveness. However, there were several strategies for facilitating liking that were not strategies for maintaining liking. These were assume control, comfortable self, nonverbal immediacy, personal autonomy, similarity, and trustworthiness. Similarly, there were several strategies for maintaining liking that were not strategies for facilitating liking. These were faithfulness, honesty, physical affection, reliability, self-improvement, shared spirituality, third party relations, and verbal affection. Thus, the study of Bell et al. provides some empirical support that similar strategies are used to initiate/escalate a relationship and to maintain a relationship. However, the results of this study also indicate that some relational development strategies are uniphasic.

Guerrero, Eloy, and Wabnik (1993) conducted a longitudinal study of dating relationships. Participants completed Stafford and Canary's (1991) measure of maintenance strategies at the beginning of the study and again 8 weeks later indicating what strategies their partner used to maintain the relationship. At Time 2, participants also indicated whether their relationship had escalated, remained stable, de-escalated, or terminated. The results of the study indicated that perceived partner frequent use of positivity strategies was related to relational maintenance or escalation. Infrequent use of these strategies was related to de-escalation or termination. Perceptions of openness and assurances increased over time in escalating relationships; whereas, perceptions of positivity, assurances, and sharing tasks decreased in de-escalating relationships. Finally, perceptions of positivity, openness, assurances, and sharing tasks remained stable in stable relationships. The results of this study indicate that relational maintenance strategies operate not only to maintain relationships but also to change them. In particular, frequent use of relationship maintenance strategies can lead to relationship maintenance and escalation. Infrequent use of relationship maintenance strategies can lead to relationship de-escalation and termination.

Dindia (1991) examined relationship development strategies across stages of relationship development. The purpose of the study was to determine the extent to which relationship development strategies are multiphasic. Participants reported the strategies they use to initiate, escalate, maintain, repair, and terminate relationships. Dindia coded the strategies into 24 categories and found that 19 of the categories were reported in two or more relational stages. For example, communication and contact, rewards, and togetherness were strategies reported to initiate, escalate, maintain, and repair relationships. Many of the strategies used to terminate a relationship were the opposite of strategies to initiate, escalate, maintain, and repair relationships. For example, avoiding communication and contact and making the relationship costly for the partner were two strategies reported to terminate relationships. A potential problem with this study is that subjects reported on all five stages of relationships and may have engaged in a "response set" in which they reported the same strategies across relationship stages.

Consequently, in a follow-up study, Dindia (1992) asked participants to choose a relationship they were currently involved in, and, depending on the stage of the relationship, describe the strategies they use to initiate, escalate, maintain, repair, de-escalate, or terminate the relationship. The results of the study were 21 strategies, all of which were multiphasic, used in two or more relational stages. For example, communication and contact, rewards, and time together/shared activities were strategies reported to initiate, escalate, maintain, and repair relationships. The results of this study also indicated that some of the strategies used to de-escalate and terminate relationships are the opposite of strategies designed to initiate, escalate, maintain, and repair relationships. For example, withdrawing from communication and contact was a strategy reported to de-escalate and terminate relationships. The results of Dindia's studies provide some empirical support for the generality and parsimony of an all-inclusive typology of relationship development strategies rather than separate typologies of relational initiation, escalation, maintenance, and termination strategies. However, one cannot conclude from the results of these studies that all relationship strategies are multiphasic. Only strategies that constituted 1% or more of the data were analyzed in Dindia's studies. Strategies that were reported less frequently may be uniphasic strategies. Thus, there may be more uniphasic relationship strategies than Dindia's results indicate.

Summary and Implications for Theory and Research

There are a number of similarities in the typologies of relationship initiation, escalation, maintenance, and termination strategies. Table 1 synthesizes these strategies and presents a typology of relationship development strategies. The relationship development strategies include: contact, avoidance, communication, metacommunication, indirectness, rewards, costs, similarity, dissimilarity, self-presentation (positive attributes), self-presentation (negative attributes), affection (verbal, nonverbal, and tokens), indifference, social networks, spontaneity/novelty, and shared tasks/responsibilities.

In general, the strategies listed in Table 1 are multiphasic. Research on relationship development strategies has found that communication and contact is used to initiate, escalate, and maintain relationships. The opposite of communication and contact, avoidance, is used to terminate relationships. Metacommunication and indirectness are used to escalate, maintain, and terminate relationships, but not to initiate relationships. Rewards, self-presentation of positive attributes, and affection are used to initiate, escalate, and maintain relationships. Their opposites, costs, self-presentation of negative attributes, and indifference, are used to terminate relationships. Similarity is reported to initiate and maintain relationships; whereas, dissimilarity is reported to terminate relationships. Social networks are used to escalate and terminate relationships. Two strategies appear to be uniphasic: spontaneity/novelty and sharing tasks/responsibilities appear to be used exclusively to maintain relationships.

It can be argued from the theoretical perspective of Morton and Douglas (1981) that many of the relationship development strategies in Table 1 are multiphasic because they are designed to influence important relationship characteristics. For example, communication, contact, affection, and avoidance may be strategies designed to influence familiarity or intimacy. Rewards, costs, self-presentation of positive attributes, self-presentation of negative attributes, similarity, dissimilarity, affection, indifference, spontaneity/

Table 1
Typology of Relationship Development Strategies[a]

Relationship dimension	Initiate	Escalate	Maintain	Terminate
Contact				
Inclusion (i.e., bring other into presence)	B & P			
Increased contact		T		
Self-inclusion (i.e., join in partner's activities)	B & D		B D & G	
Inclusion of other (i.e., include other in activities)	B & D		B D & G	
Togetherness (time & activities together)			D & B	
Avoidance				
Exclusion (i.e., avoid other)				B & P
Withdrawal				B
Behavioral de-escalation				C
Withdrawal/avoidance				B
Communication				
Communication (e.g., talk)			D & B	
Talk about your day			D & B	
Personal communication		T		
Openness	B & D		B D & G	
Openness (includes self-disclosure)			S & C	
Openness/honesty (and share feelings)			D & B	
Honesty			B D & G	
Idiomatic speech		T		
Influence perceptions of closeness (e.g., "we" idioms)	B & D		B D & G	
Sexual intimacy		T		
Metacommunication				
Metacommunication			D & B	
Openness (i.e., metacommunication)			S & C	
Relationship negotiation		T		
Direct definitional bid		T		
Accept definitional bid		T		
Directness (i.e., say you want to keep relationship at same level)			A	
Open confrontation (i.e., openly express desire to terminate)				B
State of relationship talk				B
Negotiated farewell				B
Fait accompli				B
Attributional conflict				B
Positive tone				C
Positive tone				B

(continues)

Table 1 (*Continued*)

Relationship dimension	Initiate	Escalate	Maintain	Terminate
Negative identity management				C
Justification				C
Deescalation (i.e., suggest trial separation)				C
Indirectness				
Suggestive actions		T		
Fading away (i.e., mutually let relationship fade away)				B
Pseudo-deescalation				B
Rewards				
Other enhancement (i.e., show you think highly of other)	B & P			
Self-concept confirmation (i.e., compliment/build esteem)	B & D		B D & G	
Favor-rendering	B & P			
Increase rewards		T		
Balance (i.e., balance favors)			A	
Altruism (i.e., help partner)	B & D		B D & G	
Facilitate enjoyment	B & D		B D & G	
Reward association	B & D		B D & G	
Prosocial strategies (e.g., positive, cheerful, favors)			D & B	
Positivity (i.e., being positive and cheerful)			S & C	
Ceremonies			D & B	
Concede control	B & D		B D & G	
Costs				
Cost-rendering				B & P
Cost escalation				B
Similarities				
Similarity	B & P			
Similarity	B & D			
Shared spirituality			B D & G	
Dissimilarity				
Difference				B & P
Self-presentation (positive attributes)				
Self-presentation (e.g., favorable image)	B & P			
Behavioral adaptation (i.e., favorable impression)		T		
Assume control	B & D			
Assume equality	B & D		B D & G	
Comfortable self	B & D			
Dynamism	B & D		B D & G	
Optimism	B & D		B D & G	

(continues)

Table 1 (*Continued*)

Relationship dimension	Initiate	Escalate	Maintain	Terminate
Personal autonomy	B & D			
Present interesting self	B & D		B D & G	
Trustworthiness	B & D			
Personal appearance		T		
Physical attractiveness	B & D		B D & G	
Self-improvement			B D & G	
Conversational rule-keeping	B & D		B D & G	
Self-presentation (negative attributes)				
Self-presentation (i.e., unfavorable image)				B & P
Affection				
Tokens of affection		T		
Gifts			D & B	
Verbal expressions of affection		T		
Nonverbal expressions of affection		T		
Physical affection			B D & G	
Express affection			D & B	
Verbal affection			B D & G	
Assurances (i.e., communicate commitment, love, faithfulness)			S & C	
Faithfulness			B D & G	
Warmth			D & B	
Sensitivity	B & D		B D & G	
Supportiveness	B & D		B D & G	
Listening	B & D		B D & G	
Balance (i.e., balance emotional support levels)			A	
Acquire information	B & P			
Elicit disclosure	B & D		B D & G	
Nonverbal immediacy (i.e., nonverbally communicate interest)	B & D			
Indifference				
Other negation (i.e., communicate partner not liked)				B & P
Disinterest (i.e., cease to acquire info)				B & P
Social network				
Social enmeshment (i.e., interact with partner's social network)		T		
Network (spend time together with network)			S & C	
Spend time with network			D & B	
Third party relations (i.e., demonstrate positive feelings to partner's network)			B D & G	

(*continues*)

Table 1   (*Continued*)

Relationship dimension	Initiate	Escalate	Maintain	Terminate
Social support & assistance (i.e., ask advice from network)		T		
Tasks/responsibilities				
Sharing tasks			S & C	
Reliability (i.e., dependable in carrying out responsibilities)			B D & G	
Spontaneity/novelty			D & B	
Other				
Manipulatory strategies				B
Avoidance (i.e., avoid things that would change level of relationship)			A	

[a]Key to sources: A = Ayres, 1983; B = Baxter, 1982, 1984; B & D = Bell & Daly, 1984; B D & G = Bell, Daly, & Gonzalez, 1987; C = Cody, 1982; D & B = Dindia & Baxter, 1987; S & C = Stafford & Canary, 1991; T = Tolhuizen, 1989.

novelty, and shared tasks/responsibilities may be strategies to influence attraction. Communication, contact, avoidance, shared tasks/responsibilities, and social networks may be strategies to influence interconnectedness. Thus, strategies to initiate, escalate, and maintain relationships may involve strategies to bring into existence, increase, and maintain intimacy, attraction, and interconnectedness (by communicating with and rewarding partner, etc.), respectively; whereas, strategies to terminate relationships may involve strategies to decrease or eliminate intimacy, attraction, and interconnectedness (by avoiding communication and contact, making the relationship costly for the partner, etc.).

Alternatively, interpreting the relationship development strategies from the theoretical perspectives of Lewin (1951), Levinger (1965, 1976), and Davis (1973), it can be argued that many of the relationship development strategies are multiphasic because they are designed to activate and deactivate external forces that hold a relationship together or pull it apart. Strategies to initiate, escalate, maintain, and repair relationships may be designed to activate forces that bring and hold a couple together (e.g., attraction); whereas, strategies to terminate relationships may involve strategies designed to deactivate the forces that hold a couple together and activate the forces that pull a couple apart.

Interpreting relationship development strategies according to the theoretical framework of Byrne and Murnen (1988) helps us to understand why some strategies are uniphasic, but does not explain the preponderance of multiphasic strategies. Byrne and Murnen argued that attraction is important at all stages of relationship development, but what influences attraction may differ at different stages of relationship development. They posited that similarity, habituation, and evaluation are crucial to maintaining (but not necessarily initiating) attraction and, therefore, are important for maintaining (but not necessarily initiating) relationships. However, research on relationship development strategies indicates that similarity is used to initiate and maintain relationships, whereas the opposite, dissimilarity, is used to terminate relationships.

Byrne and Murnen also asserted that "maintenance involves something beyond the mere repetition of those variables that initiated attraction in the first place and something besides the mere absence of the variables that are associated with relationship failure" (1988, p. 294). However, research on relationship development strategies indicates that many of the strategies designed to initiate and escalate relationships are also used to maintain relationships (e.g., contact, communication, rewards, affection, and self-presentation of positive attributes). Similarly, research by Bell and his colleagues (Bell 1984; Bell et al., 1987) indicates a preponderance of similar strategies to initiate and maintain affinity, a concept similar to attraction. In addition, research on relationship development strategies indicates that the opposites of several strategies to terminate relationships (e.g., dissimilarity, costs, avoidance, self-presentation of negative attributes) are used to maintain relationships (e.g., similarity, rewards, communication and contact, self-presentation of positive attributes). Finally, this research indicates that the absence of maintenance strategies is associated with the de-escalation and termination of relationships (Guerrero et al., 1993).

In support of Byrne and Murnen's position, spontaneity/novelty appears to be used exclusively to maintain relationships. This strategy is obviously designed to influence habituation and it makes sense that this strategy would only be reported to maintain relationships because habituation would only be an issue for those in the maintenance stage of a relationship. Similarly, it makes sense that sharing tasks and being reliable in carrying out responsibilities would only be a strategy for people who are maintaining relationships, which in most cases would be couples who are living together. By sharing tasks and performing household chores, partners maintain a high ratio of positive to negative feelings which maintains attraction but is generally irrelevant to initiating and escalating attraction.

Thus, existing research on relationship development strategies tends to support the theoretical perspectives of Morton and Douglas (1981), Lewin (1951), Levinger (1965, 1976), and Davis (1973). These perspectives are similar in that they argue that there are underlying dimensions of relationships—or forces that hold a relationship together/pull it apart—that generalize to all stages of relationship development. Thus, whether attraction is viewed as an underlying dimension of a relationship or a force that holds a relationship together (and its opposite, repulsion, pulls a relationship apart), strategies directed at attraction—initiating, escalating, sustaining, de-escalating, and terminating attraction—are strategies to initiate, escalate, maintain, de-escalate, and terminate relationships and these strategies are similar across stages of relationship development. Byrne and Murnen's (1988) perspective is similar in that it implicitly views attraction as the underlying dimension of a relationship or the force that holds a relationship together. However, it departs from the former perspectives in that Byrne and Murnen argue that what affects attraction differs at different stages of relationship development. In general, empirical research on relationship development strategies supports the former view, that is, what affects attraction (and the strategies that are used to affect attraction) is similar across stages of relationship development.

Conclusion

There is some theoretical and empirical support for a typology of relationship development strategies that is generalizable to all stages of relationships, including relationship maintenance. Similarly, there is some empirical support that strategies used to initiate and develop relationships are also used to maintain relationships, and that their opposites are used to terminate relationships. However, further research needs to test the degree to which relationship development strategies, in particular, relationship maintenance strategies, are multiphasic. Specifically, there needs to be research designed to test the usefulness of the proposed typology of relationship development strategies for the maintenance stage of relationships.

Although generality and parsimony are important goals of theory building, two criteria are used to judge the usefulness of a typology: exhaustiveness and mutual exclusiveness. The exhaustiveness of the proposed typology of relationship development strategies is yet to be determined. The typology may exclude important uniphasic maintenance strategies, strategies that are used only to maintain relationships. Similarly, the typology may mask important differences between similar strategies used to initiate and/or escalate relationships and strategies used to maintain relationships. For example, similarity is used to initiate and maintain relationships. However, the kinds of similarities that are emphasized at these stages probably differ. Thus, this typology may lead us to believe that relationship initiation and maintenance are more alike than is really the case. Alternatively, research based on this typology can be conducted to distinguish the types of similarities that initiate and/or escalate relationships versus maintain relationships. Research employing this typology can inform us whether certain strategies are more effective for some stages than others. Ultimately, such a typology can help us determine whether "relationship maintenance involves something beyond the mere repetition of the variables that initiated attraction in the first place and something besides the mere absence of the variables that are associated with relationship failure" (Byrne & Murnen, 1988).

References

Ayres, J. (1983). Strategies to maintain relationships: Their identification and perceived usage. *Communication Quarterly, 31*, 62–67.

Baxter, L. A. (1982). Strategies for ending relationships: Two studies. *Western Journal of Speech Communication, 46*, 223–241.

Baxter, L. A. (1984). Trajectories of relationship disengagement. *Journal of Social and Personal Relationships, 1*, 29–48.

Baxter, L. A. (1985). Accomplishing relationship disengagement. In S. Duck and D. Perlman (Eds.), *Understanding personal relationships: An interdisciplinary approach* (pp. 243–265). Beverly Hills, CA: Sage.

Baxter, L. A., & Dindia, K. (1990). Marital partners' perceptions of marital maintenance strategies. *Journal of Social and Personal Relationships, 7*, 187–209.

Baxter, L. A., & Philpott, J. (1982). Attribution-based strategies for initiating and terminating relationships. *Communication Quarterly, 30*, 217–224.

Bell, R. A., & Daly, J. A. (1984). The affinity-seeking function in communication. *Communication Monographs, 51*, 91–115.

Bell, R. A., Daly, J. A., & Gonzalez, C. (1987). Affinity-maintenance in marriage and its relationship to women's marital satisfaction. *Journal of Marriage and the Family, 49*, 445–54.

Buley, J. L. (1977). *Relationships and Communication*. Dubuque, IA: Kendall/Hunt.

Burgoon, J. K., & Hale, J. L. (1987). Validation and measurement of the fundamental themes of relational communication. *Communication Monographs, 54*, 19–41.

Byrne, D., & Murnen, S. (1988). Maintaining loving relationships. In R. Sternberg & M. Barnes (Eds.), *The Psychology of love*. New Haven, CT: Yale University Press.

Cody, M. (1982). A typology of disengagement strategies and an examination of the role intimacy, reactions to inequity, and relational problems play in strategy selection. *Communication Monographs, 49*, 148–170.

Davis, M. S. (1973). *Intimate relations*. New York: The Free Press.

Dindia, K. (1991, November). *Uniphasic versus multiphasic relational maintenance and change strategies*. Paper presented at the Speech Communication Association convention, Atlanta, GA.

Dindia, K. (1992, November). *A typology of relational maintenance and change strategies*. Paper presented at the Speech Communication Association convention, Chicago.

Dindia, K., & Baxter, L. (1987). Strategies for maintaining and repairing marital relationships. *Journal of Social and Personal Relationships, 4*, 143–158.

Dindia, K., & Emery, D. (1982, July). *Strategies for maintaining and repairing marital relationships*. Paper presented to the International Conference on Personal Relationships, Madison, WI.

Duck, S. (1988) *Relating to others*. Stratford, England: Open University Press.

Guerrero, L. K., Eloy, S. V., & Wabnik, A. I. (1993). Linking maintenance strategies to relationship development and disengagement: A reconceptualization. *Journal of Social and Personal Relationships, 10*, 273–283.

Levinger, G. (1965). Marital cohesiveness and dissolution: An integrative review. *Journal of Marriage and the Family, 27*, 19–28.

Levinger, G. (1976). A social psychological perspective on marital dissolution. *Journal of Social Issues, 32*, 21–47.

Levinger, G. (1979). A social exchange view on the dissolution of pair relationships. In R. L. Burgess & T. L. Huston (Eds.), *Social exchange in developing relationships* (169–193). New York: Academic Press.

Levinger, G. (1983). Development and change. In H. H. Kelley, E. Berscheid, A. Christensen, J. H. Harvey, T. L. Huston, G. Levinger, E. McClintock, L. A. Peplau, & D. R. Peterson (Eds.), *Close relationships* (315–359). New York: W. H. Freeman.

Lewin, K. (1951). *Field theory in social science.* New York: Harper.

Morton, T. L., & Douglas, M. A. (1981). Growth of relationships. In S. Duck & R. Gilmour (Eds.), *Personal relationships 2: Developing personal relationships.* New York: Academic Press.

Reynolds, P. D. (1971). *A primer in theory construction.* Indianapolis, IN: Bobs-Merril.

Shea, B. C., & Pearson, J. C. (1986). The effects of relationship type, partner intent, and gender on the selection of relationship maintenance strategies. *Communication Monographs, 53,* 354, 364.

Stafford, L., & Canary, D. J. (1991). Maintenance strategies and romantic relationship type, gender and relational characteristics. *Journal of Social and Personal Relationships, 8,* 217–242.

Tolhuizen, J. H. (1989). Communication strategies for intensifying dating relationships: Identification, use and structure. *Journal of Social and Personal Relationships, 6,* 413–434.

Tolhuizen, J. H. (1992, November). *The association of relational factors to intensification strategy use.* Paper presented at the convention of the Speech Communication Association, Chicago.

Social Psychological Approaches

6

The Investment Model

An Interdependence Analysis of Commitment Processes and Relationship Maintenance Phenomena

Caryl E. Rusbult
Stephen M. Drigotas
Julie Verette
Department of Psychology
University of North Carolina at Chapel Hill
Chapel Hill, North Carolina

Introduction

Over the past few decades social scientists have exerted considerable effort in their attempts to understand why some romantic relationships grow stronger with the passage of time while other relationships wither and die. Many (or most) researchers working in the close relationships field have assumed that the best route to understanding such issues is to explore the determinants and consequences of satisfaction (e.g., Berscheid, 1985; Clark & Reis, 1988). In some respects this point of view makes perfect sense; if individuals are happy with their relationships, surely they should be more likely to remain with their partners. All things considered, it is easier to stick with a line of action when things are going well than when things are going poorly. Unfortunately, simply understanding how people come to love their partners and feel satisfied with their relationships is not sufficient to explain how and why some relationships not only persist but thrive whereas others do not.

Communication and Relational Maintenance
Copyright © 1994 by Academic Press, Inc. All rights of reproduction in any form reserved.

Satisfaction ebbs and flows even in the most gratifying involvements, and most relationships at some time are threatened by tempting "greener grass"—few relationships ride an ever-increasing wave of unchallenged satisfaction. Assuming this to be so, the question becomes one of understanding why some relationships make it through both good times and bad times and why others do not.

This chapter employs interdependence theory constructs (Kelley, 1979; Kelley & Thibaut, 1978; Thibaut & Kelley, 1959) to analyze commitment processes and relationship maintenance phenomena. Hence, features of interdependence theory are first reviewed. We then present the investment model (Rusbult, 1980a, 1983): a theory of the process by which individuals become committed to their relationships as well as the circumstances under which feelings of commitment erode and relationships end. Whereas previous research has focused on satisfaction levels in trying to understand relationship stability, we propose that two additional variables—perceived quality of alternatives and quantity of investments—are also important in understanding why individuals initially become committed and how they remain committed to their relationships. Following this, we use the investment model to explain how and why relationships are maintained despite such threats as periodic declines in satisfaction, the presence of attractive and tempting alternatives, or inevitable noncorrespondent outcomes. We propose that subjective commitment is a central force in motivating a variety of relationship maintenance phenomena, defined in our work as the prorelationship activities that help relationships persist and promote healthy functioning in ongoing relationships. This section reviews research on relationship maintenance activities such as accommodative behavior, tendencies to derogate attractive and threatening alternatives, willingness to sacrifice for the good of a relationship, and tendencies toward perceived relationship superiority. In closing, we consider the functional value of commitment and relationship maintenance phenomena, and discuss fruitful directions for future research.

Dependence on a Relationship:
The Interdependence Orientation

Interdependence theory focuses on the interaction between partners as the essence of all close relationships, emphasizing that understanding behavior and feelings in relationships requires knowledge of the structure of interdependence between partners (Kelley, 1979; Kelley & Thibaut, 1978; Thibaut & Kelley, 1959). Importantly, in characterizing interdependence the authors cited here distinguish between the concepts of satisfaction and dependence. *Satisfaction level* refers to the positive versus negative emotions an individual experiences with respect to a relationship, based on the sense that a given partner and relationship gratify one's most important needs (e.g., John loves Mary because she fulfills his needs for intimacy). In contrast, *dependence level* refers to the extent to which an individual "needs" a relationship and relies primarily on a given partner and relationship for the fulfillment of important needs (e.g., John needs Mary because his needs for intimacy cannot be adequately fulfilled elsewhere).

What produces feelings of satisfaction with a relationship? In an ongoing relationship, the degree of satisfaction or dissatisfaction experienced by an individual is affected not only by that individual's own choices and behaviors, but also by the choices and behaviors of the partner. For example, consider John and Mary: John enjoys caring for the children and tending to activities at home while Mary pursues her career; Mary finds this arrangement to be highly gratifying. Both enjoy high levels of emotional openness, yet they also derive pleasure from simply engaging in everyday activities together. John and Mary gratify one another's most basic needs, and their mutual happiness is promoted by the specific sort of relationship they developed. Thus, the outcomes they enjoy as a consequence of their involvement are not only quite good on average, but are also highly correspondent—the behaviors John naturally wishes to enact are those that bring Mary pleasure, and the activities Mary prefers are those that John would be inclined to desire as well.

Interdependence theory formally represents the pleasant—and sometimes not so pleasant—experiences encountered during the course of extended interaction in terms of rewards and costs. *Rewards* are defined as "the pleasures, satisfactions, and gratifications that a person enjoys" (Thibaut & Kelley, 1959, p. 12), and *costs* are defined as "any factors that operate to inhibit or deter the performance of a sequence of behavior. Cost is high when great physical or mental effort is required, when embarrassment or anxiety accompany the action, or when there are conflicting forces or competing response tendencies of any sort" (pp. 12–13). For convenience, the rewards obtained and the costs incurred can be combined to calculate an overall "goodness of outcome" value for any given interaction. Relationships marked by a greater number or intensity of pleasurable interaction outcomes should be experienced as more satisfying.

However, the rewarding and costly interactions experienced in a relationship are not the only things that influence satisfaction level. Feelings of satisfaction are also affected by the individual's internal standard for evaluating a relationship, or *comparison level* (CL). By CL, Thibaut and Kelley (1959) refer to "the standard against which the member evaluates the 'attractiveness' of the relationship or how satisfactory it is" (p. 21). Accordingly, an individual compares the average outcomes obtained in a relationship with what he or she expects from relationships in general, based on "all outcomes known to the member, either by direct experience or symbolically" (p. 21). When obtained outcomes are better than what is expected, the individual is more likely to feel satisfied.

As noted earlier, it seems intuitively obvious that satisfying relationships should be somewhat more likely to persist than dissatisfying relationships. However, satisfaction by itself is not the whole story—simply experiencing a good number of supra-CL interactions is not enough to produce a harmonious and stable involvement. To further account for relationship stability, interdependence theory introduces the concept of dependence, which is influenced by a second comparison criterion, the *comparison level for alternatives*, or CL_{alt}. Frequently, individuals contemplate what might be experienced outside the current relationship in the best available alternative situation—in a specific alternative relationship, in multiple alternative relationships, or on one's own (i.e., in an uninvolved state, interacting with friends and relatives rather than a romantic partner). Outcomes obtained in the current relationship are compared to anticipated outcomes in the best alternative option. According to Thibaut and Kelley (1959), "the CL_{alt} can be defined informally as the lowest level of outcomes a member will accept in light of available alternative opportunities. It follows that as soon as outcomes drop below CL_{alt}, the member will leave the relationship" (p. 21).

Thus, dependence on a relationship is stronger—and the odds of remaining in that relationship are greater—when the outcomes experienced in a relationship are perceived to be better than what might be obtained elsewhere. Dependence on a relationship is thus defined in terms of the discrepancy between outcomes obtained in the current relationship and those anticipated from alternative relationships. In essence, dependence refers to the degree to which an individual relies on a partner and relationship for fulfilling important needs—the degree to which the needs that are satisfied in a given relationship cannot be gratified elsewhere. When level of satisfaction with the current relationship is quite high and the quality of available alternatives is perceived to be poor, dependence is strong. When individuals believe that they are obtaining the best possible "deal" in their relationship—however poor the relationship may be in an absolute sense—they are more dependent on the relationship, and are likely to remain together.

Clarifying and Extending Interdependence Theory: The Investment Model

What does the experience of dependence "feel like" to involved partners? The investment model suggests that dependence is subjectively represented as feelings of commitment (Rusbult, 1980a, 1983). Accordingly, the investment model is consonant with other work emphasizing commitment (e.g., Johnson, 1991), cohesion (e.g., Levinger, 1979a, 1979b), and other factors that compel people to maintain their relationships (e.g., "barriers"; see Attridge, this volume). *Commitment level* represents long-term orientation toward a relationship, and includes intentions to remain in the relationship as well as feelings of attachment (Johnson, 1982; Rosenblatt, 1977). Because highly committed individuals need their relationships, feel connected to their partners, and have a more extended, long-term time perspective, they are more likely to remain in their relationships and engage in a wide variety of relationship maintenance behaviors.

The investment model suggests that the interdependence theory explanation of the causes of dependence does not account for the full picture in explaining why some relationships persist. If feelings of commitment and decisions to remain in a relationship were determined solely by a comparison of the satisfactions derived from a current relationship to those anticipated in alternative relationships, few relationships would endure—a relationship would quickly (or eventually) falter on the occasion of poor outcomes or the appearance of an appealing alternative. In reality, it would seem that some relationships survive even when an attractive alternative is available, and even when outcomes in the relationship fall below what partners feel they deserve. How can we explain such persistence in the face of tempting alternatives and fluctuating satisfaction?

The investment model asserts that feelings of commitment are influenced not only by *satisfaction level* and perceived *quality of alternatives*, but also by a third factor, *investment size*. Investments are the resources that become attached to a relationship and would decline in value or be lost if the relationship were to end. In the developing stages of a relationship partners begin to learn about one another through the course of ongoing interaction. The time that is spent with a partner represents the most basic form of investment in a relationship—time is a resource that is "put into" a relationship that could not be recovered if the relationship were to end. As interaction with a given partner progresses, partners continue to invest directly in their relationship through mechanisms such as self-disclosure, effort expenditure, and the binding of their identities to the relationship. Moreover, some investments are indirect, and occur when originally extraneous resources such as mutual friends, children, or shared material possessions become attached to a relationship. Thus, a variety of concrete and abstract resources may become tied to an ongoing relationship, and such investments can serve as powerful psychological inducements to continue a relationship (see also Attridge, this volume).

In summary, the investment model proposes that dependence on a relationship is subjectively experienced as a sense of commitment, and that commitment is enhanced when individuals feel satisfied with their relationships, when they perceive their alternatives to be of poor quality, and when they have invested numerous important resources in their relationships. Feelings of commitment subjectively summarize the net effects of satisfaction, alternatives, and investments, and directly mediate individuals' decisions to remain in versus end their relationships (see Figure 1). Is strong commitment a good thing or a bad thing? In short, both. Of course, large investments and poor alternatives can trap individuals in unhappy relationships, but individuals may also actively employ these processes to produce enhanced stability. In relationships that are generally gratifying, individuals may burn available bridges and throw in their lot with partners, in part as a means of holding a relationship together through difficult times.

Empirical Support for the Investment Model

A good deal of research has supported the investment model and its theoretical claims (e.g., Rusbult, 1980a, 1983; Duffy & Rusbult, 1986; Rusbult, Johnson, & Morrow, 1986b). Empirical studies using a variety of participant populations and diverse methodologies have consistently demonstrated that commitment level is positively associated with satisfaction level and investment size, and that it is negatively associated with perceived quality of alternatives. Correlations between commitment and each of the three components typically range from .30 to .70 or so. Each of the three variables contributes independently to predicting commitment, and collectively the variables account for 50 to 90% of the variance in feelings of commitment. Moreover, causal modeling techniques have revealed findings consistent with the claim that commitment partially or wholly mediates the effects of satisfaction, alternatives, and investments on decisions to remain in versus end a relationship. Compared to less committed persons, highly committed individuals are substantially more likely to remain with their partners.

For example, Rusbult (1983) conducted a 7-month longitudinal study of dating relationships. Every 17 days participants completed questionnaires that tapped each model component. Trend analyses revealed patterns of

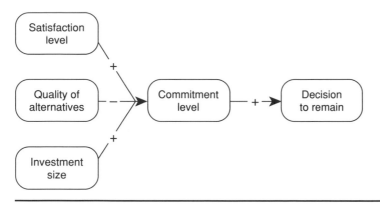

Figure 1

The investment model of commitment processes.

change over time that were consistent with investment model predictions: Increases over time in commitment were associated with increasing satisfaction level, declining alternative quality, and increasing investments. Also, analyses differentiating between participants who remained in their relationships (Stayers), participants who voluntarily ended their relationships (Leavers), and participants whose partners' ended their relationships (the Abandoned) revealed that commitment increased over time for Stayers, declined for Leavers, and was intermediate for the Abandoned. Furthermore, whereas Stayers' reports of satisfaction level and investment size increased over time, alternatives were judged to become less and less attractive. The opposite was true for those who voluntarily left their relationships (Leavers), while the Abandoned once again exhibited scores between those two extremes. Finally, causal modeling analyses revealed that decisions to remain in or end a relationship were strongly—albeit partially—mediated by changes over time in commitment.

Many studies have provided good direct or indirect support for investment model predictions. For example, feelings of commitment and decisions to maintain a relationship are associated with satisfaction level constructs such as degree of love for a partner, self-reported satisfaction, and "marital comparison level index," a measure of the degree to which outcomes in marriage exceed expectations (Buunk, 1987; Drigotas & Rusbult, 1992; Duffy & Rusbult, 1986; Felmlee, Sprecher, & Bassin, 1990; Lin & Rusbult, 1992; Lund, 1985; Rusbult, 1980a; Rusbult et al., 1986b; Rusbult, Verette, Whitney, Slovik, & Lipkus, 1991; Sabatelli, 1984; Sabatelli & Cecil-Pigo, 1985; Simpson, 1987). Also, commitment and decisions to persist in a relationship are related to alternative quality constructs, including measures of dissolution barriers and items designed to tap the best available alternative, best imagined alternative, and ease of finding an alternative partner (Drigotas & Rusbult, 1992; Duffy & Rusbult, 1986; Felmlee et al., 1990; Lin & Rusbult, 1993; Rusbult, 1980a; Rusbult et al., 1986b; Rusbult et al., 1991; Sabatelli & Cecil-Pigo, 1985; Simpson, 1987). Finally, commitment and decisions to remain in a relationship are related to investment size constructs such as personal investment in a relationship, support from the surrounding social network, duration of relationship, and exclusivity of relationship (Duffy & Rusbult, 1986; Felmlee et al., 1990; Lin & Rusbult, 1993; Lund, 1985; Rusbult, 1980a; Rusbult et al., 1986b; Rusbult et al., 1991; Simpson, 1987).

The generalizability of this model has been documented. The investment model has been shown to predict commitment and relationship stability not only in dating relationships (Rusbult, 1980a, 1983), but also in more extended adult relationships (Rusbult et al., 1986b), in both heterosexual and homosexual relationships (Duffy & Rusbult, 1986), and in the relationships of young adults residing in the United States, Taiwan, and the Netherlands (Buunk, Engels, Ponjee, & Vaessen, 1993; Lin & Rusbult, 1993). Also, this model has been used as a means of understanding commitment in highly distressed relationships, such as abusive relationships; compared to women who leave battering partners, those who remain with their partners exhibit far greater investments in their relationships and have exceedingly poor alternatives, and accordingly feel committed despite the fact that their relationships are tremendously dissatisfying (Rusbult & Martz, 1993; Strube, 1988). Moreover, in addition to its applications to the study of romantic relationships, the investment model has been employed to study commitment processes in friendships (Rusbult, 1980b) as well as in organizational settings (i.e., job commitment and turnover; Farrell & Rusbult, 1981; Rusbult & Farrell, 1983).

The Investment Model
and Relationship Maintenance Processes

Thus far, we have implied that the ultimate consequence of commitment is whether a relationship endures or terminates. However, to remain in a relationship is but the minimum requirement for relationship maintenance. At one time or another most relationships suffer problems such as periodic declines in satisfaction, the presence of attractive and tempting alternatives, or the simple ravages of time. It is not enough to know *whether* relationships endure or terminate during such periods. A complete scientific understanding of behavior in relationships necessitates delineating *how* relationships persist through such periods. Thus, we turn to a discussion of relationship maintenance phenomena.

We take it as given that partners in ongoing relationships invariably confront situations that are potentially harmful to the longevity of their involvement—situations in which they must solve mutual problems of interdependence (e.g., periods of dissatisfaction, the presence of tempting alternatives). Moreover, the relationship-maintaining solution to such interdependence problems typically entails some cost in the form of personal sacrifice or effort expenditure. For example, it is typically beneficial to a relationship to accommodate rather than retaliate when a partner behaves badly, but doing so may produce costs for the accommodator such as feelings of resentment or lowered self-esteem. With repeated exposure to particular classes of interdependence dilemmas, stable response orientations may evolve (Mellen, 1981; Rusbult & Verette, 1991). Some individuals may routinely engage in prorelationship behaviors and endure whatever costs are involved, and others may typically act in accordance with their direct and immediate self-interest. Holmes (1981) suggests that such stable response tendencies are guided by macromotives—by the relatively enduring, internalized attitudes that emerge in the context of a given relationship.

We suggest that commitment is a central macromotive in relationships, and that feelings of commitment serve to (1) subjectively summarize the nature of an individual's dependence on a relationship; (2) direct reactions to both familiar and novel interdependent situations; and (3) shape tendencies to engage in relationship maintenance behaviors, even when such actions may be costly, effortful, or otherwise contrary to the individual's immediate self-interest. Why should this be so? First, given that commitment encompasses the net effects of other dependence-enhancing variables—satisfaction, alternatives, and investments—feelings of commitment should exert profound and general motivational effects on behavior. Commitment represents extended time orientation, and highly committed individuals should accordingly behave in ways that are consistent with this perspective, acting to ensure that their relationships endure and are healthy. In a general sense, highly committed individuals have a vested interest in the well-being of their partners as well as in the future of their relationships, and should accordingly act to protect such investments. Second, for highly committed partners, engaging in prorelationship behaviors on earlier occasions may yield direct benefits for the individual on later occasions. Given the strength and adaptive utility of reciprocity norms, earlier cooperative acts are likely to yield later reciprocal cooperation from one's partner, especially in the context of an extended interdependent relationship (Axelrod, 1983, 1984). Third, by engaging in personally costly, prorelationship behaviors, a committed individual may communicate to the partner his or her cooperative, long-term orientation. When people behave in ways that are inconsistent with their immediate self-interest (e.g., sacrificing for the good of a relationship) they provide their partners with relatively unambiguous evidence of their feelings, attitudes, and intentions (Kelley, 1979).

Figure 2 displays our expanded model of relationship maintenance phenomena, and represents our claims regarding the links between three primary dependence-enhancing variables (satisfaction, alternatives, investments), feelings of commitment, and maintenance activities such as willingness to accommodate or the inclination to derogate attractive and threatening alternative partners. The following sections of the chapter review each relationship maintenance mechanism in turn. In each instance, we discuss the nature of the interdependence dilemma confronted by involved partners, explaining how pro-relationship behavior frequently may stand in opposition to the pursuit of direct and immediate self-interest. Also, we review empirical evidence in support of the claim that each maintenance phenomenon is promoted by feelings of commitment to a relationship.

Tendencies to Accommodate

When individuals confront dissatisfying incidents in their relationships, one possible reaction is to terminate the relationship. However, leaving the

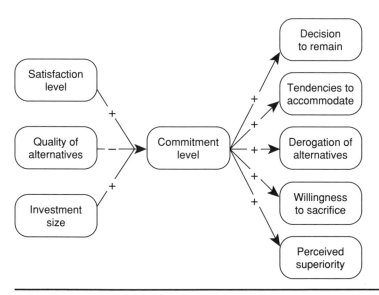

Figure 2

A model of relationship maintenance phenomena.

partner is obviously just one of a host of possible reactions. According to Rusbult and Zembrodt (1983), potential reactions to dissatisfaction differ from one another along two dimensions: responses are either *active or passive* with respect to the problem at hand (i.e., responses differ in the extent to which they actively address the problem); and responses are either *destructive or constructive* with respect to the broader relationship (i.e., responses either harm or help the relationship). Using these two dimensions, we can describe four characteristic modes of response to dissatisfaction.

As displayed in Figure 3, the *exit* category includes behaviors that are actively destructive to the future of a relationship such as "separating, moving out of a joint residence, actively abusing one's partner, getting a divorce, threatening to leave, or screaming at one's partner" (Rusbult et al., 1991, p. 54). *Neglect* behaviors passively allow conditions in a relationship to deteriorate through avoidance reactions such as "ignoring the partner or spending less time together, avoiding discussing problems, treating the partner poorly (being cross with him or her), criticizing the partner for things unrelated to the real problem, or just letting things fall apart" (p. 54). It should be clear that in the destructive response categories, the enacted behaviors are likely to be detrimental to a relationship.

In contrast, two additional categories of response address dissatisfying incidents in a manner that is relatively more constructive. *Voice* responses are active attempts to improve conditions in a relationship, and include behaviors such as "discussing problems, seeking help from a friend or therapist, suggesting solutions, changing oneself, or urging the partner to change" (Rusbult et al., 1991, p. 54). *Loyalty* reactions are essentially a matter of optimistically waiting for positive change, as illustrated by behaviors such as "waiting and hoping that things will improve, supporting the partner in the face of criticism, or praying for improvement" (pp. 53–54). Thus, although loyalty reactions are relatively passive, they are constructive in that they are associated with benign thoughts and positive intentions—the passive response is intended to benefit the relationship by means that are indirect yet supportive (e.g., standing by a partner during difficult times, avoiding escalation, and hoping that conditions will improve).

Early research employing the exit–voice–loyalty–neglect typology demonstrated that particular interdependent patterns of response to dissatisfaction were associated with superior functioning in relationships. To begin with, we obtained evidence of a "good manners" model of couple functioning: relationships exhibited superior overall functioning to the extent that they engaged in lower levels of exit and neglect (Rusbult, Johnson, & Morrow, 1986a). But beyond this, when one individual in a relationship engaged in either of the two destructive reactions (exit or neglect), thus creating a situation that was potentially harmful to couple functioning, relationship distress was reduced when the individual's partner was inclined to inhibit

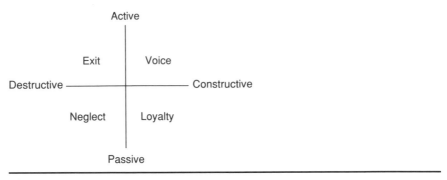

Figure 3

A model of responses to dissatisfaction in close relationships.

inclinations to react in kind (i.e., to inhibit exit or neglect), instead biting the bullet and responding constructively, with voice or loyalty (Rusbult et al., 1986a; see also Gottman et al., 1976; Jacobson, Follette, & McDonald, 1982; Margolin & Wampold, 1981). This interdependent pattern of responding is termed *accommodation*.

The simple message in this body of research is straightforward: partners should retain their good manners even during dissatisfying incidents—or perhaps especially during dissatisfying incidents—and would do well to behave constructively under all circumstances. Unfortunately, partners do not behave well under all circumstances. And when a partner engages in exit or neglect responses, the individual is faced with a dilemma: being treated in an inconsiderate manner generates a natural impulse to behave inconsiderately in turn (i.e., to fight fire with fire). For example, Yovetich and Rusbult (in press) asked participants to recall incidents when their partners engaged in potentially destructive acts, and to report both their initial, private response inclinations and their actual, public reactions. Compared to their actual responses, private inclinations were substantially more negative. Also, Rusbult and her colleagues (Rusbult et al., 1991) found that participants were less likely to react constructively to a partner's destructive act when operating under conditions of reduced social concern. Compared to their response tendencies under conditions of normal social concern, when participants were asked to report how they would respond if they were not concerned about their partner's reaction, the future of their relationship, or their public image or self-concept, participants were far more likely to react destructively to a partner's potentially destructive acts.

These findings suggest that accommodation is experienced as a costly or effortful reaction; that is, accommodating rather than retaliating when a partner behaves poorly is not the individual's immediate response inclination. However, accommodation is clearly in the best interest of the relationship. When confronted with such an "accommodative dilemma," what is it that makes individuals willing to react with voice or loyalty, inhibiting inclinations to react with exit or neglect? Prior research demonstrates that tendencies to accommodate are greater among individuals who are more committed to their relationships, feel more satisfied with their relationships, perceive their alternatives to be of poor quality, have invested numerous important resources in their relationships, and perceive their relationships to be central to what is most meaningful in their lives, as well as among individuals with greater psychological femininity and greater tendencies toward partner perspective-taking. However, causal modeling analyses revealed that once the impact of commitment level is accounted for, the influence of each of these factors on accommodation is reduced or eliminated. That is, consistent with our model of relationship maintenance processes, commitment to a relationship appears to be the primary mediating variable in promoting willingness to accommodate, partially or wholly accounting for the influence of other dispositions and features of interdependent relationships.

Derogation of Alternatives

Even when a relationship is going smoothly, attractive alternatives may come onto the scene. Moreover, it is clear that the temptation to enjoy such alternatives can sometimes be acute; desire to engage in extrarelationship sexual involvement is related to the presence of a realistic and attractive alternative partner (Buunk, 1980a) as well as to the desire for new experiences and personal growth (Atwater, 1982). Although temptation to enjoy the potential benefits of an alternative may be great, to the degree that involvement in a current relationship is strong, the costs involved in enjoying an alternative relationship are also likely to be acute. The most acute possible cost is termination of the current relationship. When the gratifications provided by the current relationship cannot match those anticipated in an alternative relationship (e.g., entering a thrilling new relationship filled with wild abandon), some individuals may choose to terminate the current relationship and enjoy what the alternative has to offer. But other types of possible cost obviously exist. For partners who do not wish to end their relationships, the enjoyment of an alternative relationship by one or both partners may generate rather serious problems, such as feelings of guilt or shame, the pain of jealousy or insecurity, reduced feelings of love, or intense conflict. Therefore, it is understandable that many relationship maintenance activities represent solutions to the interdependence problems associated with threatening alternatives.

Of course, there are several ways to deal with threatening alternatives. Lucky partners may never have to directly confront such threats. As Kelley (1983) notes, when alternatives are aware of an individual's commitment to his or her partner, they may "take themselves out of the running and look elsewhere for associations" (p. 305). Also, individuals who are committed to monogamous involvement may attempt to "drive away" potential alternatives by wearing conspicuous symbols of their commitment (e.g., a wedding ring) or by making it implicitly or explicitly clear that they do not wish to initiate extrarelationship sexual or romantic involvement (e.g., reacting in a cool manner to flirtatious behavior). Furthermore, some partners may either comply with existing cultural norms or develop their own norms as a means of governing extradyadic behavior and minimizing the negative impact of such involvements (Buunk, 1980b). Typically, such rules specify the precise circumstances under which extrarelationship involvements are permissible (e.g., "only brief contacts are acceptable"), as well as the conditions under which such involvements are not acceptable (e.g., "I would be devastated if you were to fall in love with another").

Yet another means of dealing with the threat occasioned by the presence of a tempting and available alternative is to *derogate alternative partners*, "taking a 'sour grapes' attitude toward the rewarding aspects of the interaction or by emphasizing the negative, cost-increasing aspects of it" (Thibaut & Kelley, 1959, p. 175). Indeed, questionnaire responses obtained from individuals involved in ongoing dating relationships revealed that among individuals whose relationships persisted, the judged attractiveness of alternative partners declined substantially over time (Rusbult, 1983). Moreover, Johnson and Rusbult (1989) reasoned that if the tendency toward derogation of alternatives is a motivated maintenance phenomenon, then derogation tendencies should be most pronounced when the alternative partner is most threatening: when commitment to the current relationship is strongest; when the alternative clearly is available as a potential dating partner; and when the alternative is exceptionally attractive. Consistent with this line of reasoning, in the context of a "computer dating study," these authors observed increasing tendencies toward derogation of potential alternatives as a function of increasing commitment to the current relationship. And importantly, the link between commitment and derogation was stronger to the extent that the alternative was more physically attractive, and when participants judged alternatives under conditions of realistic threat (i.e., the alternative might be an actual computer-assigned date) rather than making hypothetical judgments about alternatives. Similar findings have been obtained by other authors (e.g., Simpson, Gangestad, & Lerma, 1990; Verette, 1989).

Thus, although alternatives may sometimes be quite tempting, enjoyment of the alternative may pose a serious threat for the stability of an ongoing relationship. To deal with such threat and reduce the perceived costs of foregoing alternative involvements, committed individuals exhibit a tendency to derogate attractive alternatives—to convince themselves that the alternative is really not so attractive after all. Some research also suggests an additional strategy for dealing with threatening alternatives: Verette (1989) obtained some evidence that among highly committed persons, the presence of threatening alternatives can sometimes yield bolstering of the current relationship (i.e., tendencies to evaluate the current partner and relationship in a more favorable light; see section on perceived relationship superiority, below).

Willingness to Sacrifice

Sometimes, partners in close relationships are forced to decide whether to pursue their immediate self-interest or to pursue the best interest of their relationship. That is, it is inevitable that on some occasions, self-interest will be at odds with what is best for one's partner or relationship. Individuals sometimes react to such noncorrespondence of outcomes with an important relationship maintenance mechanism termed *willingness to sacrifice*. In essence, sacrifice represents the willingness to solve dilemmas of noncorrespondent outcomes by sacrificing self-interest for the good of a relationship, by engaging in behaviors that one otherwise might not wish to enact, or by foregoing behaviors that one otherwise might find desirable. Once again, we assert that this maintenance mechanism should be more probable to the extent that an individual is highly committed to his or her relationship—to the extent that the individual takes a broader time perspective with regard to the partner and relationship.

Three studies of willingness to sacrifice explored this prediction (Van Lange, Rusbult, & Drigotas, 1993). In all three studies, willingness to sacrifice was positively correlated with commitment level, satisfaction level, and investment size, and was negatively correlated with perceived quality of alternatives. Importantly, causal modeling analyses revealed results consistent with the claim that commitment mediates the effects on sacrifice of other investment model constructs: In all three studies, subjective commitment accounted for a good deal of the variability in willingness to sacrifice; also, commitment substantially mediated the effects of satisfaction, alternatives, and investments. Once again, these findings provide good support for claims regarding the centrality of subjective commitment in accounting for tendencies to incur costs or exert effort for the well-being of a relationship.

Perceived Relationship Superiority, or Relationship-Enhancing Illusion

One of the more important determinants of the manner in which individuals experience and evaluate their lives comes in the form of social comparison

(Festinger, 1954). When objective evidence that might form the basis for self-evaluation is not available, individuals tend to evaluate their current circumstances through comparison to similar others. Such comparisons not only offer a basis for *self-evaluation*, but may also be employed as a means of *relationship evaluation*. Indeed, Buunk, Van Yperen, Taylor, and Collins (1991) found that when faced with uncertainty in the evaluation of their marriages, participants exhibited enhanced desire to interact with others, especially with individuals in well-functioning marriages. Ostensibly, those in well-functioning marriages serve as standards for comparison.

Does such social comparison yield accurate impressions? A growing literature suggests that individuals frequently exhibit self-serving biases in information processing, and that they may engage in social comparison, at least in part, as a means of bolstering impressions of themselves and their ongoing relationships (Buunk & Van Yperen, 1989, Collins, Taylor, Van Yperen, & Dakof, 1990; Martz et al., 1993; Taylor & Brown, 1988; Titus, 1980). For example, in research employing a thought-listing technique, Van Lange and Rusbult (in press) found that participants held a greater number and proportion of positive beliefs regarding their own relationships than others' relationships (i.e., positive superiority), and that they held a greater number and proportion of negative beliefs regarding others' relationships than their own (i.e., negative superiority). Subjects were also asked to rate each quality in their lists for degree of positivity. These data further revealed that participants' evaluative judgments of their own relationships were more positive—and less negative—than were their evaluations of others' relationships. Moreover, these authors found that positive information dominated participants' thoughts and beliefs about their own relationships (i.e., own relationship positivity), whereas negative information dominated thoughts and beliefs about others' relationships (i.e., other relationship negativity). Collectively, these tendencies are termed *perceived relationship superiority*.

Logically, it is not possible for all individuals to have relationships that far exceed others' relationships. We cannot all be princes surrounded by fools. Thus, it would seem that at least part of the tendency to perceive one's relationship as superior to others' relationships may be due to biased processing of relationship information (see also Stafford & Reske, 1990). And of course, such biased processing to some extent is costly and effortful—it requires some degree of effort to focus primarily on the qualities for which one's own relationship actually does excel, to locate poorly functioning comparison relationships to which to compare one's own relationship, to selectively encode or recall negative information about others' relationships, or to selectively attend to positive information regarding one's own relationship.

Rusbult, Van Lange, Verette, and Yovetich (1993) reasoned that the ability to incur such cognitive costs in order to protect a favorable view of one's relationship might stand as yet another relationship maintenance activity, arguing that perceived superiority accordingly should be related to feelings of commitment to one's ongoing relationship. These authors conducted a two-wave panel study of ongoing dating relationships, and found that perceived relationship superiority is a fairly stable phenomenon: Time-1 and Time-2 measures of perceived superiority were strongly correlated. Moreover, causal modeling analyses revealed that Time-1 commitment level fully mediated the effects of satisfaction level, alternative quality, and investment size on Time-2 perceived superiority. These findings suggest that perceived relationship superiority stands as a relationship maintenance mechanism. And once again, the willingness and ability to engage in this potentially effortful maintenance behavior is largely mediated by feelings of commitment to a relationship.

The Functional Value of Commitment and Relationship Maintenance Phenomena

Throughout this chapter, we have implied that commitment has adaptive value, and we have asserted that so-called relationship maintenance phenomena promote healthy functioning in ongoing relationships. In some sense, these assertions seem self-evidently true: It is difficult to argue with the claim that highly committed relationships are "good" relationships in other respects as well. And it seems implausible that healthy functioning is not promoted by "maintenance" phenomena such as tendencies to accommodate, derogation of alternatives, willingness to sacrifice, and perceived relationship superiority. Nevertheless, such assertions call out for empirical evidence.

The first question that arises in discussions of healthy functioning is What is "healthy" in the context of an ongoing relationship? We have employed two main criteria for "health" in our work. First, much of our work examines the link between predictor variables and actual decisions to remain in versus terminate a relationship. But as noted earlier, surely the mere persistence of a relationship should be regarded as a rather minimal requirement for relationship health. Accordingly, in many of our studies we have obtained a second measure of "relationship health," asking participants to complete the Dyadic Adjustment Scale (Spanier, 1976), a frequently employed measure of adjustment that taps aspects of healthy functioning such as quality and quantity of time spent together, the expression of affection and approval, degree of agreement regarding major life activities (e.g., religious matters, major life decisions), and the gratifications enjoyed from emotional and sexual intimacy.

Abundant evidence suggests that when individuals are more dependent on their relationships—that is, when they are more committed, more satisfied, more heavily invested, and perceive that their alternatives are poor—their relationships are more likely to persist over time (Buunk, 1987; Drigotas & Rusbult, 1992; Felmlee et al., 1990; Lund, 1985; Rusbult, 1983; Rusbult & Martz, 1993; Simpson, 1987; Van Lange et al., 1993). In addition, prior research has demonstrated a link between overall commitment level and scores on the Dyadic Adjustment Scale (Van Lange et al., 1993). Importantly, this relationship exists even when the Dyadic Adjustment Scale is purged of commitmentlike items such as "How often do you discuss or have you considered separation, or terminating your relationship?" Moreover, recent evidence demonstrates that even when we first account for the impact on Dyadic Adjustment of each partner's individual commitment level, the mutuality of their commitment further predicts couple adjustment (Rusbult, Verette, & Drigotas, 1993). That is, the hallmark of effective couple functioning is (1) a strong commitment that is (2) experienced equally by the partners.

Thus, it seems clear that strong commitment has good adaptive value for couples. But is it equally true that the maintenance phenomena just described "pay off" for couples as predicted? In the few longitudinal studies that have addressed such issues, it has been demonstrated that couples are more likely to persist to the extent that one or both partners exhibit high levels of sacrifice (Van Lange et al., 1993) and exhibit strong tendencies toward perceived relationship superiority (Rusbult et al., 1993). It has also been demonstrated that among relationships that persist, perceived quality of alternatives declines substantially over time (Johnson & Rusbult, 1989). However, whether this decline results from the active *derogation* of attractive alternatives or other causes (e.g., alternatives taking themselves out of the running) is not yet clear. Finally, couples that persist have been shown to exhibit greater levels of accommodation when their partners behave poorly— specifically, in relationships that endure, individuals exhibit particularly strong tendencies to react to negative partner behaviors with voice, and exhibit particularly weak tendencies to meet fire with fire by engaging in destructive exit behaviors (Verette, Drigotas, Rusbult, & Van Lange, 1993).

Some studies have also examined the link between relationship maintenance behaviors and Dyadic Adjustment scores. As previously noted, any scale items directly related to the maintenance behavior in question were deleted from the Dyadic Adjustment score in examining relationships with that behavior (e.g., conflict items were eliminated when performing analyses concerning accommodation). This work, too, suggests that relationship maintenance phenomena are associated with good functioning in relationships; both concurrent Dyadic Adjustment scores and Dyadic Adjustment scores obtained at later occasions are greater in relationships in which individuals exhibit greater tendencies toward accommodation (Drigotas, Whitney, & Rusbult, 1993; Verette et al., 1993) and in which individuals exhibit greater perceived relationship superiority (Rusbult et al., 1993). A positive relationship between Dyadic Adjustment and willingness to sacrifice has also been observed, but this positive association was significant only at one time interval (Van Lange et al., 1993).

Thus, in general, it appears that relationship health is promoted by both strong commitment and by greater tendencies toward the relationship maintenance mechanisms discussed herein. The important point here is that it is not enough to know that specific relationship maintenance behaviors are promoted by strong commitment. It is important to demonstrate that strong commitment to a relationship serves a positive function in that relationship; that is, feelings of commitment not only help keep a couple together, but also help keep a couple well adjusted.

Directions for Future Research

Although the research conducted thus far on commitment processes and relationship maintenance phenomena has served an important purpose in helping us understand how and why relationships sometimes persist and thrive, many questions remain to be answered. Although the answers to some of these questions are currently under investigation, others remain to be addressed in future research. One important direction for the future concerns the emphasis in most extant research on the perspective of one individual's feelings and behavior in his or her relationship. Most of the existing work on interdependence in relationships essentially examined one-half of an interdependent relationship—one partner's feelings of commitment, one partner's willingness to accommodate, and so on. Research employing this emphasis has obviously provided good support for predictions derived from interdependence theory. However, experiences in relationships frequently are a function of *both* partners' feelings and behaviors. Accordingly, in future work, it might be fruitful to take account of *both* partners' feelings of commitment, and *both* partners' inclinations to engage in relationship maintenance behaviors. For example, in recent research we have found that mutuality of commitment—the degree to which partners feel equally committed to their relationship—predicts Dyadic Adjustment above and beyond variance accounted for by each individual's absolute commitment level (Rusbult, Verette, & Drigotas, 1993).

In a related vein, it would be interesting to determine whether partner mutuality in levels of each maintenance mechanism (e.g., voice and loyalty; derogation of alternatives) can predict overall couple functioning better than individual levels of each mechanism. We expect that when costly or effortful maintenance behaviors are borne largely by one partner alone, overall relationship functioning is impaired. Indeed, prior research has provided some support for the assertion that greater mutuality in partners' willingness to accommodate is associated with greater couple functioning (Rusbult et al., 1991). Also, in current work, we are attempting to determine whether non-mutuality in levels of accommodation may produce negative consequences—in the form of reduced self-esteem, lowered general life satisfaction, or poor emotional and physical well-being—for the partner who is the "accommodation expert" (Rusbult, Verette, Drigotas, Agnew, Arriaga, & Cox, 1993).

Yet another related research topic currently under investigation concerns levels of correspondence in partners' perceptions of one another's commitment levels. This work is based on the reasoning that when partners are either unsure of—or inaccurately perceive—one another's commitment levels, they are likely to expend a fair amount of time and energy dealing with problems such as feelings of uncertainty and insecurity, guilt and the sense of unwanted responsibility, and so forth. When partners accurately perceive one another's commitment levels, time and energy is freed for partners to work toward improving their relationship, increasingly care for one another's needs, or simply have fun together. Recent research on correspondence in perceptions of partner commitment has demonstrated the power of this construct in predicting Dyadic Adjustment above and beyond both absolute commitment level and mutuality of commitment (Drigotas, 1993).

Another direction for future work involves broad questions concerning causality. The model of commitment and relationship maintenance presented in Figures 1 and 2 suggests that dependence-enhancing variables (satisfaction, alternatives, investments) influence feelings of commitment, which in turn promotes relationship maintenance. Over the course of an extended relationship, surely there are feedback loops whereby the maintenance behaviors influence variables that are represented in our model as distal causes. For example, it seems probable that when individuals are strongly inclined to derogate attractive and tempting alternatives, they may come to perceive available alternatives as being generally poorer in quality. Such a shift should yield stronger commitment, which once again should produce enhanced tendencies toward derogation of alternatives and so on and so on in an extended feedback loop. In the future, it would be exciting to conduct the experimental work and extended longitudinal investigations that might enable us to explore such bidirectional causation.

Finally, it would be illuminating to explore the precise means by which individuals come to engage in relationship maintenance behaviors. For example, what thoughts, attributional interpretations, or emotional reactions accompany the willingness to sacrifice for the well-being of a partner or relationship? In recent work, we have begun to explore how the thoughts and emotions experienced at the time of a dissatisfying incident influence tendencies to accommodate. Early work has demonstrated that more committed individuals experience more benevolent emotions and develop more benign explanations for their partners' potentially destructive acts, and accordingly exhibit greater willingness to accommodate (Verette, Rusbult, & Schmidt, 1993). Toward the broad goal of fully understanding the means by which relationships are maintained, it would be quite useful to perform similar micro-level analyses of the other maintenance behaviors discussed in this chapter. This would help to delineate precisely how feelings of commitment lead individuals to behave in ways that promote healthy functioning in their relationships.

Conclusions

This chapter employed interdependence theory constructs and propositions to the goal of understanding how and why some relationships persist and thrive whereas other promising relationships wither and die. Importantly, interdependence theory distinguishes between satisfaction with a relationship and dependence on a relationship. The investment model adopts this distinction, arguing that the state of dependence is subjectively represented as commitment to a relationship. Also, we have summarized evidence in support of the claim that stronger commitment is promoted by higher satisfaction level, greater investment size, and lower perceived quality of alternatives. The investment model is a robust theory of commitment processes that has proven to be effective in predicting feelings of commitment in a diverse range of interdependent relationships (e.g., in romantic involvements, friendships, and organizational settings). Furthermore, strong commitment appears to encourage a variety of behaviors that promote improved overall functioning in relationships, including the willingness to accommodate rather than retaliate when a partner has behaved badly, the tendency to sacrifice one's immediate self-interest for the good of a relationship, the inclination to derogate potentially threatening alternative partners, and the tendency to perceive one's relationship as superior to the relationships of other individuals. Collectively, this work demonstrates the utility of interdependence theory in providing a rich and relatively comprehensive understanding of behavior in ongoing relationships. The interdependence orientation thus contributes a key element to our understanding of close relationships, adding much to a literature that has focused primarily on phenomena such as attraction and satisfaction and suggesting that our knowledge of close relationships phenomena may be importantly extended through an analysis of both the nature and functions of interdependence in ongoing relationships.

Acknowledgments

Preparation of this chapter was supported in part by grants awarded to the first author—by Grant BSR-1-R01-MH-45417 from the National Institute of Mental Health, and by Grant BNS-9023817 from the National Science Foundation.

References

Atwater, L. (1982). *The extramarital connection*. New York: Irvington.

Axelrod, R. (1983). The emergence of cooperation among egoists. *American Political Science Review*, 75, 306–318.

Axelrod, R. (1984). *The evolution of cooperation*. New York: Basic Books.

Berscheid, E. (1985). Interpersonal attraction. In G. Lindzey & E. Aronson (Eds.), *Handbook of social psychology* (3rd ed., Vol. 2, pp. 413–484). New York: Random House.

Buunk, B. (1980a). Extramarital sex in the Netherlands: Motivations in social and marital context. *Alternative Lifestyles*, 3, 11–39.

Buunk, B. (1980b). Sexually open marriages: Ground rules for countering potential threats to marriage. *Alternative Lifestyles*, 3, 312–328.

Buunk, B. (1987). Conditions that promote breakups as a consequence of extradyadic involvements. *Journal of Social and Clinical Psychology*, 5, 271–284.

Buunk, B. P., Collins, R. L., Taylor, S. E., Van Yperen, N. W., & Dakof, G. A. (1990). The affective consequences of social comparison: Either direction has its ups and downs. *Journal of Personality and Social Psychology*, 59, 1238–1249.

Buunk, B. P., Engels, Ponjee, & Vaessen (1993). *Commitment processes among young Dutch adults*. Unpublished manuscript, University of Groningen, The Netherlands.

Buunk, B. P., & Van Yperen, N. W. (1989). Social comparison, equality, and relationship satisfaction: Gender differences over a ten-year period. *Social Justice Research*, 3, 157–180.

Buunk, B. P., & Van Yperen, N. W. (1991). Referential comparisons, relational comparisons, and exchange orientation: Their relation to marital satisfaction. *Personality and Social Psychology Bulletin*, 17, 709–717.

Buunk, B. P., Van Yperen, N. W., Taylor, S. E., & Collins, R. L. (1991). Social comparison and the drive upward revisited: Affiliation as a response to marital stress. *European Journal of Social Psychology*, 21, 529–546.

Clark, M. S., & Reis, H. T. (1988). Interpersonal processes in close relationships. *Annual Review of Psychology*, 39, 609–672.

Drigotas, S. M. (1993). *Perceptions of commitment and relationship stability*. Dissertation research in progress, University of North Carolina at Chapel Hill.

Drigotas, S. M., & Rusbult, C. E. (1992). Should I stay or should I go?: A dependence model of breakups. *Journal of Personality and Social Psychology*, 62, 62–87.

Drigotas, S. M., Whitney, G. A., & Rusbult, C. E. (1992). *On the peculiarities of loyalty: A diary study of responses to dissatisfaction in everyday life.* Unpublished manuscript, University of North Carolina at Chapel Hill.

Duffy, S., & Rusbult, C. E. (1986). Satisfaction and commitment in homosexual and heterosexual relationships. *Journal of Homosexuality, 12,* 1–23.

Farrell, D., & Rusbult, C. E. (1981). Exchange variables as predictors of job satisfaction, job commitment, and turnover: The impact of rewards, costs, alternatives, and investments. *Organizational Behavior and Human Performance, 27,* 78–95.

Felmlee, D., Sprecher, S., & Bassin, E. (1990). The dissolution of intimate relationships: A hazard model. *Social Psychology Quarterly, 53,* 13–30.

Festinger, L. (1954). A theory of social comparison processes. *Human Relations, 7,* 117–140.

Gottman, J. M., Notarius, C., Markman, H., Bank, S., Yoppi, B., & Rubin, M. E. (1976). Behavior exchange theory and marital decision making. *Journal of Personality and Social Psychology, 34,* 14–23.

Holmes, J. G. (1981). The exchange process in close relationships: Microbehavior and macromotives. In M. J. Lerner and S. C. Lerner (Eds.), *The justice motive in social behavior* (pp. 261–284). New York: Plenum.

Jacobson, N. S., Follette, W. C., & McDonald, D. W. (1982). Reactivity to positive and negative behavior in distressed and nondistressed married couples. *Journal of Consulting and Clinical Psychology, 50,* 706–714.

Johnson, D. J., & Rusbult, C. E. (1989). Resisting temptation: Devaluation of alternative partners as a means of maintaining commitment in close relationships. *Journal of Personality and Social Psychology, 57,* 967–980.

Johnson, M. P. (1982). Social and cognitive features of the dissolution of commitment to relationships. In S. Duck (Ed.), *Personal relationships 4: Dissolving personal relationships* (pp. 51–73). New York: Academic Press.

Johnson, M. P. (1991). Commitment to personal relationships. In W. H. Jones & D. W. Perlman (Eds.), *Advances in personal relationships* (Vol. 3, pp. 117–143). London: Jessica Kingsley.

Kelley, H. H. (1979). *Personal relationships: Their structures and processes.* Hillsdale, NJ: Lawrence Erlbaum.

Kelley, H. H. (1983). Love and commitment. In H. H. Kelley, E. Berscheid, A. Christensen, J. H. Harvey, T. L. Huston, G. Levinger, E. McClintock, L. A. Peplau, & D. R. Peterson (Eds.), *Close relationships* (pp. 265–314). New York: W. H. Freeman.

Kelley, H. H., & Thibaut, J. W. (1978). *Interpersonal relations: A theory of interdependence.* New York: Wiley.

Levinger, G. (1979a). A social exchange view on the dissolution of pair relationships. In R. L. Burgess & T. L. Huston (Eds.), *Social exchange in developing relationships* (pp. 169–193). New York: Academic Press.

Levinger, G. (1979b). A social psychological perspective on marital dissolution. In G. Levinger & O. C. Moles (Eds.), *Divorce and separation: Context, causes, and consequences* (pp. 37–60). New York: Basic Books.

Lin, Y. H. W., & Rusbult, C. E. (1993). *Commitment to dating relationships and cross-sex friendships in America and China: The impact of centrality of relationship, normative support, and investment model variables.* Unpublished manuscript, University of North Carolina at Chapel Hill.

Lund, M. (1985). The development of investment and commitment scales for predicting continuity of personal relationships. *Journal of Social and Personal Relationships, 2,* 3–23.

Margolin, G., & Wampold, B. E. (1981). Sequential analysis of conflict and accord in distressed and nondistressed marital partners. *Journal of Counseling and Clinical Psychology, 49,* 554–567.

Martz, J. M., Verette, J., Arriaga, X. B., Slovik, L. F., Cox, C. L., & Rusbult, C. E. (1993). *Positive illusion in close relationships*. Unpublished manuscript, University of North Carolina at Chapel Hill.

Mellen, S. L. W. (1981). *The evolution of love*. Oxford, England: Freeman.

Rosenblatt, P. C. (1977). Needed research on commitment in marriage. In G. Levinger & H. L. Raush (Eds.), *Close relationships: Perspectives on the meaning of intimacy* (pp. 73–86). Amherst, MA: University of Massachusetts.

Rusbult, C. E. (1980a). Commitment and satisfaction in romantic associations: A test of the investment model. *Journal of Experimental Social Psychology, 16*, 172–186.

Rusbult, C. E. (1980b). Satisfaction and commitment in friendships. *Representative Research in Social Psychology, 11*, 96–105.

Rusbult, C. E. (1983). A longitudinal test of the investment model: The development (and deterioration) of satisfaction and commitment in heterosexual involvements. *Journal of Personality and Social Psychology, 45*, 101–117.

Rusbult, C. E., & Farrell, D. (1983). A longitudinal test of the investment model: The impact on job satisfaction, job commitment, and turnover of variations in rewards, costs, alternatives, and investments. *Journal of Applied Psychology, 68*, 429–438.

Rusbult, C. E., Johnson, D. J., & Morrow, G. D. (1986a). Impact of couple patterns of problem solving on distress and nondistress in dating relationships. *Journal of Personality and Social Psychology, 50*, 744–753.

Rusbult, C. E., Johnson, D. J., & Morrow, G. D. (1986b). Predicting satisfaction and commitment in adult romantic involvements: An assessment of the generalizability of the investment model. *Social Psychology Quarterly, 49*, 81–89.

Rusbult, C. E., & Martz, J. (1993). *Remaining in an abusive relationship: An analysis of nonvoluntary commitment*. Unpublished manuscript, University of North Carolina at Chapel Hill.

Rusbult, C. E., Van Lange, P. A. M., Verette, J., & Yovetich, N. A. (1993). *Perceived superiority and well-being in close relationships*. Unpublished manuscript, University of North Carolina at Chapel Hill.

Rusbult, C. E., & Verette, J. (1991). An interdependence analysis of accommodation processes in close relationships. *Representative Research in Social Psychology, 19*, 3–33.

Rusbult, C. E., Verette, J., & Drigotas, S. M. (1993). *Absolute commitment level, mutuality of commitment, and adjustment in marital relationships*. Manuscript in preparation, University of North Carolina at Chapel Hill.

Rusbult, C. E., Verette, J., Drigotas, S. M., Agnew, C. R., Arriaga, X. B., & Cox, C. L. (1993). *A longitudinal study of accommodation processes in marriage*. Research in progress, University of North Carolina at Chapel Hill.

Rusbult, C. E., Verette, J., Whitney, G. A., Slovik, L. F., & Lipkus, I. (1991). Accommodation processes in close relationships: Theory and preliminary empirical evidence. *Journal of Personality and Social Psychology, 60*, 53–78.

Rusbult, C. E., & Zembrodt, I. M. (1983). Responses to dissatisfaction in romantic involvements: A multidimensional scaling analysis. *Journal of Experimental Social Psychology, 19*, 274–293.

Sabatelli, R. M. (1984). The marital comparison level index: A measure for assessing outcomes relative to expectations. *Journal of Marriage and the Family, 46*, 651–662.

Sabatelli, R. M., & Cecil-Pigo, E. F. (1985). Relational interdependence and commitment in marriage. *Journal of Marriage and the Family, 47*, 931–937.

Simpson, J. A. (1987). The dissolution of romantic relationships: Factors involved in relationship stability and emotional distress. *Journal of Personality and Social Psychology, 53*, 683–692.

Simpson, J. A., Gangestad, S. W., & Lerma, M. (1990). Perception of physical attractiveness: Mechanisms involved in the maintenance of romantic relationships. *Journal of Personality and Social Psychology, 59*, 1192–1201.

Spanier, G. B. (1976). Measuring dyadic adjustment: New scales for assessing the quality of marriage and similar dyads. *Journal of Marriage and the Family, 38*, 15–28.

Stafford, L., & Reske, J. (1990). Idealization and communication in long-distance premarital relationships. *Family Relations, 39*, 274–279.

Strube, M. J. (1988). The decision to leave an abusive relationship: Empirical evidence and theoretical issues. *Psychological Bulletin, 104*, 236–250.

Taylor, S. E., & Brown, J. D. (1988). Illusion and well-being: A social psychological perspective on mental health. *Psychological Bulletin, 103*, 193–210.

Thibaut, J. W., & Kelley, H. H. (1959). *The social psychology of groups.* New York: Wiley.

Titus, S. L. (1980). A function of friendship: Social comparisons as a frame of reference for marriage. *Human Relations, 33*, 409–431.

Van Lange, P. A. M., & Rusbult, C. E. (in press). My relationship is better than—and not as bad as—yours is: The perception of superiority in close relationships. *Personality and Social Psychology Bulletin.*

Van Lange, P. A. M., Rusbult, C. E., & Drigotas, S. M. (in press). Willingness to sacrifice in close relationships. *personality and Social Psychology Bulletin.*

Verette, J. (1989). *Reactions to threatening alternatives: Bolstering the current partner as a function of degree of commitment to one's current relationship.* Unpublished master's thesis, University of North Carolina at Chapel Hill.

Verette, J. (1992). *Understanding partner intentions in conflict situations: A test of the inference model.* Unpublished doctoral dissertation, University of North Carolina at Chapel Hill.

Verette, J., Drigotas, S. M., Rusbult, C. E., & Van Lange, P. A. M. (1993). *The consequences of accommodation for couple functioning and relationship stability: A two-wave panel study.* Unpublished manuscript, University of North Carolina at Chapel Hill.

Verette, J., Rusbult, C. E., & Schmidt, G. W. (1993). *Emotions and attributional interpretations as proximal mediators of willingness to accommodate in close relationship.* Unpublished manuscript, University of North Carolina at Chapel Hill.

Yovetich, N. A., & Rusbult, C. E. (in press). Accommodation behavior in close relationships: Exploring transformation of motivation. *Journal of Experimental Social Psychology.*

7

Barriers to Dissolution of Romantic Relationships

Mark Attridge
Department of Psychology
University of Minnesota
Minneapolis, Minnesota

Introduction

Based on *United States Current Population Reports* data from 1985, demographers Martin and Bumpass (1989) estimate that approximately two-thirds of all first marriages are likely to fail. Yet, in spite of such pessimistic predictions, the vast majority of people do get married (U.S. Bureau of the Census, 1990). Further, of those who divorce most remarry within a few years (Spanier & Thompson, 1984). The paradoxical frequency of both marriage and divorce has generated considerable interest among the lay public and from researchers in varied disciplines in trying to figure out how to maintain marital relationships and, if need be, how to repair those risking dissolution.

This chapter explores how the social–psychological concept of barriers to ending a relationship can add to our understanding of relationship maintenance and repair. The principal conceptual model to address this topic has considered barriers, or restraining forces, to "affect one's behavior only if one wishes to leave the relationship" (Levinger, 1976, pp. 24–25). However, a review of other conceptual models (Lund, 1985; Johnson, 1982; Rusbult, 1983) suggests that various kinds of barriers may influence the behavior of romantic partners when they are happy with the relationship as well as when they are dissatisfied. This expanded view of barrier influence allows for investigation of how different kinds of barriers are linked to relationship maintenance and repair strategies. It is the primary thesis of this chapter that acknowledgment of these barriers provides insights into the manner in which romantic relationships are maintained. Specifically, I hold that romantic relationships are sustained and restored to the extent partners desire and create barriers to dissolution.

This chapter is organized into four sections. Presented first is a discussion of the conceptual framework. Four models illustrate the centrality of barriers. This is followed by a survey of the research literature examining the hypothesized deterrent effect of different kinds of barriers on relationship stability. This reveals that the presence and strength of internal psychological and external structural barriers are correlated with greater relationship satisfaction and commitment and are predictive of greater relationship stability in longitudinal tests of premarital and marital relationships. A third section notes recent changes that have occurred in society resulting in the weakening of barrier forces for many couples. The final section discusses the creation and strengthening of barriers as a strategy for relationship maintenance. Comments to direct further research are also offered.

Conceptual Framework

Several conceptual models include barrier forces as factors important to the stability of romantic relationships. The earliest and most influential model, the marital cohesiveness model proposed by Levinger (1965, 1976) is reviewed first. This is followed by the commitment model (Johnson, 1982), the investment model (Rusbult, 1983), and the barrier model (Lund, 1985). Common themes and differences between the models are then briefly discussed.

Levinger's Model of Marital Cohesiveness

Integrating the ideas of field theory (Lewin, 1951) and group psychology (Festinger, Schachter, & Black, 1950), Levinger (1965, 1976) developed a model for understanding marital cohesiveness and divorce that considers marriage as a special instance of social groups in general. According to this model, the strength of a marital relationship is "a direct function of the attractions within and barriers around the marriage, and an inverse function of such attractions and barriers from other [alternative] relationships" (Levinger, 1965, p. 19).

Attractions, broadly defined to correspond to Lewin's (1951) concept of "driving forces," include: (1) the positive attributes of the partner, (2) the pleasures gained from interacting with the partner, (3) the ability of the partner to improve one's social status, or (4) other extrinsic goals. One can experience negative attractions (or repulsions) toward the partner as well. A relationship partner can feel attractions toward his or her primary partner as well as toward *alternative* partners. (Note that ending the current relationship and then having no relationship at all is also an alternative.) Levinger (1965) has proposed that *barriers* against relationship dissolution, corresponding to Lewin's (1951) concept of "restraining forces," come from such sources as "the emotional, religious, and moral commitments that a partner feels toward his marriage or toward his children; the external pressures of kin and community, of the law, the church, and other associational memberships" (p. 20). Levinger also notes obligations to maintain associations with people other than the spouse, such as one's parents, children, friends, employers, other lovers, and so on. Whether maintaining these outside relationships is compatible with maintaining the primary relationship is a critical issue. When commitment to alternative relationships excludes the spouse, these third-party relationships may threaten the cohesiveness of the marriage.

It is important to consider the conditions under which barriers are conceptualized to influence the cohesiveness of the marital relationship. According to Levinger (1965), "the strength of barriers matters little if the partners' attraction is high enough" (p. 20). It is when a partner's attraction to the relationship is low that the barriers to leaving the relationship become important. At such a time, the costs associated with overcoming the barriers must then be considered and weighed against the desire to end the relationship. If in addition to being dissatisfied with the relationship, one also has strong alternative attractions, then the barriers to breakup become even more important because the potential outcomes offered by the alternative cannot be fully realized without ending the current relationship.

Johnson's Model of Commitment to the Relationship

In stating that "people stay in relationships for two major reasons: because they want to; and because they have to," Johnson (1982, pp. 52–53) addresses factors of relationship stability similar to those in Levinger's model. Johnson, however, places more emphasis on the operation of constraint in relationship dissolution than on attractions to the relationship. In this model, romantic relationship stability is hypothesized to be primarily a function of two factors: personal commitment and structural commitment. *Personal commitment* stems from the following three components: (1) the satisfaction one gets from participating in the relationship, (2) the extent to which one's definition of self includes aspects associated with being in the relationship, and (3) an internalized sense of moral commitment to the maintenance of the relationship. Once a relationship partner experiences a significant decline in these aspects of personal commitment to the relationship, then "the process of relationship dissolution becomes salient and the social and cognitive consequences of the structural commitments must be faced" (Johnson, 1982, p. 54). *Structural commitments* are the conditions which make it difficult to leave the relationship, regardless of one's personal commitment to it. Four types of structural commitments are deemed important: (1) irretrievable investments (time, energy, other relationships, career choices, forgone alternatives, etc.), (2) social pressures to maintain the relationship, (3) the quality of available alternatives, and (4) the costs of specific relationship termination procedures (social, economic, legal, practical, etc.). The self-identity component of personal commitment to the relationship is perhaps the most distinguishing feature of this model.

Rusbult's Investment Model

Using interdependence theory (Kelley & Thibaut, 1978) as a starting point and building on Levinger's (1979) later work, Rusbult (1980, 1983) has developed and empirically tested the investment model to account for the satisfaction and stability of interpersonal relationships (see also Rusbult, Drigotas, & Verette, this volume). This model addresses the same main factors as those in Levinger's cohesiveness model but emphasizes the mediating role of psychological commitment to the relationship. According to the investment model, relationship stability is determined by the level of commitment to the relationship and commitment is hypothesized to be a function of three interrelated factors: (1) the level of *satisfaction* with the relationship (e.g., the radio of rewards to costs), (2) the quality of its *alternatives*, and (3) the size of *investments* in the relationship. Rusbult (1983, p. 103) states that "investments increase commitment and help to 'lock the individual into his or her relationship' by increasing the costs of ending it—to a greater or lesser degree, to abandon a relationship is to sacrifice invested resources." Rusbult makes a distinction between intrinsic and extrinsic kinds of investments. Intrinsic investments include the resources that are put directly into the relationship, such as time, emotional effort, and self-disclosure. Extrinsic investments include extraneous resources that have become connected to the relationship as it has developed over time, such as mutual friends, shared memories, shared material possessions, and the activities/persons/objects/events that are uniquely associated with the relationship. Note that in Levinger's (1976) model, restraining forces are largely a function of the costs that come from actions to end the relationship (e.g., social stigma, legal fees, change in living arrangement, parental or moral guilt, etc.), whereas in the Rusbult model, it is more the *potential* of losing what one already has that builds commitment to the relationship. This difference makes it possible to explore how "investments" influence relationship partners at points other than just when facing dissolution.

Lund's Barrier Model

Lund's (1985) "barrier model," which is grounded in process models of relationship development and research on attitude change, was developed to predict relationship stability. According to this model, barriers to ending a relationship develop from the interaction over time of increasing behavioral investments and increasing commitment to making the relationship last. Even though no specific rationale is provided (other than referring to Levinger's work) for the particular behaviors included as items on her "investment scale," almost all of the behaviors are ones that have been included in the preceding conceptual models. The distinction made in the other models between commitment and alternatives, is not made in Lund's work. What is most interesting about Lund's (1985) barrier model is the timing of when barriers are relevant to relationship partners. Lund proposes that both barriers and commitment increase over time and increases in one lead to increases in the other. This same prediction is made in Rusbult's investment model. Lund's second hypothesis is that barrier forces are more strongly linked to relationship commitment than are the rewards received from the relationship. Lund hypothesized and found that the level of commitment and the strength of barriers are better predictors of romantic relationship stability than are love and rewards in the relationship.

Integration of Conceptual Models

Although each of these four models has its distinctive aspects, there are more similarities than differences between them. In one manner or another, all models include attractions to the relationship, attractions to alternatives, and restraints on leaving the relationship as factors that influence relationship stability. There is also some consistency across the models in the specific factors considered to represent barriers to dissolution. These factors can be subsumed into two broad classes: internal psychological barriers and external structural barriers. *Internal psychological barriers* include personal commitment to maintaining the relationship, obligation to the marital bond, religious or moral beliefs about the importance of commitment, considering the relationship an important part of one's self-identity, irretrievable personal investments, and parental obligations. *External structural barriers* include legal costs, financial considerations (e.g., sharing a residence, possessions, assets, debts), financial dependence on partner, and social network pressures.

The division of barriers into an internal/external classification is found to varying degrees in the conceptual models of Levinger (1979), Rusbult (1983), and Johnson (1982). A similar distinction is made by Kelley (1983) in his assessment of the types of commitments to relationships. This distinction is also supported in factor analytic research. In two samples of married couples and using items representing most of the previously mentioned barriers except for self-identity and irretrievable investments, Bagarozzi and Pollane (1983) found that these kinds of barriers loaded onto two orthogonal factors. One factor, called Willingness to Separate/Divorce and Internal Psychological Barriers, included the unwillingness to separate or divorce, obligation to marriage vows, religious beliefs, and obligations to children. The other factor, called External Circumstantial Barriers, included financial considerations, job concerns, legal costs of separating, and pressures from friends, neighbors, and relatives.

A point about the timing of when barriers influence relationship partners must be made. The idea that barriers (particularly external ones) are only relevant to partners when they are dissatisfied and exploring their alternatives (Levinger, 1965, 1976) is based on the conceptualization of barriers as representing "costs" that inhibit dissolution. Although this view has merit, it may be too limiting. For example, when satisfaction with the relationship is high, certain barrier factors may be viewed not so much as "potential costs" but more as sources of attraction to the relationship. It is later on when the relationship begins to sour that these same factors are likely to be reinterpreted as forces that restrain partners from leaving. For example, getting legally married could be an attraction early on, but later makes it difficult to break up. Indeed, Levinger (1976, p. 44) has acknowledged a problem in the lack of distinctiveness among the three components of attraction, barriers, and alternative attraction in his model of marital cohesiveness and states that it is possible to "interpret the same empirical variable (e.g., home ownership or religious precept) as a source of both attraction and of barrier forces." Similarly, Rusbult (1983) notes the possibility that different investments can be interpreted as being either rewarding or costly depending on the particular relationship.

Further, there is empirical evidence that barriers are associated with greater attractions and fewer alternatives and that barriers increase with relationship development. For example, stronger barriers correlate positively with greater love for one's partner in samples of dating relationships (Lund, 1985) and in heterosexual cohabiting and married couples (Kurdek & Schmitt, 1986). Greater investments also correlate positively with greater commitment to the relationship in dating partners (Rusbult, 1980, 1983; Lund,

1985), in cohabitating heterosexual couples (Kurdek & Schmitt, 1986), and in marital relationships (Kurdek & Schmitt, 1986; Sabatelli & Cecil-Pigo, 1985). A comparison of individuals in romantic relationships at different stages of development (Lund, 1985) reveals a linear association between barriers and level of relationship development, such that barriers become increasingly stronger with escalating involvement. Thus, it appears that relationship partners' attempts to increase their barriers coincides with their satisfaction and commitment to the relationship.

The four models reviewed strongly suggest that barriers act as powerful forces in the preservation of romantic relationships. Moreover, the internal/external distinction indicates that barriers involve elements central to the individual's self-concept as well as social structural factors. Moreover, the strength of barrier forces (along with attractions to the relationship and alternatives) should represent a significant influence on relationship stability. If barriers do keep romantic partners together, then it would make sense for men and women in romantic relationships to try to strengthen existing barriers and/or create additional barriers as a strategy for relationship maintenance or repair. But before advocating such a view, it is necessary to first determine the validity of barriers in terms of their effect on relationship stability.

Research on Barriers as Deterrents to Dissolution

The 1965 and 1976 reviews of the empirical literature by Levinger are perhaps the best sources of past work documenting that marital stability is often enhanced under conditions of high attraction to the relationship, poor alternatives, and strong barriers. More recent comprehensive reviews of the research literature on premarital (Surra, 1990) and marital relationships (Kitson, Babri, & Roach, 1985; White, 1990) continue to find general support for these factors. This analysis has focused on barriers, what follows is a selective but representative survey of studies that have examined the deterrent effects of internal and external barriers.

Internal Psychological Barriers

Commitment and Obligations to the Marital Bond

Obligation to marriage can take several forms. Believing that divorce is morally wrong is associated with greater marital commitment (Sabatelli & Cecil-Pigo, 1985) and with staying married (Booth, Johnson, White, & Edwards, 1985). Obligation, expressed behaviorally as length of courtship prior to marriage and the number of years together once married, is associated with lower rates of divorce (Kitson et al., 1985; Levinger, 1965, 1976; White, 1990). Past experiences with failure to uphold marital vows (i.e., prior own divorce or parental divorce) may also predict marital instability. Professing commitment to continuing the relationship is associated with greater stability over time for premarital relationships (Lund, 1985; Rusbult, 1983; Surra, 1990).

Religious Beliefs

Because many organized religions encourage marital union and do not support divorce, the greater one's commitment is to religion, the greater should be one's commitment to marriage. Several studies provide support for this association (Booth et al., 1985; Kitson et al., 1985; Levinger, 1965, 1976; White, 1990). For example, Glenn and Supancic (1984) examined cross-sectional data from seven U.S. national surveys conducted in the 1970s and 1980s (representing over 8,800 married men and women), and found a significant negative association between religiosity and rate of marital dissolution. White men and women who said they "never" attended church had a divorce rate two to three times higher than those who attended church "every week or more." In addition, compared to those belonging to a particular religious denomination, those who said they had "no religion" had the highest divorce rate. Similar results have been found in a study of cohort data from nearly 4,000 Canadian women (Balakrishnan, Rao, Lapierre-Adamcyk, & Krotki, 1987).

Self-Identity

Duck (1984, p. 178) has argued that the "repair of relationships must take into consideration the complexity of the individual's life context, including an understanding of issues of self-definition. This is important because partners are usually attached not only to one another but also to their roles as partners." Empirical support for the integration of marital roles into the self-concept of spouses comes from a study of a large sample of Iowa residents (Mulford & Salisbury, 1964) in which 29% of men and 41% of women referred in some way to their roles as husbands and wives when asked to provide responses to the Twenty Statements Test (i.e., answering the question "Who am I?").

Aron and his colleagues (Aron & Aron, 1986; Aron, Aron, Tudorr, & Nelson, 1991) have recently articulated a conceptual model of "including the other in the self" that describes the ways in which relationship partners come to view themselves as being defined through their associations with each other. According to this perspective, the more the relationship partner is incorporated into the self-identity, the more difficult it is to end the relationship because of the psychological costs that would result from having to restructure the self-identity to remove those aspects associated with the partner. Preliminary support for this idea has been obtained in a study of dating relationships (Aron, Aron, & Smollan, 1992).

The model of social identity proposed by Sarbin and Scheibe (1983) asserts that a person's self-identity is formed through inferential processes that integrate the various social roles enacted by the person and by interaction with others in the social world. According to this model, self-identity is shaped most by social roles that have high status (granted and/or attained) and high involvement, and are positively valued. Business executives, doctors, or other professionals are examples of high status roles. High involvement roles include those that demand a lot of energy and personal initiative, such as a research scientist, writer, or artist. Positively valued roles can take many forms depending on the social climate, but often such roles require the person to contribute toward the betterment of self and/or others—teachers, public servants, or members of the clergy are some examples. Sarbin and Scheibe (1983) suggest that positive changes in identity occur through processes of "upgrading" that include commendation and promotion, whereas negative changes in identity occur through processes of "degradation" that include derogation and demotion. This model has implications for barriers to relationship termination. If being a spouse or romantic partner is perceived by the individual as being a high status role that is very involving and positively valued, then to end the relationship would result in a possible degradation of identity and loss of that important role (at least until another partner could be found).

Other theorists (Higgins, 1987; Markus & Nurius, 1986) consider self-identity to be a constellation of several dimensions, including positive and negative selves, as well as possible or future selves. These different aspects of the self are thought to be motivating factors that shape behavior toward the prospect of forming a particular desired self sometime in the future and also toward avoiding the "undesired self." This view has implications for understanding how self-identity can represent either a barrier to breakup *or* a catalyst for relationship termination, depending on the individual. First, if ending the current relationship would result in losing valued aspects of one's positive self, then those aspects of the self that are influenced by being in the relationship constitute a barrier to ending the relationship. It is also possible, though, that if by leaving one's partner one could then begin a process of redefining one's self-identity to include the realization of a desired future self and/or the purging of negative aspects of the undesired self, then self-identity could be a motivating factor for ending the relationship.

Reis and Shaver's (1988) model of intimacy processes emphasizes each partners' responsiveness to the other in regard to feeling understood, validated, and cared for. Thus, this model invokes the importance of the self in proposing that intimacy is partly dependent on one's self-identity being validated by the relationship partner. Along similar lines, Knudson (1985) considers marital compatibility to derive from spouses' attempts to develop a shared consensually valid definition of each other, of the relationship between them, and of the place of their relationship in the broader network of relationships in which they live.

Irretrievable Personal Investments
Several studies have found that spending time together with one's relationship partner and engaging in a wide range of activities with the partner predict the stability of dating relationships (Attridge, Berscheid, Simpson, & Creed, 1992; Berscheid, Snyder, & Omoto, 1989; Simpson, 1987). Experiencing frequent positive emotions in the relationship and self-disclosure to one's partner have also been predictive of romantic relationships that continue over time (Attridge et al., 1992).

Children
Morgan and Rindfuss (1985) suggest that "a marital birth serves to inhibit marital disruption by imposing strong legal, financial, and emotional barriers against disruption" (p. 1070). Indeed, longitudinal panel studies and cross-sectional studies of national census data consistently indicate that having a child seems to function as a barrier to marital disruption (Glick & Norton, 1978; Kitson et al., 1985; White, 1990). One longitudinal analysis of a national probability sample of nearly 1,800 women over a 15-year period (from 1968 to 1983), found that women with "no children in the household were more than six times as likely to experience a marital disruption as women with two children, who in turn were about twice as likely as women with three or more children" (Greenstein, 1990, p. 673). In another study that involved over 11,000 Californian families, the deterrent effect of the presence of children on divorce was found even when controlling for spouses' education, age at marriage, previous divorce, race, length of stay in California, and spouse filing for divorce (Rankin & Maneker, 1985).

External Structural Barriers

Legal Barriers
Presumably, the legal status of being married serves as a barrier to relationship dissolution. In almost all cases, the costs (financial, procedural, emotional, etc.) associated with obtaining a divorce are greater than those associated with ending a nonmarital relationship (Blumberg, 1985). The shift to no-

fault divorce laws that occurred in the 1980s has not produced the expected jump in divorce rates in the United States, but seems to have produced a temporary increase in Canadian divorces (Balakrishnan et al., 1987). To avoid the barriers of legal matrimony, romantic partners can opt instead to live together out of wedlock. But couples who cohabitate tend to break up more often than do those who marry (Kitson et al., 1985; Thornton, 1988; White, 1990). The causal link between cohabitation and relational instability is difficult to determine given that the kinds of people who choose to cohabitate may differ from those who choose to marry in ways that make the former more prone to relationship breakup.

Financial Barriers

In addition to legal fees accompanying separation or divorce, the longer two people are together, the greater the likelihood they will accrue mutually owned assets (and debts) that would be difficult to divide in the event of separation or divorce. In a longitudinal study of a representative national sample of married men and women, Booth et al. (1985) found that jointly owning a home and having valuable joint family assets predicted those who stayed married versus those whose relationships ended over a 3-year period. In many cases, there are the additional, and continuing, financial costs of alimony and child support.

Lack of economic self-sufficiency is also likely to be a barrier to breakup. If a partner wants to leave his or her spouse but lacks the financial resources to do so, then that partner is economically dependent on the other partner; this economic insolvency constitutes a barrier to ending a relationship. Given that in the majority of married couples the female earns less than the male (U.S. Bureau of the Census, 1990), lack of independent income represents a stronger barrier to divorce for females than for males. Women at high risk for divorce are also more likely to be in the labor force, to have higher wages, and to work more hours than women in low-divorce risk groups (Green & Quester, 1982; Voydanoff, 1990). Further, Greenstein's (1990) analysis spanning 15 years and representing nearly 1,800 American women, found that wives who earned less than 25% of their total family income during the course of their marriage were the least likely to experience a marital disruption, whereas wives who earned more than 75% of their total family income were the most likely to divorce.

Social Barriers

Often the friends and family of one or both partners exert some form of influence on the relationship partners through their participation as members of the couples' shared social network. Members of the social network may be motivated to assist in keeping the couple together so that they themselves avoid social disruption. "If the couple is at the center of its own support structure, then a crack in the relationship threatens a fracture of the network" (Cobb & Jones-Cobb, 1984, p. 62). When Johnson (1982) asked over 400 college students to construct a list of people whose opinions of their personal life were important to them and then to report how each of the persons on that list would feel if the respondent's current dating relationship were to end, network disapproval of a breakup was clearly associated with level of romantic involvement. The percentage of people in the network disapproving of the breakup was 19% for occasionally dating relationships, 50% for regular dating relationships, 63% for exclusive dating relationships, and 86% for engaged relationships.

In addition to pressures to stay together, friends, family and in-laws may contribute monetary or material resources (e.g., loans, a place to live, furniture, etc.) to the couple as well as offering acceptance, social status, and the opportunity for inclusion in social activities. A breakup could entail the loss of these kinds of tangible and interpersonal benefits provided by the shared social network of the couple. In a study of recently divorced men and women who gave retrospective accounts of their past and present social networks, Rands (1988) found that the turnover of people in these networks had changed dramatically after divorce. For example, approximately 2 years after marital separation only 51% of the initial network associates remained, with the person's own relatives and own first acquaintances (rather than the spouse's) being the most stable members of the social network. In general, the social network of divorced men and women became smaller, less dense, and more segmented following marital separation.

Declining Barriers in a Changing Society

In an address given to researchers interested in the study of relationships, Levinger (1990) called for more investigation of the interplay of the micro-level events that occur within relationships and the macro-level societal conditions in which relationships are embedded. Because barriers to dissolution have been conceptualized to have both internal and external sources, they are particularly appropriate for such investigation.

Recent analysis of historical trends in sociological, psychological, and census data suggests that compared to past generations, large numbers of men and women in romantic relationships in contemporary society are less likely to experience multiple and strong barriers to relationship termination (Attridge & Berscheid, in press; Berscheid & Campbell, 1981; Levinger, 1979,

1990). Advances made in earnings and education have contributed to a large scale reduction of economic dependency barriers for many women, especially younger women. With greater numbers of couples cohabitating out of wedlock and the adoption of no-fault divorce laws across the land, legal barriers to relationship termination have also diminished. Barriers associated with children are also less prevalent today than in the past, due to decreasing family size, increasing childlessness in couples, and the growing prominence of single parenting and remarriage. As greater numbers of people are without a religious preference and the impact of religion on individuals has declined, so have barriers to breakup associated with religion. Many forms of social and attitudinal barriers also have declined in recent years as people are becoming more accepting of divorce in society.

Moreover, there has been a parallel increase over the same period in the availability and attractiveness of alternative relationship partners and of alternative lifestyles (Attridge & Berscheid, in press; Berscheid & Campbell, 1981; Levinger, 1979, 1990). For example, with more women in higher education and the workforce there is now more contact between men and women for extended periods of time when they are not with their romantic partners. Not only has the opportunity to interact with potential alternative partners increased, but the outcomes that these alternative partners can offer has increased because gains in education and employment experience generally lead to greater earning power (although women still lag behind men in average income). In addition, sexual relations between relationship partners prior to marriage is now expected and considered normative for many people (especially young adults).

Use of Barriers for Relationship Maintenance

The empirical evidence reviewed in the previous sections suggests that romantic relationship stability is often influenced by different internal and external factors that have been conceptualized as barriers to ending a relationship, but the influence of barriers has historically weakened in a changing society that also offers increasingly available and tempting alternatives. What implications does this have for understanding relationship maintenance? One implication is that there exists both reason to, and need for, romantic partners to adopt relationship maintenance strategies that include attempts to strengthen the barriers available to them.

Presented first in this section is a description of ways to create and strengthen different kinds of barriers. Also discussed is how the presence of strong or weak barriers can influence the kinds of responses people have when they become dissatisfied with their relationship. This section ends with a discussion of motivational and environmental factors that limit the use of barrier-based relationship maintenance strategies.

Creating New Barriers
and Making Existing Barriers Stronger

Even though there are conceptual and empirical reasons to suggest that creating and/or strengthening barriers is an effective strategy for relationship maintenance, if people themselves do not believe that barriers help to keep a relationship together, then it is unlikely such a strategy will be adopted. Attridge and Witt (1993) conducted an exploratory investigation of this issue. The study addressed three basic questions: (1) Do people believe that barrier forces help to maintain their relationships?; (2) Do people want barriers to be a part of their relationships?; and (3) Do people communicate about barriers with their relationship partners?

Attridge and Witt (1993) found that most people in their sample believed that barriers would help to some degree to maintain the relationship. As a group, the internal barriers were judged as helping to maintain the relationship to a greater degree than were the external barriers. The barriers with the highest ratings were personal commitment, investments (time, energy, affection), and the support of friends, family, and other people; the barriers of joint financial assets, joint debt, and financial dependence on partner had the lowest ratings. Doing rewarding and positive things with one's relationship partner was rated as the best way to maintain the relationship. To a lesser degree, avoiding doing costly or negative behaviors, avoiding significant contact with people who could be (or are) alternative romantic partners, and emphasizing how the current partner is relatively better than the available alternatives were also rated as being helpful to maintaining the relationship. The mean value for each strategy in response to the second and third questions (i.e., wanting barriers to be a part of the relationship in the future and communicating to the partner about barriers) were also toward the high end of the scale. This indicates that people wanted more barriers, more attractions, and less alternatives, and that they also communicated about these strategies with their partners. In short, this study provides preliminary evidence that relational partners hold the subjective belief that strengthening barriers helps to maintain their relationships.

According to the results of this study, individuals in romantic relationships should be motivated to strengthen barriers to breakup. But how should they go about it? There are many ways to increase barriers to breakup and most of them are interrelated, with changes in one kind of barrier influencing the presence and strength of other barriers. Because individuals have more personal control over the formation of internal barriers, these may be the first to be strengthened when relational partners want the relationship to continue. One way to create greater costs to breakup would be to develop stronger personal and moral obligations to maintaining the relationship. This could be done through self-examination of the virtues of commitment and of staying with what has been started (Johnson, 1982). Partners could renew their pledge to stay together and in so doing include a symbolic gift or experience to mark the event. Partners can also strive to deepen their religious experiences through reading or talking with knowledgeable others about religion and what it says about marital commitment and maintaining relationships. Relatedly, one could go to church or temple more often (such activity may also strengthen social network barriers as well).

Increasing the degree to which the relationship partner is included in one's self-identity could prove an especially effective strategy for long-term relationship maintenance because of the importance of the self in mediating and regulating a wide range of behavior (Markus & Wurf, 1987). An individual could think of how his or her relationship partner affects the different temporal aspects of self-identity—past, present, and future—and of ways to increase the influence of that partner. Roles can also be examined and changed to reflect the importance and influence of the relationship. For example, a partner could think of how much pleasure and pride is derived from being an economic provider, a lover, a care-giver, a parent, or some other role and how difficult it would be to enjoy the same role if the relationship were to end. Further, the development of relationship-based roles that require coordination of actions between partners could be encouraged. Similarly, self-identity can be expanded to include the partner more by figuring out ways that the partner is able to help in striving toward important personal goals, such as success at work, relating to family members, or personal development. On a more pragmatic level, partners could increase the amount of time they spend alone with each other doing the things they find pleasurable and that produce positive emotional experiences. Even doing mundane tasks (household chores, shopping, cleaning, etc.) together rather than separately could increase a sense of commitment to the relationship.

External structural kinds of barriers can also be the target of change efforts. Making a legal commitment to each other through marriage is of course a significant barrier that can create a host of related costs if the marital bond must be broken later on. Couples can also enter into other legally binding arrangements, most of them financial (e.g., a rental lease, starting a business, taking out loans together) that make it more difficult to break up. The accumulation of shared possessions and material objects that would be difficult to divide after a relationship split is an additional method for increasing barriers. The quest to establish various external barriers can also provide an opportunity for couples to work together; for example, romantic partners could communicate about the kind of home they want, the kinds of possessions and property they hope to obtain in the near (or distant) future, the kind of marriage they want, what the ceremony would be like, and so on. Partners could search for information regarding the best way to go about moving in together, having a wedding, buying a house, sharing their money, and so on. Although such activities do not produce immediate external barriers, the effort expended by the couple in planning and engaging in the process of developing external barriers should lead to greater internal barriers through increased psychological commitment.

Relationship partners can also try to establish a social network in which others interact with them as a couple, in contrast to each partner having extradyadic relationships in which the other partner is excluded. The friends of each partner could be brought into the lives of the couple so that both partners may interact with friends who were previously known only to one partner. A couple could also start to build new friendships with other couples or with those people who know both members of the couple and respect their union. Family members (parents, siblings, etc.) of each partner could also be included in the life of the couple. Going to family events together and encouraging family members to learn about and appreciate the qualities of the partner could promote a strong social support network. A couple could also increase their joint participation in the neighborhood or community work. Having other people respond to them as a "couple" (e.g., the newlyweds in the corner house) can foster roles that each partner can use to feel more committed to the relationship. Not only is each person a "wife" or a "husband," but also the additional roles enacted through social participation with friends, family, and the community.

Having children so that they would constitute a barrier to ending the relationship is arguably the most complex of all barrier-related maintenance behaviors. Given the multitude of consequences (for both relationship partners and for the child) commonly associated with starting a family, it seems unlikely that anyone would consider children solely as a means of creating a barrier to relationship termination. Reflecting this complexity are findings that the barrier effect of children on marital dissolution is qualified by whether parenthood occurs before or after marriage; birth of a child prior to marriage increases the chances of subsequent divorce (White, 1990), whereas birth of a first child after the couple is married is associated with a divorce rate of virtually zero for the year immediately following the birth (Waite, Haggstrom, & Kanouse, 1985). Interestingly, one study of married couples suggests that children present more of a barrier to marital termination for husbands than for wives (Sabatelli & Cecil-Pigo, 1985). A potential explanation for this finding is that the risk of losing the children is less for women than for men because women retain primary custody of the children in the majority of divorces.

Level of Existing Barriers and Response to Dissatisfaction

In what way does the initial strength of barrier forces in a relationship, prior to attempts at making them stronger, influence how romantic partners respond to dissatisfaction with the relationship? Rusbult's (1987) exit–voice–loyalty–neglect typology describes how the level of investments (or barriers to breakup) affects the type of reactions made to dissatisfaction. According to this typology, *exit* reactions involve actually ending or threatening to end the relationship, *voice* responses involve actively and constructively expressing one's dissatisfaction with the intent of improving conditions, *loyalty* involves passive but optimistic waiting for conditions to improve, and *neglect* involves passively allowing the relationship to atrophy. In this framework it is hypothesized that partners with high relational investments have the most to lose if the relationship were to end, and therefore should be motivated to respond to being dissatisfied in a constructive manner (through loyalty or voice) so that the relationship can be repaired and maintained. In contrast, partners with low investments in the relationship have little to keep them in the relationship and thus when they become dissatisfied they are apt to react to problems with exit or neglect responses. Thus, an absence of significant barriers to keep a partner from leaving the relationship means that it is less likely that the partner will initiate constructive behaviors to repair the relationship. By implication, to develop stronger barriers should then increase the chances of responding to dissatisfaction with the constructive behaviors of voice or loyalty, rather than with the destructive behaviors of exit or neglect. Use of constructive behaviors should contribute to returning the relationship to a more satisfying experience. Rusbult (1987) reviews several studies offering support for these predictions.

Motivation to Strengthen Barriers: Three Types of Couples

Use of a relationship maintenance or repair strategy is limited to when one or both partners want to maintain the relationship. The potential for effective use of strengthening barriers to breakup as a means of preventing dissolution should be greatest when *both* partners in the couple want the relationship to continue. In this type of couple, each partner is motivated to help the relationship continue and thus could try to strengthen their own internal barriers as well as working with the other partner to create stronger external barriers that require their joint efforts.

But how effective can strengthening barriers be for the type of couple that is divided in their motivation to stay together, with one partner wanting to continue and the other one wanting to end the relationship? Trying to strengthen barriers that require the joint efforts of both partners (e.g., moving in together, getting married, buying a home, etc.) does not appear to be an option when one of the partners refuses to participate. Moreover, the internal psychological barriers that can be constructed independently of the partner (e.g., increasing personal or moral obligations, deepening religious beliefs, and changing self-identity) are effective at preventing breakup only if they are made by the person most wanting to leave, because it is that individual who must weigh the desire to leave against the costs of leaving.

The third type of couple is characterized by both partners lacking the motivation to continue the relationship. If the desire to end the relationship is strong enough for both partners, then neither one should be interested in trying to repair or maintain the relationship. Thus, for the men and women in this type of couple, trying to increase their barriers to ending the relationship is at odds with their goal of breaking up. This is not to say that barriers are irrelevant to such couples. Presumably, when both partners want out of the relationship then they both must be willing to bear whatever costs are associated with the breakup. It is possible, however, that in spite of their feelings of dissatisfaction with the relationship, neither one is able to bear the costs of breaking up posed by a high level of barriers (e.g., staying together for the sake of the children), and so they remain together. This situation has been referred to as an "empty-shell" marriage (Levinger, 1965).

Barrier Deprivation

For the couple who wants to have stronger barriers but because of limited resources, or other reasons, is unable to do so, what are the implications for satisfaction and stability? Is failure to obtain desired barriers associated with relationship distress? Whereas some men and women may be content to participate in relationships characterized by weak barriers (e.g., a couple at the early stages of romantic attraction), others instead may want to have stronger barriers to breakup only to find they are unable to create them. Several factors can limit the ability of couples to develop the barriers (particularly external barriers) that they want.

Compared to partners who live in the same place, partners who live in different geographic locations from each other (e.g., the commuter marriage or "long-distance romance"—25% of the sample in Attridge & Witt, 1993) have less time to spend together, which makes it relatively more difficult to experience irretrievable investments of shared interaction and frequent exchanges of affection. It is likely that each person in this situation will, to some degree, develop a new network of friends in the place where they live, with the consequence being a diluting of couples' shared social network. Further, it may be more difficult for these couples to secure financial and structural barriers because they may postpone consolidating their possessions and homes (e.g., each renting an apartment rather than buying a house). Other couples, perhaps for educational or employment reasons, may live in the same place but it is not where the relatives of one or both partners live. This condition reduces the opportunity for building a strong social network.

Even relationship partners who live in the same town and have family nearby can be deprived of barriers for economic reasons. If couples want to develop certain barriers (e.g., home ownership, shared assets, living closer to a strong family or social network) but lack the financial resources to do so then they could be labeled as "barrier deprived" couples. In a review of economic distress and family relations, Voydanoff (1990) notes that many young couples today are experiencing economic deprivation. For example, young families had substantially lower adjusted family income in 1986 than in 1970. Voicing a similar concern, *BusinessWeek* magazine recently featured a cover story on the lack of prosperity among young adults and described how the American dream is now out of reach for many in the under-30 generation ("Young Americans," 1991). Similarly, a cover story for *U.S. News and World Report* (Boroughs, Hage, Black, & Newman, 1992) offered a troubling account of how the economic recession of the early 1990s has forced many couples to forestall their plans to marry, buy a home, or start a family until the economic situation improves. Thus, a threatening economic climate for a substantial (and growing) subpopulation of young couples may restrict the opportunity to develop and strengthen financially related barriers to relationship termination.

Conclusions and Future Directions

This chapter has examined the social–psychological construct of barriers to relationship termination as applied to romantic relationship maintenance and repair strategies. Themes were identified across several conceptual models as to the role of barriers in keeping partners from leaving a relationship once the factors of attraction to the relationship and to its alternatives are considered. Internal and external barrier factors were identified. Internal barriers include commitment and the obligation to the marital bond, religious beliefs, self-identity, irretrievable investments, and obligations to children. External barriers include legal costs, financial considerations, and social network pressures.

Empirical evidence was reviewed suggesting that these factors representing barriers to breakup are often associated with greater marital stability, but the influence of many of these barriers has declined with recent historical changes in society. Based on these findings, it was argued that there now exists both reason to, and need for, couples who want to maintain or repair their relationship to strengthen whatever barriers are available to them. The Attridge and Witt (1993) study suggests that people had a high level of subjective belief in the ability of barriers (particularly internal barriers) to help maintain a relationship, that people wanted to strengthen barriers, and that partners often communicated about barriers.

Several conceptual issues were raised that require further attention. A critical factor in determining the effectiveness of strengthening barriers to preventing relationship dissolution is the relative difference between relationship partners' motivations. Are the efforts of one partner to strengthen his or her barriers to leaving the relationship effective when the other partner does not follow suit? Because it takes two people to maintain a relationship, but only one to end it, the within-couple agreement in their motivation to establish barriers needs to be examined in more detail. The level of existing barrier strength in a couple is also important. It is argued that higher barriers are more likely to foster efforts to maintain or repair the relationship in a constructive manner than are lower barriers. The experience of "barrier deprivation" is also of interest. The consequences of a desire for stronger barriers but an inability to attain them could have important implications for romantic partners, especially younger or low socioeconomic status couples. Relevant to this idea, tests of Higgins' (1987) self-discrepancy theory have found that negative emotional experiences are associated with cognitive conditions of the actual self being discrepant from the ideal self. If romantic partners hold the view that their ideal self includes being in a relationship that is characterized by strong and multiple barriers to termination, then it is plausible that failure over time to secure those barriers would result in an ideal self/real self discrepancy that could lead to negative emotional experiences. This possibility awaits further investigation.

Finally, although many studies have examined different factors representing barriers to dissolution, each study used its own measure of barriers. A comprehensive scale for the assessment of barriers would add needed consistency to future research and would make it easier to interpret and integrate research findings. Such a measure could include assessment of not only the current level of barriers but also the desire for a kind of barrier at a point in time. The perceived effectiveness of each barrier at maintaining the relationship could also be assessed. Interest in the measurement of specific barriers could be extended to determining the relative strength of different kinds of barriers as deterrents to breakup.

An interesting study would be one that includes a sampling of relationships that differ in the level of existing barriers (e.g., dating, engaged, newlyweds, and married) and in which the assessment of barriers and other relevant conceptual factors (e.g., attractions, alternatives, etc.) would be obtained from both partners in each couple. This kind of data could be used to explore patterns of within-couple agreement on use of barrier strategies. If this kind of information was collected at several points over a significant time period, then it would be possible to examine longitudinal trends in the desire for and creation of barriers in relation to other factors like relationship satisfaction. Measures obtained at the initial time point could also be used to predict relationship outcomes that occurred later, such as the status of the relationship (together or not), the level of satisfaction with the relationship, and the like. A study that incorporates these considerations would be able to add substantially to our conceptual understanding of the role of barriers in relationship maintenance.

Acknowledgments
The helpful comments of Kara Witt, Kathryn Dindia, George Levinger, Dan Canary, Laura Stafford, and an anonymous reviewer are gratefully acknowledged.

References
Aron, A., & Aron, E. N. (1986). *Love as the expansion of self: Understanding attraction and satisfaction.* New York: Hemisphere.

Aron, A., & Aron, E. N., & Smollan, D. (1992). The inclusion of the other in the self scale and the structure of interpersonal closeness. *Journal of Personality and Social Psychology, 63,* 596–612.

Aron, A., Aron, E. N., Tudorr, M., & Nelson, G. (1991). Close relationships as including the other in the self. *Journal of Personality and Social Psychology, 60,* 241–253.

Attridge, M., & Berscheid, E. (in press) Entitlement in romantic relationships in the United States: A social exchange perspective. In M. Lerner & G. Mikula (Eds.), *Entitlement and the affectional bond.* New York: Plenum.

Attridge, M., Berscheid, E., Simpson, J., & Creed, M. (1992, July). *Predicting the stability of romantic relationships from individual versus couple data.* Paper presented at the biannual meeting of the International Society for the Study of Personal Relationships, Orono, Maine.

Attridge, M., & Witt, K. F. (1993, June). *Beliefs about barriers to relationship dissolution: Issues of validity, desirability, and communication.* Paper presented at International Network of Personal Relationships conference, Milwaukee, WI.

Bagarozzi, D. A., & Pollane, L. (1983). A replication and validation of the spousal inventory of desired changes and relationship barriers (SIDCARB): Elaboration and diagnostic and clinical utilization. *Journal of Sex and Marital Therapy, 9,* 303–315.

Balakrishnan, T. R., Rao, K. V., Lapierre-Adamcyk, E., & Krotki, K. J. (1987). A hazard model analysis of the covariates of marriage dissolution in Canada. *Demography, 24,* 395–406.

Berscheid, E., & Campbell, B. (1981). The changing longevity of heterosexual close relationships: A commentary and forecast. In M. J. Lerner & S. C. Lerner (Eds.), *The justice motive in social behavior* (pp. 209–234). New York: Plenum.

Berscheid, E., Snyder, M., & Omoto, A. (1989). The relationship closeness inventory: Assessing the closeness of interpersonal relationships. *Journal of Personality and Social Psychology, 57,* 792–807.

Blumberg, G. (1985). New model of marriage and divorce: Significant legal developments in the last decade. In K. Davis (Ed.), *Contemporary marriage.* New York: Sage.

Booth, A., Johnson, D., White, L., & Edwards, J. (1985). Predicting divorce and marital separation. *Journal of Family Issues, 6,* 331–346.

Boroughs, D. L., Hage, D., Black, R. F., & Newman, R. J. (1992, October 19). Love and money: The dark shadow of recession is contributing to the breakup of hearts and homes all across America. *U.S. News and World Report,* pp. 54–60.

Cobb, S., & Jones-Cobb, J. M. (1984). Social support, support groups and marital relationships. In S. W. Duck (Ed.), *Personal relationships 5: Repairing personal relationships* (pp. 47–66). New York: Academic Press.

Duck, S. (1984). A perspective on the repair of personal relationships: Repair of what, when? In S. W. Duck (Ed.), *Personal relationships 5: Repairing personal relationships* (pp. 163–184). New York: Academic Press.

Festinger, L., Schachter, S., & Back, H. (1950). *Social pressures in informal groups.* New York: Harper.

Glenn, N. D., & Supancic, M. (1984). The social and demographic correlates of divorce and separation in the United States: An update and reconsideration. *Journal of Marriage and the Family, 46,* 563–75.

Glick, P. C., & Norton, A. J. (1978). Marrying, divorcing, and living together in the U.S. today. *Population Bulletin,* Vol. 32, No. 5. Washington: Population Reference Bureau.

Green, W. H., & Quester, A. O. (1982). Divorce risk and wives' labor supply behavior. *Social Science Quarterly, 63,* 16–27.

Greenstein, T. N. (1990). Marital disruption and the employment of women. *Journal of Marriage and the Family, 52,* 657–676.

Higgins, E. T. (1987). Self-discrepancy: A theory relating self and affect. *Psychological Review, 94,* 319–340.

Johnson, M. P. (1982). Social and cognitive features of the dissolution of commitment to relationships. In S. Duck (Ed.), *Personal relationships 4: Dissolving personal relationships* (pp. 51–74). New York: Academic Press.

Kelley, H. H. (1983). Love and commitment. In H. H. Kelley, E. Berscheid, A. Christensen, J. H. Harvey, T. L. Huston, G. Levinger, E. McClintock, L. A. Peplau, & D. R. Peterson. *Close relationships* (pp. 265–312). San Francisco: Freeman.

Kelley, H. H., & Thibaut, J. W. (1978). *Interpersonal relations: A theory of interdependence.* New York: Wiley-Interscience.

Kitson, G. C., Babri, K. B., & Roach, M. J. (1985). Who divorces and why: A review. *Journal of Family Issues, 6,* 255–293.

Knudson, R. M. (1985). Marital compatibility and mutual identity confirmation. In W. Ickes (Ed.), *Compatible and incompatible relationships* (pp. 233–251). New York: Springer-Verlag.

Kurdek, L. A., & Schmitt, J. P. (1986). Relationship quality of partners in heterosexual married, heterosexual cohabitating , and gay and lesbian relationships. *Journal of Personality and Social Psychology, 51,* 711–720.

Levinger, G. A. (1965). Marital cohesiveness and dissolution: An integrative review. *Journal of Marriage and the Family, 27,* 19–28.

Levinger, G. A. (1976). A social psychological perspective on marital dissolution. *Journal of Social Issues, 3*, 21–47.

Levinger, G. A. (1979). A social exchange view on the dissolution of pair relationships. In R. L. Burgess & G. Levinger (Eds.), *Social exchange in developing relationships* (pp. 169–193). New York: Academic Press.

Levinger, G. A. (1990, July). Figure versus ground: Micro and macro perspectives on personal relationships. Invited Address to Fifth International Conference on Personal Relationships, Oxford University.

Lewin, K. (1951). *Field theory in social sciences.* New York: Harper.

Lund, M. (1985). The development of investment and commitment scales for predicting continuity of personal relationships. *Journal of Social and Personal Relationships, 2*, 3–23.

Markus, H., & Nurius, P. (1986). Possible selves. *American Psychologist, 41*, 954–969.

Markus, H., & Wurf, E. (1987). The dynamic self-concept: A social psychological perspective. *Annual Review of Psychology, 38*, 299–337.

Martin, T. C., & Bumpass, L. L. (1989). Recent trends in marital disruption. *Demography, 26*, 37–51.

Morgan, S. P., & Rindfuss, R. R. (1985). Marital disruption: Structural and temporal dimensions. *American Journal of Sociology, 90*, 1055–1077.

Mulford, H. A., & Salisbury, W. W., II. (1964). Self-conceptions in a general population. *The Sociological Quarterly, 5*, 35–46.

Rands, M. (1988). Changes in social networks following marital separation and divorce. In R. M. Milardo (Ed.), *Families and social networks* (pp. 127–146). Beverly Hills, CA: Sage.

Rankin, R. P., & Maneker, J. S. (1985). The duration of marriage in a divorcing population: The impact of children. *Journal of Marriage and the Family, 47*, 43–52.

Reis, H., & Shaver, P. (1988). Intimacy as an interpersonal process. In S. Duck (Ed.), *Handbook of personal relationships: Theory, research, and interventions* (pp. 367–389). New York: Wiley.

Rusbult, C. E. (1980). Commitment and satisfaction in romantic associations: A test of the investment model. *Journal of Experimental and Social Psychology, 16*, 172–186.

Rusbult, C. E. (1983). A longitudinal test of the investment model: The development (and deterioration) of satisfaction and commitment in heterosexual involvements. *Journal of Personality and Social Psychology, 45*, 101–117.

Rusbult, C. E. (1987). Responses to dissatisfaction in close relationships: The exit–voice–loyalty–neglect model. In D. Perlman & S. Duck (Eds.), *Intimate relationships: Development, dynamics, and deterioration* (pp. 209–238). Newbury Park, CA: Sage.

Sabatelli, R. M., & Cecil-Pigo, E. F. (1985). Relational interdependence and commitment to marriage. *Journal of Marriage and the Family, 47*, 931–938.

Sarbin, T. R., & Scheibe, K. E. (1983). A model of social identity. In T. R. Sarbin & K. E. Scheibe (Eds.), *Studies in social identity* (pp. 5–30). New York: Praeger.

Simpson, J. A. (1987). The dissolution of romantic relationships: Factors involved in relationship stability and emotional distress. *Journal of Personality and Social Psychology, 53*, 683–692.

Spanier, G. B., & Thompson, L. (1984). *Parting: The aftermath of separation and divorce.* Newbury Park, CA: Sage.

Surra, C. A. (1990). Research and theory on mate selection and premarital relationships in the 1980s. *Journal of Marriage and the Family, 52*, 844–865.

Thornton, A. (1988). Cohabitation and marriage in the 1980s. *Demography, 25*, 497–505.

U.S. Bureau of the Census. (1990). *Statistical abstract of the United States: 1990.* Washington, D.C.: U.S. Government Printing Office.

Voydanoff, P. (1990). Economic distress and family relations: A review of the eighties. *Journal of Marriage and the Family, 52*, 1099–1115.

Waite, L., Haggstrom, G., & Kanouse, D. (1985). The consequences of parenthood for the marital stability of young adults. *American Sociological Review, 50,* 850–857.

White, L. K. (1990). Determinants of divorce: A review of research in the eighties. *Journal of Marriage and the Family, 52,* 904–912.

Young Americans. (1991, August 19). What happened to the American dream? *Business Week* (pp. 80–85).

8

Maintaining Marital Satisfaction and Love

Anita L. Vangelisti
Department of Speech Communication
The University of Texas at Austin
Austin, Texas

Ted L. Huston
Department of Human Ecology
The University of Texas at Austin
Austin, Texas

Introduction

Willard Waller (1938), exercising a penchant for hyperbole, suggested that "all young lovers know that their passion is without parallel in the history of the human race, and that their marriage will be like no other, but their life together usually turns out to be just another marriage like all the rest" (p. 313). In spite of the high hopes that many couples undoubtedly bring to marriage, scholars have found that most spouses fail to maintain the relatively high levels of satisfaction they feel during courtship. In fact, some researchers have argued that spouses typically experience a linear decline in their marital satisfaction so that the longer partners are married, the more dissatisfied they become with their relationship (Blood & Wolfe, 1960; Lewis & Spanier, 1979). Theoretically, this decline has been linked to a variety of factors, including spouses' tendency to change, as individuals, over time (Pineo, 1961), partners' increasing awareness of areas in which they differ from one another (Waller, 1938), and modifications in the ways spouses view themselves and their relational needs (Graziano & Musser, 1982). Empirically, however, the causal associations between declines in marital satisfaction and various qualities of marriage remain tenuous.

To investigate the changes that spouses experience in satisfaction and love during the early years of marriage, Huston and his colleagues have followed 168 couples over a 2-year period, beginning 2 months after they were married to just after their second wedding anniversary. Consistent with previous work (see Spanier, Lewis, & Cole, 1975), these data indicate that on average, partners experience declines over time in both their marital satisfaction and their love for one another (Huston, McHale, & Crouter, 1986). Furthermore, declines in both satisfaction and love occur equally for parents and nonparents (MacDermid, Huston, & McHale, 1990). In other words, for this sample, parenthood, per se, did not influence spouses' marital satisfaction and love for one another.

What is it then, about marriage, that makes couples less content with their relationship as time passes? Burr (1970) suggests that since spouses seek a variety of goals in their marital relationship, partners may be simultaneously satisfied with one aspect of their marriage and dissatisfied with another aspect. In short, spouses' feelings for one another and about their relationship are likely influenced by their feelings about a number of different aspects of their marriage. Scholars have long recognized that marriage is both a "working partnership" and an affectional relationship—that it involves both instrumental activities, on the one hand, and affective behaviors on the other (Kotlar, 1962; Wills, Weiss, & Patterson, 1974). However, little is known about the relative contribution of satisfaction with specific aspects of marriage to partners' general evaluations of their relationship.

Many conceptions of relational maintenance identify specific interaction strategies and provide a rationale for why those strategies are likely to be associated with marital satisfaction. Studies conducted by Dindia and Baxter (1987) and Ayres (1983), for instance, empirically explore the linkages between particular types of interaction behaviors and marital satisfaction. These works and others (e.g., Bell, Daly, & Gonzalez, 1987; Shea & Pearson, 1986) look to the literature on marriage to identify aspects of the marriage that should be important to spouses' marital happiness. They then presume that the roots of marital distress lie, for example, in the couples' style of interaction rather than in other kinds of concerns such as finances, or the absolute amount of time spouses have for one another. Given the growing body of research demonstrating an association between communication and marital satisfaction (see Noller & Fitzpatrick, 1990; Noller & Guthrie, 1991 for reviews), the presumption that couples' interaction behaviors are often an important part of relational maintenance is well founded. However, having noted this, it is also important to add that there are other domains of marriage that contribute to maintaining marital satisfaction and love. For instance, Stafford and Canary (1991) found that couples who share tasks exhibit more mutual control, like each other more, and are more committed to and satisfied with their relationship.

In contrast to most views of relational maintenance, our approach is empirical in that we ask spouses to evaluate various domains of their marriage and we then connect those evaluations to (1) spouses' overall levels of marital satisfaction and love, and (2) the extent to which the relatively positive feelings that characterize couples' relationships when they are newlyweds are maintained over the first 2 years of their marriage. Once we identify the domains that predict changes in spouses' marital satisfaction and love, we explore the behavior patterns that contribute to partners' evaluations of those domains. Our conceptualization of relational maintenance, in other words, involves identifying the features that account for the stability of marital satisfaction and love over time.

In this chapter, we identify and describe eight different domains of married life that may influence spouses' marital satisfaction and love. These domains include not only the quality of communication—which has been the focus of much of the research on the maintenance of marriage—but also other aspects of how couples organize their lives together, including such matters as how they divide household work, the quality of their sexual relationship, and the extent of their involvement with friends and kin. We report how partners' assessments of these domains relate to their general evaluations of their marriage when both the domains and the general evaluations are measured concurrently. Subsequently, we examine whether spouses' evaluations of the domains early in marriage account for changes in their satisfaction and love, and we explore some of the behavioral features of the marriage that account for these changes. We conclude the chapter by offering four critical distinctions that should be considered in studying maintenance processes in marriage.

Identifying Domains of Marriage

Several strategies were used to identify domains of marriage that might be associated with spouses' relational satisfaction and love. First, we examined theories and research focused on the correlates of marital satisfaction to identify potentially problematic aspects of marriage. This literature search revealed a loose association between scholars' disciplinary roots and the marital issues they considered. Thus, for example, communication scholars and clinical psychologists generally focus on patterns of interpersonal behaviors, spotlighting in particular how couples differing in marital satisfaction work through disagreements (e.g., Christensen & Heavey, 1990; Fitzpatrick, 1988; Gottman, 1979). Sociologists, in contrast, have emphasized matters such as economic hardship (Conger et al., 1990; Liker & Elder, 1983), division of labor (Parmelee, 1987), and power and influence (Gray-Little & Burks, 1983) as factors affecting marriage.

Our second strategy was to examine the literature on divorce to identify the kinds of issues people who have been divorced provide as reasons for the demise of their marriage. Most of the reasons centered on interpersonal problems, including communication difficulties (Bloom, Hodges, & Caldwell, 1983; Cupach & Metts, 1986; Kitson & Sussman, 1983), sexual incompatibilities (Burns, 1984; Thurnher, Fenn, Melichar, & Chiriboga, 1983), lack of companionship (Hays, Stinnett, & DeFrain, 1980), conflicts over gender roles (e.g., division of labor) (Cupach & Metts, 1986), and concerns centering on control or influence (Hays et al., 1980). Of the situational factors contributing to divorce, financial problems were reported most frequently (Albrecht, Bahr, & Goodman, 1983).

Third, and finally, because our view of marriage is anchored in interdependence theory (Kelley & Thibaut, 1978), we recognized that marital partners vary in the extent to which they are able to pursue the activities they like in the context of their marriage. Thus, for example, partners may react negatively to such matters as a lack of time to pursue activities together as a couple, being cut off from the opportunity to pursue the leisure activities they most enjoy, or feeling isolated from either friends or family. Indeed studies have demonstrated that the amount of time spouses spend together and the number of activities they engage in together are often positively associated with their marital satisfaction (Marini, 1976; Surra & Longstreth, 1990). Successful relationships, according to interdependence theory, require couples to coordinate their activities. Such coordination not only places a premium on communication, but also emphasizes the importance of spouses' abilities to organize their time together. In addition, because conflicts of interests inevitably arise when spouses attempt such coordination, partners who feel they are heard—that is, those who feel they have influence—are more likely to feel satisfied.

Taken together, this threefold search suggested eight different domains of marriage, loosely grouped into three categories. The first two categories pertain to the character of the marital relationship itself, whereas the third category relates to factors that impinge on the relationship. First, marital relationships can be described in terms of recurring microbehavioral processes that take place during interaction. For example, marriages may differ in how frequently spouses initiate sex, how often they criticize each other, how much they disclose, and how consistently they validate each other. The first category, therefore, focuses on partners' *interaction* with one another. The domains of marriage we studied that fell under this general heading were communication, influence, and sex.

Marital relationships also may be described in terms of more macro-behavioral activity patterns. Some couples, for instance, may create a "parallel" pattern of marriage with highly differentiated roles and limited companionship; other couples, in contrast, may develop an "interactional" pattern, a pattern that involves role sharing and a highly companionate marital lifestyle (Bernard, 1964). The second general category thus emphasizes the *macrobehavioral organization* of the couple's marriage. The ways partners were able to spend their own leisure time, the amount of time spouses had to spend together as a couple, and the division of household labor comprised this category. Finally, circumstances and associations that impinge on the relationship and potentially influence how spouses feel about their marriage, make up the third category. These *contextual factors* included the amount of time partners spend with members of their social network and the partners' financial situation.

The PAIR Project[1]

To assess spouses' satisfaction with these eight domains, face-to-face interviews were conducted with each of the 168 couples followed by Huston and his colleagues over the first 2 years of their marriage (Huston, McHale, & Crouter, 1986; Huston, Robins, Atkinson, & McHale, 1987). Couples were initially identified through marriage license records, available in the courthouses of four predominantly rural counties in central Pennsylvania. The sample was largely of a working-class background.

All of the couples who participated in the first phase of the study were interviewed within 3 months of their wedding and all were in their first marriage. The second and third phases of data collection were timed to take place at yearly intervals, shortly after couples' first and second wedding anniversaries. Two primary data collection procedures were used each year. First, each couple was interviewed, usually in the couple's home, by a male and

---

[1]PAIR is an acronym. It stands for "Processes of Adaptation in Intimate Relationships," and captures the larger purpose of a longitudinal study of newlyweds, intensively studied over the first 2 years of marriage.

female interviewer. These face-to-face interviews were followed by a series of phone interviews designed to gather data about the activities that the partners carried out in their day-to-day life.

Most of the data summarized in the present chapter are taken from the face-to-face interviews with the couples who stayed married and participated in all three phases of data collection. During the face-to-face interviews, couples were told that some aspects of their marriage may be more satisfying than others and were asked to think about each area separately from the others. Partners were then asked to rate the extent of their satisfaction with each domain on a 9-point scale, ranging from *very dissatisfied* (1) to *very satisfied* (9). In every case, the spouses were interviewed separately to avoid any influence that a co-present spouse might have on reports of satisfaction.

Table 1 contains the eight domains as well as the items used to assess each. The couples were asked to evaluate the eight domains twice during the first 2 years of their marriage. The first occasion took place just after their first anniversary. During these interviews, spouses were asked to evaluate how satisfied they were with each domain over the past 2 months of their marriage. They were also asked to provide retrospective assessments of their satisfaction with each domain when they were newlyweds. Partners' final evaluation of the domains took place just after their second anniversary.

Changes in Domains of Satisfaction over Time

Spouses' satisfaction with most of the domains decreased over time. Both husbands and wives became less satisfied with the quality of their communication, with the amount of influence they had in the marriage, and with their sexual relationship. These declines in satisfaction were equally evident for couples who became parents and for those who remained childless. Spouses became less satisfied with much of the behavioral organization of their relationship. Their satisfaction with the way they themselves spent their leisure time significantly decreased, particularly for wives who became mothers. Couples also were less satisfied with the amount of time they had to spend together as a couple; however, spouses who became parents were even less satisfied, both before and after they made the transition to parenthood. The patterns of change in satisfaction with the division of labor were different for husbands and wives and depended not only on whether couples became parents, but also on whether they made the transition to parenthood during their first or second year of marriage. Satisfaction with the way household tasks were divided did not change over time for couples who remained childless. Wives who gave birth prior to their first wedding anniversary, however, showed a sharp decline in satisfaction after a year of marriage, with the decline continuing between the couples' first and second anniversaries. Wives

Table 1
Items Used to Assess the Domains of Marriage[a]

Domain	Item
	Interaction
Communication	. . . the way you and your partner have been communicating with one another
Influence	. . . the amount of influence you've had on making decisions that matter to both of you
Sex	. . . your sexual relationship with your partner
	Behavioral Organization
Own Leisure	. . . the way you yourself have been spending your free time
Division of Household Tasks	. . . the way jobs around the house have been divided between you and your partner
Time Together	. . . the amount of time that you and your partner have been spending together—just the two of you
	Context
Network	. . . the amount of time you yourself have been spending with your own friends and relatives
Finances	. . . you and your partner's financial situation

[a]Subjects were asked, "During the past two months, how satisfied or dissatisfied have you been with . . ."

who had children between the couples' first and second wedding anniversaries, however, did not show a decline in their satisfaction with the division of labor subsequent to becoming mothers; their husbands, in contrast, became less satisfied with how work around the house was divided subsequent to becoming a father. The only domain in which satisfaction did not change over time had to do with the couples' financial situation.

Given the retrospective nature of spouses' newlywed evaluations of the eight domains, it is certainly possible that the differences in satisfaction between the newlywed and first year assessments were influenced by partners' tendency to contrast their satisfaction at one time with their satisfaction at another (different) time. It is important to note, however, the changes in the domain evaluations are consistent with the changes in spouses' overall assessments of their marital satisfaction and love and that these more general measures were taken concurrently, at all three time periods (see Huston et al., 1986).

As a whole, the pattern of changes in spouses' assessments of their domain satisfaction reinforces the notion that most partners enter marriage with extraordinarily positive views of their relationship, perhaps views that are unrealistically positive. Over time, as spouses become more accustomed to their marriage, they also become more familiar with their partner's shortcomings. The idealism often associated with courtship inevitably fades (Waller, 1938). Having said this, it is important to recognize that couples differ in the extent to which their love and marital satisfaction vary over time (Huston et al., 1986; MacDermid et al., 1990; McHale & Huston, 1985). Some spouses experience substantial declines in their positive feelings for each other and may even go so far as to end their marriage. Others are able to maintain comparatively high levels of marital satisfaction and love.

While the data presented up to this point provide some initial indications of spouses' perceptions of the various domains of their marriage over time, they do not tell us about the relative importance of those domains to partners' overall marital satisfaction and love for one another. There is reason to believe from the literature, for instance, that women may pay more attention to socioemotional factors and men to instrumental issues in marriage (Kotlar, 1962; Wills et al., 1974). Moreover, research suggests that women's relational satisfaction is more closely associated with their spouse's communication than is men's satisfaction (Acitelli, 1992). It may be the case, therefore, that wives who are dissatisfied with the communication in their marriage also tend to become generally dissatisfied with their marital relationship. In contrast, husbands may become unhappy with their marriage when they feel dissatisfied with instrumental issues, such as the division of household tasks. To explore concerns such as these, we examined the associations between the eight marital domains and spouses' more general evaluations of their relationship—their marital satisfaction and their love for one another.

Which Domains of Marriage Are Reflected in Marital Satisfaction and Love?

Our conception of marital satisfaction is based on the approach taken by researchers studying the correlates of life satisfaction (Campbell, Converse, & Rodgers, 1976). Scholars studying life satisfaction have been far more careful than researchers studying marital satisfaction to avoid including items in their measures that pertain to potential causes or consequences. The Marital Opinion Questionnaire used by Huston and his colleagues (Huston et al., 1986) addresses this issue by requiring respondents to indicate the extent to which their marriage creates feelings that can be evaluated along positive and negative continua (e.g., enjoyable–miserable, rewarding–disappointing, hopeful–discouraging). The scale thus makes no reference to the behavioral patterns that might be associated with these feelings. In contrast, many scales used to measure marital satisfaction include items assessing behaviors or activities that are relevant to specific domains of marriage. For example, the Locke-Wallace Marital Adjustment Scale (Locke & Wallace, 1959) requires respondents to indicate whether disagreements are resolved through a mutu-al give-and-take between spouses. Because such items assess spouses' percep-tions of behaviors in specific realms of their marriage, any associations found between these measures of marital quality and spouses' evaluations of various aspects of their marriage (e.g., their communication, their leisure activities, the division of household tasks) are questionable (see Fincham & Bradbury, 1987a; Huston *et al.*, 1986; Norton, 1983 for full discussions of this issue).

In addition to completing the Marital Opinion Questionnaire at yearly intervals, the couples followed by Huston and his colleagues completed a measure of love designed by Braiker and Kelley (1979). Although the love and satisfaction measures are correlated (husbands: Phase 1 $r = .65$, Phase 2 $r = .72$, Phase 3 $r = .77$; wives: Phase 1 $r = .56$, Phase 2 $r = .69$, Phase 3 $r = .73$), the two scales assess different aspects of spouses' general marital evalua-tions.

Because satisfaction involves the pleasure or enjoyment spouses derive from their relationship, marital satisfaction is likely to fluctuate with positive and negative events, regardless of whether the causes of those events are attributable to intrinsic qualities of the partner or the relationship. Thus, for example, spouses may become dissatisfied when their work schedules tempo-rarily prevent them from spending as much time together as they would like or when they are experiencing difficulties communicating their wants and desires to each other. For instance, one respondent, who was very much in love with her husband, reported that she was quite dissatisfied with her marriage. Her dissatisfaction centered on the fact that her husband worked overtime and that she was taking care of a new baby. She was unhappy with the lack of time she and her husband had to enjoy together. Things were not going well for her in the marriage, but she did not feel that her husband was to blame.

Distinct from marital satisfaction, love is best described as an attitude—a stance that each partner takes in terms of feeling drawn toward (or away from) the other (see also Marston & Hecht, this volume). As a consequence, the love that partners feel toward each other is likely to be linked to their perceptions of their partner's intrinsic qualities. Similarly, the domains of marriage that are most closely associated with love should be those which are seen as most influenced by stable qualities of the partner and of the relation-ship. For instance, spouses who are dissatisfied with their sexual relationship as newlyweds may feel less love for one another as time passes. The intense personal nature of individuals' sexual behavior, in combination with the com-mon assumption that sex should be at its best in the early years of marriage, may encourage partners to associate a satisfying sexual relationship with feelings of love for one another.

Because love and marital satisfaction are correlated, special procedures were followed to ensure that spouses' evaluations of love were not confounded by their marital satisfaction, and vice versa. To examine the associations between spouses' assessments of the eight domains of marriage and their marital satisfaction and love, a series of hierarchical regressions were conducted. When spouses' marital satisfaction was the dependent variable of interest, their love scores were entered into the regression equations prior to entering the relevant predictor variables. Conversely, when spouses' love for one another served as the dependent variable, their marital satisfaction was entered into the regression equations in the first step. This procedure created measures of marital satisfaction and love that were independent of each other.

Cross-Sectional Findings

Figure 1 summarizes the associations between the eight domains of marriage and spouses' marital satisfaction and love. As can be seen from the figure, the aspects of the marriage that pertain to qualities of the couples' interpersonal relationship were most consistently related to spouses' evaluations of their marriage. Husbands' and wives' assessments of their communication were particularly relevant predictors of their more general marital satisfaction. In fact, the association between communication and marital satisfaction was present for husbands and wives in four of the six regressions. Communication emerged as a significant predictor of satisfaction during the second year of marriage, and remained significant for both husbands and wives during the third year of marriage.

A more specific examination of the links between spouses' marital satisfaction and the eight areas of marriage at each time period reveals some interesting differences between the domains that were linked to marital satisfaction and love for wives and husbands at the three time periods. Marital satisfaction for newly married wives was largely tied to the sociability of their lifestyle; the more satisfied they were with the amount of time they had available to spend with friends and relatives (their social network), and the more satisfied they were with the amount of time they had to spend doing things with their husbands as a couple, the more satisfied they were overall. During the second year of marriage, wives' assessments of communication, as well as their evaluations of their sexual relationship, became positively associated with their overall marital satisfaction. By the beginning of the couples' third year of marriage, however, wives' marital happiness was associated with communication and the amount of influence they felt they had in the marriage; satisfaction with their sexual relationship was no longer associated with their marital satisfaction (though it was associated with their love). In addition, wives who made more positive assessments of their satisfaction with the division of household tasks also reported relatively high levels of marital satisfaction during the third year of marriage.

DOMAIN	SATISFACTION						LOVE					
	Husbands			Wives			Husbands			Wives		
	1	2	3	1	2	3	1	2	3	1	2	3
Interaction												
Communication	•	•		•	•		+	+				
Influence	•			•								
Sex				•			•	+	+			•
Behavioral Organization												
Own Leisure										•		
Division of Household Tasks					•							
Time Together			•									
Context												
Network			•									
Finances							+	•				

Figure 1

Associations between the eight domains of marriage and spouses' marital satisfaction and love. Bullets, $p \le .05$; plus signs, $p \le .08$.

None of the eight domains of marriage were significantly associated with marital satisfaction for the husbands when the couples were newlyweds. Shortly after the couples' first anniversary, husbands who were more satisfied with communication and with the amount of influence they had felt significantly more satisfied with their marriage. After 2 years, satisfaction with communication was the only one of the eight domains that significantly covaried with husbands' marital happiness.

The most common correlate of love was partners' evaluations of their sexual relationship. The associations between spouses' love for one another and their assessments of their sexual relationship were not as strong as those between satisfaction and assessments of communication, however. For husbands, during the first year of marriage, satisfaction with their sexual relationship was positively associated with the love they felt for their wives. Marginally significant associations were found between husbands' evaluations of their sexual relationship and their love at the beginning of their second and third years of marriage. At the beginning of the second year of marriage, marginally significant associations also emerged between husbands' love and their assessments of both the quality of their communication with their wives and their evaluations of their financial situation. With regard to the latter, husbands who were *less* satisfied with their finances tended to be more in love. This inverse association became stronger by the beginning of the couples' third year of marriage.

For wives, the pattern of results was slightly different. As newlyweds, none of the eight domains were significantly associated with their love for their husbands. After a year of marriage, wives who were more satisfied with the way they, themselves, had been spending their free time were significantly more in love with their husbands. By the beginning of the third year of marriage, wives who were more satisfied with their sexual relationship tended to report stronger feelings of love.

Longitudinal Findings

Figure 2 shows the results of the longitudinal analyses. The pattern of findings summarized in Figure 2 suggests that changes in spouses' love and marital satisfaction were associated with different domains of marriage for husbands and for wives. As we might guess from the literature (Acitelli, 1992; Wills et al., 1974), changes in wives' love and marital satisfaction over the first 2 years of marriage were linked to interaction variables. In contrast, changes in husbands' marital evaluations were predicted by a comparatively instrumental aspect of the way spouses organize their behavior. More specifically, wives' assessments of the communication in their marriage were associated with changes in their love for their husband—the more satisfied wives were with their marital communication, the more stable their love. In addition, wives who indicated a high level of satisfaction with influence during the first year of marriage became less satisfied with their relationship over time; however, wives who were more satisfied with influence also tended to report more stable love for their husband over the first 2 years of marriage. These seemingly paradoxical findings suggest that wives' satisfaction with influence plays a very complex role in marriage. Wives may be more happy with their marital relationship when their husbands take charge of decisions, but may feel closer to husbands when they, themselves, take a role in decision making.

Changes in husbands' love were predicted by husbands' assessments of the division of household labor during the first year of marriage. Husbands who were relatively happy with the way household tasks were divided also tended to report more stable feelings of love for their wives. The only association

DOMAIN	CHANGE IN SATISFACTION		CHANGE IN LOVE	
	Husbands	Wives	Husbands	Wives
Interaction				
Communication				●
Influence	+	●		●
Sex				
Behavioral Organization				
Own Leisure				
Division of Household Tasks			●	
Time Together				
Context				
Network				
Finances				

Figure 2

Results of longitudinal analyses. Bullets, $p \leq .05$; plus signs, $p \leq .08$.

between the eight domains of marriage and changes in husbands' marital satisfaction involved a marginally significant link between husbands' satisfaction with influence and changes in their more general marital satisfaction.

Although the pattern of longitudinal findings is consistent with previous research that posits a gender difference in spouses' attention to the socioemotional and instrumental aspects of their marital relationship (Huston & Vangelisti, 1991; Kotlar, 1962; Wills et al., 1974), it also raises an interesting question. If changes in wives' love are predicted by their assessments of their marital communication and changes in husbands' love are predicted by their evaluations of the division of household tasks, what are the behavioral and attitudinal correlates of spouses' assessments of these two critical variables early in marriage? To probe this question, two additional analyses were conducted. First, given the gender differences found in the predictors of husbands' and wives' love, we examined the influence of spouses' attitudes toward women (Atkinson & Huston, 1984; Spence & Helmreich, 1978) on the association between the predictors and both marital satisfaction and love. We reasoned that wives who hold relatively egalitarian sex-role attitudes might be particularly sensitive to the quality of communication and that husbands who tended toward traditionalism in sex-role attitudes might respond negatively to pressure to become involved in household work. To do these analyses, spouses' attitudes toward women and the other predictor variables were entered together into the regression first, followed by the interaction between attitudes toward women and the relevant predictor variable (either satisfaction with communication or with division of labor). The results of these analyses indicated that for both husbands and wives, neither attitudes toward women nor the interaction between attitudes toward women and the relevant predictor variables significantly affected the association between the predictor variables and marital satisfaction or love.

The second set of additional analyses involved identifying behavioral correlates of the relevant predictor variables. For wives, their assessment of communication was the critical variable in predicting changes in their love. For husbands, satisfaction with the division of household tasks was the critical variable. Our goal in conducting these additional analyses was to identify (1) whether wives' satisfaction with the quality of communication was anchored in the extent to which their husbands were affectionate or negative, and (2) whether husbands' satisfaction with division of labor covaried with either their own or their spouse's level of participation.

To predict wives' satisfaction with communication during the first year of marriage, we examined the extent to which their husbands reportedly behaved affectionately (outside of sexual intercourse) and communicated negative feelings. These data were gathered via a series of nine phone interviews, spaced out over a 2- to 3-week period. A total of 104 couples participated in the interviews. The wives were asked to indicate the extent to which their husbands enacted several affectional behaviors and negative behaviors over the 24-hour period ending at 5 p.m. the evening of the call (see Huston & Vangelisti, 1991). The data were aggregated over the nine telephone interviews to provide more reliable indicators of affectional expression and negativity. To predict husbands' evaluations of the division of household tasks early in marriage, we looked at the number of household tasks that husbands and wives performed as newlyweds. Information about participation in household work was gathered during the telephone interviews. Spouses were asked to report how often, if at all, they performed each of 26 household tasks during each 24-hour period. As with the positive and negative behaviors, the data were aggregated over the nine telephone interviews to provide a more reliable measure of participation. Because we thought that the impact of these behavioral patterns on ratings of satisfaction might depend on spouses' sex-role attitudes, we considered the interaction between the relevant behaviors and spouses' sex-role attitudes as well.

Results indicated that wives' satisfaction with communication during the first year of marriage was predicted by their husbands' expression of positive feelings. Neither spouses' negative communication nor the interaction between wives' attitudes toward women and spouses' communication predicted wives' satisfaction with communication during the first year of marriage. To predict husbands' assessments of the division of household tasks, we looked at husbands' ratings of the number of household tasks performed by each spouse during the first year of marriage. Analyses revealed that the more household tasks husbands performed when they were newlyweds, the less satisfied husbands were with the division of labor. However, the number of household tasks performed by wives was not a significant correlate. Furthermore, the interaction between husbands' attitudes toward women and the number of household tasks performed by spouses failed to predict husbands' evaluations of the division of household tasks.

Conclusions and Future Directions

Maintaining high levels of satisfaction and love in marriage is problematic. The literature suggests that although most spouses enter their marital relationships with extraordinarily high levels of satisfaction and love, these feelings dwindle as time passes (Blood & Wolfe, 1960; Graziano & Musser, 1982; Pineo, 1961). Spouses become more familiar with their relationship and, at the same time, become more aware of their partner's faults and foibles. Whatever idealized expectations they may have had for a "perfect" marriage typically fade. Because of the loss of their original hopes for their relationship, Waller (1938) notes that spouses often have to "struggle against disillusionment" in order to maintain a happy marriage.

Our fundamental purpose was to understand why some couples succeed in this struggle and are able to maintain a happy and loving union, while others fail to come to terms with their partner and become increasingly disillusioned. We were in a position to track spouses' love and satisfaction from when they were newlyweds—a time when couples are most apt to be enchanted with each other—to shortly after their second wedding anniversary. By the second year of marriage, couples have been forced to react to the reality of their relationship and as a consequence for some, disenchantment will have surfaced. Couples who are able to maintain strongly positive feelings toward each other through this period of adjustment may be in a particularly advantageous position to maintain their relationship over the longer haul.

The approach we took was largely inductive. We sought to identify the features of marriage and the contexts that were associated with satisfaction and love each year over the first 2 years of marriage; in addition, we sought to identify features that accounted for the stability of love and satisfaction over time.

Our results suggest at least four important conceptual issues or distinctions that should be considered in studying relational maintenance. First, researchers need to distinguish between (and examine) various domains of marriage. Although the findings of our study support previous investigations suggesting that spouses' assessments of their interaction behavior are associated with their marital happiness, our results also point to the potential importance of other marital domains in maintaining relatively high levels of marital satisfaction and love. For instance, during the first year of marriage, wives' evaluations of the amount of time they had to spend with family and friends, and the amount of time they had available to spend with their husbands were positively associated with their marital satisfaction. Furthermore, newlywed wives who were satisfied with the amount of time they had to engage in their own leisure activities also tended to report more love for their husbands. Whereas some of these domains certainly involve interaction between spouses, the focal point of the evaluation is not on spouses' interaction behaviors, but on the ways couples organize their lives (e.g., the amount of time they have to spend together) and on the various contextual factors (e.g., the amount of time spent with members of the network). The same can be said for the associations between husbands' evaluations of various aspects of their married life and their love for their wives. During the second and third years of marriage, for instance, husbands who were less happy with their financial situations reported higher levels of love for their wives. Whether these negative associations are due to the husbands' increased feelings of dependence or to increased efforts on the part of the wives to reassure their husbands, the area is one that is often ignored by scholars who study relational maintenance. Granted, contextual factors such as a couple's financial situation are typically seen as less controllable than spouses' interaction behaviors. They may, as a consequence, fall outside the realm of maintenance "strategies." However, because marriage is situated within a context and because contextual factors affect partners' relational satisfaction and love, scholars might be wise to attend to these issues. Contextual factors, such as economic hardship, can put a strain on couples, making it particularly important that they have well-developed problem solving skills (cf. Conger et al., 1990).

A second point raised by our study is that researchers need to distinguish between marital satisfaction and love when studying relational maintenance. In spite of the fact that marital satisfaction and love are correlated, our findings suggest that these two types of relational evaluations are associated with very different domains of marriage. For instance, after partialling out the variance due to spouses' love for one another, we found that partners' marital satisfaction was cross-sectionally associated with their evaluations of communication during the second and third years of marriage. In contrast, after partialling out the effects due to marital satisfaction, partners' assessments of their sexual relationship were more often linked to love than were their evaluations of the communication in their marriage. Because love is characterized, in part, by spouses' tendency to feel drawn toward each other, the association between partners' perceptions of their sexual relationship and their feelings of love was not surprising. Sex is not only an expression of one person's attraction to another, it is also a relatively personal domain of marriage—one that spouses might assume is connected to the intrinsic qualities of their partner. Further, the notion that the association between love and spouses' perceptions of their sexual relationship is more stable for husbands than it is for wives is supported by previous research suggesting that men typically rate sex as a more important part of their romantic relationships than do women (Schenk, Pfrang, & Rausche, 1983).

Marital satisfaction, as distinguished from love, is based primarily on the pleasure or sense of fulfillment that spouses derive from their marriage. As a consequence, marital satisfaction is less likely than love to be associated with marital domains that are linked to spouses' perceptions of their partner's intrinsic qualities. Instead, marital satisfaction should fluctuate with spouses' positive and negative behaviors, regardless of whether those behaviors are seen as reflective of their partner's personality or due to external factors (such as a hectic work schedule or illness). Given the potential importance of spouses' attributions about the causes of behavior patterns (Fincham & Bradbury, 1987b), an interesting extension of this research would be to examine spouses' reasons for making the evaluations they do about the various aspects of their marriage.

The third issue that became apparent from our results is that researchers need to continue to distinguish between wives' and husbands' assessments of their marriage. Our longitudinal findings may provide the most vivid illustration of this point (although our cross-sectional analyses revealed a number of differences between spouses as well). Changes in wives' love for their husbands were predicted by wives' assessments of the communication in their marriage and of the amount of influence they felt they had in making decisions. Both of these domains fall under the larger category of spouses' interaction behaviors. In contrast, changes in husbands' love were predicted by husbands' evaluations of the division of household tasks, an aspect of the behavioral organization of their marriage. Thus, whereas changes in wives' love were linked to the interpersonal aspects of their relationship, changes in husbands' love were more strongly associated with an instrumental domain. This pattern of results fits nicely within a growing body of literature that has found consistent differences in the extent to which husbands and wives focus on the instrumental and interpersonal domains of their relationship (Acitelli, 1992; Canary & Stafford, 1992; Wills et al., 1974).

The fourth and final issue suggested by our study is that scholars need to clearly distinguish between data that describe fixed states (at a single point in time) and those that account for change (over time). The term *maintenance* implies that the object being maintained (in this case, the marital relationship) exists over a period of time—that it is more than momentary. In our view, maintaining a relationship suggests that spouses are able to hold certain qualities of that relationship relatively constant. The qualities examined by most researchers interested in relational maintenance are marital satisfaction and love (for an exception see Canary & Stafford, 1992). Thus, those who study relational maintenance should be focusing on the tendency of spouses to maintain the relatively high levels of marital satisfaction and love they experience as newlyweds. Although examining cross-sectional correlates of marital satisfaction and love certainly provides us with important information concerning the factors that may influence spouses' marital happiness, such examinations should not be mistaken for the type of study necessary to determine the factors that influence the maintenance of marital satisfaction and love over time. It may very well be the case that behavioral patterns that covary with levels of marital satisfaction or love reflect the partners' feelings for each other rather than (independently) account for the development and maintenance of such feelings.

The differences between our cross-sectional and longitudinal findings underline the importance of this issue. Cross-sectionally, both husbands' and wives' assessments of their communication were associated with their satisfaction during the second and third years of marriage. However, neither husbands' nor wives' evaluations of their communication predicted changes in their marital satisfaction over time. In this case, assuming that the cross-sectional findings might serve as a barometer to indicate the nature and/or direction of the longitudinal results would obviously lead the researchers to erroneous conclusions. Similarly, the cross-sectional findings concerning spouses' love for one another indicate that partners' assessments of their sexual relationship were linked to their feelings of love with some consistency. The longitudinal results, however, reveal that changes in wives' love were predicted by their evaluations of their influence and of the communication in their marriage, whereas changes in husbands' love were predicted by their assessments of the division of household labor. Again, the cross-sectional correlations differ substantially from the longitudinal findings.

Conceptualizing relational maintenance as a relative lack of change in marital satisfaction and love over time not only frames maintenance as an ongoing process, but also provides scholars with a means to investigate factors that may impinge on or influence that process. For instance, numerous studies have suggested that parenthood has a negative impact on spouses' marital satisfaction (e.g., Belsky, Spanier, & Rovine, 1983; Glenn & McLanahan, 1982; Miller & Sollie, 1980). Some have argued, however, that these studies confound postpartum decreases in satisfaction with the declines in satisfaction that naturally occur over the first few years of marriage (McHale & Huston, 1985; MacDermid et al., 1990; White & Booth, 1985). By examining changes in spouses' satisfaction and love over time, and by comparing the declines in satisfaction and love experienced by parents and nonparents, researchers have demonstrated that the birth of a child is not necessarily associated with decreases in the spouses' marital satisfaction, at least in the short run. Similar procedures might be used to examine the influence of other "turning points" (Baxter & Bullis, 1986; Surra, 1987) on the maintenance of spouses' marital satisfaction and love.

Some facets of marriage that we found were associated with declines in love and satisfaction may reflect nothing more than the spouses coming to terms with the realities of marriage, along with its inevitable responsibilities and constraints. Even Romeo and Juliet, wrote Waller (1938), would no doubt have had their differences had they lived together. How much is the decline in love and satisfaction experienced by spouses the result of spouses replacing an idealized image of their partner with a more realistic one? And to what extent do early declines in love and satisfaction, as well as problems surfacing in particular aspects of marital life, reflect underlying marital problems and, as a result, foretell a cloudy future for the marriage? These are important questions to which future research must be directed.

References

Acitelli, L. K. (1992). Gender differences in relationship awareness and marital satisfaction among young married couples. *Personality and Social Psychology Bulletin, 18,* 102–110.

Albrecht, S., Bahr, H. T., & Goodman, K. (1983). *Divorce and remarriage: Problems, adaptations, and adjustments.* Westport, CT: Greenwood.

Atkinson, J., & Huston, T. L. (1984). Sex role orientation and division of labor early in marriage. *Journal of Personality and Social Psychology, 46,* 330–345.

Ayres, J. (1983). Strategies to maintain relationships: Their identification and perceived usage. *Communication Quarterly, 31,* 62–67.

Baxter, L. A., & Bullis, C. (1986). Turning points in developing romantic relationships. *Human Communication Research, 12,* 469–493.

Bell, R. A., Daly, J. A., & Gonzalez, C. (1986). Affinity-maintenance in marriage and its relationship to women's marital satisfaction. *Journal of Marriage and the Family, 49,* 445–454.

Belsky, J., Spanier, G., & Rovine, M. (1983). Stability and change in marriage across the transition to parenthood. *Journal of Marriage and the Family, 45,* 567–577.

Bernard, J. (1964). The adjustment of married mates. In H. T. Christensen (Ed.), *Handbook of marriage and the family* (pp. 675–739). Chicago: Rand McNally.

Blood, R. O., & Wolfe, D. M. (1960). *Husbands and wives: The dynamics of married living.* New York: Free Press.

Bloom, B., Hodges, W., & Caldwell, R. (1983). Marital separation: The first eight months. In E. Callahan & K. McCluskey (Eds.), *Life-span developmental psychology: Nonnormative life events.* New York: Academic Press.

Braiker, H., & Kelley, H. (1979). Conflict in the development of close relationships. In R. Burgess & T. Huston (Eds.), *Social exchange and developing relationships* (pp. 135–168). New York: Academic Press.

Burns, A. (1984). Perceived causes of marriage breakdown and conditions of life. *Journal of Marriage and the Family, 46,* 551–562.

Burr, W. R. (1970). Satisfaction with various aspects of marriage over the life cycle: A random middle class sample. *Journal of Marriage and the Family, 32,* 29–37.

Campbell, A., Converse, P. E., & Rodgers, W. L. (1976). *The quality of American life: Perceptions, evaluations, and satisfaction.* New York: Russell Sage foundation.

Canary, D. J., & Stafford, L. (1992). Relational maintenance strategies and equity in marriage. *Communication Monographs, 59,* 243–267.

Christensen, A., & Heavey, C. L. (1990). Gender and social structure in the demand/withdrawal pattern of marital conflict. *Journal of Personality and Social Psychology, 59,* 73–81.

Conger, R. D., Elder, G. H., Lorenz, F. O., Conger, K. J., Simons, R. L., Whitback, L. B., Huck, S., & Melby, J. N. (1990). Linking economic hardship to marital quality and instability. *Journal of Marriage and the Family, 52,* 643–656.

Cupach, W. R., & Metts, S. (1986). Accounts of relational dissolution: A comparison of marital and non-marital relationships. *Communication Monographs, 53,* 311–334.

Dindia, K., & Baxter, L. (1987). Strategies for maintaining and repairing marital relationships. *Journal of Social and Personal Relationships, 4,* 143–158.

Fincham, F. D., & Bradbury, T. (1987a). The assessment of marital quality: A reevaluation. *Journal of Marriage and the Family, 49,* 797–809.

Fincham, F. D., & Bradbury, T. (1987b). The impact of attributions in marriage: A longitudinal analysis. *Journal of Personality and Social Psychology, 53,* 510–517.

Fitzpatrick, M. A. (1988). *Between husbands and wives: Communication in marriage.* Newbury Park, CA: Sage.

Glenn, N., & McLanahan, S. (1982). Children and marital happiness: A further specification of the relationship. *Journal of Marriage and the Family, 49,* 63–72.

Gottman, J. M. (1979). *Marital interaction.* New York: Academic Press.

Gray-Little, B., & Burks, N. (1983). Power and satisfaction in marriage: A review and critique. *Psychological Bulletin, 93,* 513–518.

Graziano, W. G., & Musser, L. M. (1982). The joining and the parting of the ways. In S. W. Duck (Ed.), *Personal relationships. 4. Dissolving relationships* (pp. 75–106). New York: Academic Press.

Hays, M., Stinnett, N., & DeFrain, J. (1980). Learning about marriage from the divorced. *Journal of Divorce, 4,* 23–29.

Huston, T. L., McHale, S., & Crouter, A. (1986). When the honeymoon's over: Changes in the marriage relationship over the first year. In R. Gilmour & S. Duck (Eds.), *The emerging field of personal relationships* (pp. 109–132). Hillsdale, NJ: Lawrence Erlbaum.

Huston, T. L., Robins, E., Atkinson, J., & McHale, S. (1987). Surveying the landscape of marital behavior: A behavioral self-report approach to studying marriage. In S. Oskamp (Ed.), *Family process and problems: Social psychological aspects* (pp. 45–72). Newbury Park, CA: Sage.

Huston, T. L., & Vangelisti, A. L. (1991). Socioemotional behavior and satisfaction in marital relationships: A longitudinal study. *Journal of Personality and Social Psychology, 41,* 721–733.

Kelley, H. H., & Thibaut, J. W. (1978). *Interpersonal relations: A theory of interdependence.* New York: Wiley.

Kitson, G., & Sussman, M. (1982). Marital complaints, demographic characteristics, and symptoms of mental distress in divorce. *Journal of Marriage and the Family, 44,* 87–101.

Kotlar, S. L. (1962). Instrumental and expressive marital roles. *Sociology and Social Research, 46,* 186–194.

Lewis, R. A., & Spanier, G. (1979). Theorizing about the quality and stability of marriage. In W. R. Burr, R. Hill, F. I. Nye, & I. Reiss (Eds.), *Contemporary theories about the family* (Vol. 1, pp. 268–294). New York: Free Press.

Liker, J. K., & Elder, G. H. (1983). Economic hardship and marital relations in the 1930s. *American Sociological Review, 48,* 343–359.

Locke, H. J., & Wallace, K. M. (1959). Short marital-adjustment and prediction tests: Their reliability and validity. *Marriage and Family Living, 21,* 251–255.

MacDermid, S. M., Huston, T. L., & McHale, S. M. (1990). Changes in marriage associated with the transition to parenthood: Individual differences as a function of sex-role attitudes and changes in the division of household labor. *Journal of Marriage and the Family, 52,* 475–486.

Marini, M. (1976). Dimensions of marriage happiness: A research note. *Journal of Marriage and the Family, 38,* 443–337.

McHale, S. M., & Huston, T. L. (1985). The effect of the transition to parenthood on the marriage relationship: A longitudinal study. *Journal of Family Issues, 6,* 409–433.

Miller, B., & Sollie, D. (1980). Normal stresses during the transition to parenthood. *Family Relations, 29,* 459–465.

Noller, P., & Fitzpatrick, M. A. (1990). Marital communication in the eighties. *Journal of Marriage and the Family, 52,* 832–843.

Noller, P., & Guthrie, H. H. (1991). Studying communication in marriage: An integration and critical evaluation. In W. Jones & D. Perlman (Eds.), *Advances in personal relationships* (Vol. 3, pp. 37–73). London: Jessica Kingsley.

Norton, R. (1983). Measuring marital quality: A critical look at the dependent variable. *Journal of Marriage and the Family, 45,* 141–151.

Parmelee, P. A. (1987). Sex role identity, role performance, and marital satisfaction of newlywed couples. *Journal of Social and Personal Relationships, 4,* 429–444.

Pineo, P. C. (1961). Disenchantment in the later years of marriage. *Journal of Marriage and Family Living, 23,* 3–11.

Schenk, J., Pfrang, H., & Rausche, A. (1983). Personality traits versus the quality of the marital relationship as determinants of marital stability. *Archives of Sexual Behavior, 12,* 31–42.

Shea, B. C., & Pearson, J. C. (1986). The effects of relationship type, partner intent, and gender on the selection of relationship maintenance strategies. *Communication Monographs, 53,* 354–364.

Spanier, G. B., Lewis, R. A., & Cole, C. L. (1975). Marital adjustment over the family life cycle: The issue of curvilinearity. *Journal of Marriage and the Family, 37,* 263–275.

Spence, J. T., & Helmreich, R. L. (1978). *Masculinity and femininity: Their psychological dimensions, correlates, and antecedents.* Austin, TX: University of Texas Press.

Stafford, L., & Canary, D. J. (1991). Maintenance strategies and romantic relationship type, gender and relational characteristics. *Journal of Social and Personal Relationships, 8,* 217–242.

Surra, C. A. (1987). Reasons for changes in commitment: Variations by courtship type. *Journal of Social and Personal Relationships, 4,* 17–34.

Surra, C. A., & Longstreth, M. (1990). Similarity of outcomes, interdependence, and conflict in dating relationships. *Journal of Personality and Social Psychology, 59,* 501–516.

Thurnher, M., Fenn, C., Melichar, J., & Chiriboga, D. (1983). Sociodemographic perspectives on reasons for divorce. *Journal of Divorce, 6,* 25–35.

Waller, W. (1938). *The family: A dynamic interpretation.* New York: Cordon.

White, L. K., & Booth, A. (1985). The transition to parenthood and marital quality. *Journal of Family Issues, 6,* 435–449.

Wills, T. A., Weiss, R. L., & Patterson, G. R. (1974). A behavioral analysis of the determinants of marital satisfaction. *Journal of Consulting and Clinical Psychology, 42,* 802–811.

Love Ways

An Elaboration and Application to Relational Maintenance

Peter J. Marston
Department of Speech Communication
California State University, Northridge
Northridge, California

Michael L. Hecht
Department of Communication
Arizona State University
Tempe, Arizona

Introduction

We live in a society where traditional social conventions governing the experience of love and the conduct of romantic relationships are no longer clearly defined and are increasingly seen as irrelevant. The social environment that frames the love experience seems to be in an irrevocably emergent and reactive state. In the recent past, this environment has been defined not in terms of an accepted social tradition, but in terms of social shifts and turns. The very expression, the "sexual revolution," emphasizes a break with the past, a break that ventured into largely uncharted territory. In the last few years, we have seen the expressions "love in the age of AIDS" and "the new monogamy" applied to the current romantic environment, and these expressions, too, emphasize a movement into the unknown. The result is that love

Communication and Relational Maintenance
Copyright © 1994 by Academic Press, Inc. All rights of reproduction in any form reserved.

and romantic relationships are increasingly experienced in a context of confusion, doubt, and apprehension.

Indeed, even the connection between love and romantic relationships itself seems increasingly confused. It is not at all unusual to hear a friend state that she loves someone deeply but that she cannot continue to have a relationship with that person, or to hear another friend state that he is putting off any "serious" relationship until he finds someone he truly loves. It is, of course, beyond the scope of this chapter—or this book—to resolve these confusions and set the world right. The best we can hope for is to present a theoretical conception of romantic love and its maintenance in romantic relationships that recognizes the increasingly subjective nature of the love experience, for if any model or theory of love is to be salient to today's lovers, it must admit this basic assumption. Specifically, we will address three tasks. First, we will describe our concept of "love ways" (Marston, Hecht, & Robers, 1987; Marston & Hecht, 1989). Here we will focus on the theoretical and philosophical assumptions that underlie this concept. Second, we will outline a theory of the maintenance of love in romantic relationships that is derived from the love ways concept. Finally, we will discuss some practical implications of this model for improving lovers' success in maintaining their loveships.

Love Ways and the Subjective Experience of Romantic Love

A number of scholars have proposed theoretical models of romantic love (e.g., Berscheid & Walster, 1978; Hazan & Shaver, 1987; Hendrick & Hendrick, 1986; Lee, 1973; Rubin, 1973; Sternberg, 1986; Swensen, 1972). Some of these theories seek to explain love in terms of a specific realm of human experience such as physiological arousal (Berscheid & Walster, 1978), expressive behaviors (Swensen, 1972), attachment styles (Hazan & Shaver, 1987), and attitude/belief structures (Hendrick & Hendrick, 1988). Other theories have presented more comprehensive conceptions of love through the development of multidimensional models, the most prominent of which have been advanced by Rubin (1973), Lee (1973), and Sternberg (1986).

Rubin (1973) argues that love consists of three interpersonal attitudes: attachment, caring, and intimacy. In Rubin's model, *attachment* is conceived as a need to be affiliated with and dependent on one's partner; *caring* is conceived as a predisposition to help one's partner; and *intimacy* is conceived as closeness, exclusiveness, and absorption. According to this view, love is present when an individual holds these particular attitudes toward his or her partner.

Lee (1973), on the other hand, contends that there are different styles of love that can be derived from three basic types of love behaviors: eroticism, game-playing, and friendship. In Lee's model, *eroticism* includes sexual and passionate behaviors associated with strong physical attraction. *Game-playing* includes behaviors associated with the conquest dimension of dating: keeping secrets, getting the other to fall in love, and so on. *Friendship* includes caring for and sharing with the other. From Lee's perspective, these three types of love may exist alone or in various combinations, resulting in a typology of nine styles of romantic love.

Finally, Sternberg (1986) proposes a "triangular" theory of love, in which love is conceived as the product of three component forces: intimacy, passion, and commitment. In Sternberg's model, *intimacy* consists of feelings of close- ness and connectedness; *passion* consists of the drives that lead to physical attraction and sexual consummation; and *commitment* consists of the decision that one loves another and the commitment to maintain a loving relationship. The absolute and relative strengths of these forces in a given lover's experi- ence determine, respectively, the "amount" and the kind of love experienced (for example, infatuated love is passion without intimacy or commitment, and companionate love is intimacy and commitment without passion).

Recently, we have proposed an alternative conception of romantic love as a holistic subjective experience. From this view, love is conceptualized as a set of polyvalent and interdependent perceptions involving cognitions, feelings, and behaviors (Marston et al., 1987). In order to clarify and elaborate this position, we will outline in detail the theoretical bases for a holistic concep- tion of love and discuss the relationship of this conception to other theoret- ical approaches.

Five underlying theoretical assumptions inform our conception of roman- tic love. First, like many other complex emotions, love cannot be reduced to a single realm of human experience, be it cognitive, affective, or behavioral. In the subjective experience of romantic love, these realms are all interdepen- dent; therefore, any unilateral assessment of love in terms of cognitions, affects, or behaviors will offer, at best, an incomplete view of love. This assumption is recognized, at least implicitly, by theorists who have advanced multidimensional models of romantic love in that such models typically in- clude constructs that are associated with more than one realm of experience. Sternberg's triangular theory of love (1986), for example, includes forces that combine affective and behavioral elements (i.e., passion), and cognitive and behavioral elements (i.e., intimacy and commitment). Rubin (1973) defines love as a set of attitudes, but acknowledges that his conception is much broader than the traditional conception of attitudes as evaluative cognitive structures. Indeed, he describes the "attitude" of love as an "invisible package of thoughts, feelings and behavioral predispositions" (Rubin, 1973, p. 212).

Second, a given individual's experience of love is holistic. The love experience is characterized by the construction of a subjective relational gestalt from a wide range of polyvalent perceptions and meanings. To say that the perceptions and meanings associated with love are *polyvalent* means two things: (1) these perceptions vary in their importance in the experience of different lovers; and (2) these perceptions may combine in any number of ways within the subjective experience of a given lover. For example, whereas a feeling of anxiety or anticipation may be central to one lover's experience of love, it may not be salient to another's. Similarly, one lover may experience love when she tells her partner "I love you," whereas another may experience love during physical contact or while doing favors for her partner. From a holistic perspective, love is the combination of such particular perceptions into a generalized experience of or orientation toward one's partner.

Although other theorists have not employed the term polyvalent to describe this aspect of romantic love, the notion that constructs and perceptions associated with love vary in their importance and combinations in the subjective experience of lovers has gained some acceptance in the area of love research. For example, in their recent reconceptualization of Lee's love styles, Hendrick and Hendrick (1987, 1988) acknowledge the value of viewing love-related constructs as polyvalent. They argue that although originally conceived as distinct *types* or *categories* of love, the various styles may be viewed more accurately as variables that may appear in novel configurations within given relationships.

The third theoretical assumption follows directly from a view of love as a holistic experience: namely, that there are no particular cognitive, affective, or behavioral elements that are necessarily common to all love experiences. This assumption marks perhaps the clearest distinction between a holistic approach to the study of love and more traditional approaches which have focused on the development of *analytic* definitions of love—definitions that maintain that love consists of some set of particular and necessary component constructs (see, for example, Berscheid & Walster, 1978; Lee, 1973; Rubin, 1973; Sternberg, 1986). Certainly, there are many constructs that are germane to the study of romantic love: arousal, passion, intimacy, caring, and attachment, to name only a few. Further, it is likely that some of these constructs are common to the experiences of many lovers. But to *define* love in terms of these constructs presents two problems in both the conceptualization and measurement of romantic love. First, it is problematic to assume that the most common elements of love are, therefore, the most important or salient elements. Second, such definitions may obscure an understanding of romantic love *as it is experienced* by actual lovers in that such definitions may devalue perceptions that may be important to a given lover's experience of love but that are not components of the analytic definition.

In contrast to this analytic approach, a holistic approach emphasizes the *synthesis* of thoughts, feelings, and behaviors that lovers recognize and experience as love. From this perspective, establishing necessary and/or sufficient components of love is less important than examining the subjective gestalts that both identify and frame various perceptions as love in the experience of individual lovers. Indeed, given the nature of romantic love as a relational gestalt, it is possible that two individuals may share no specific perceptions in their experiences of love, but that nonetheless, both will be able to recognize their own experiences *as* love. For one lover, love may consist primarily of doing things for his partner, discussing the future with his partner, and feeling anxious when he and his partner are separated; another lover might view love as the feeling of connectedness she experiences when she is with her partner and in terms of the public commitment she has made to the relationship.

Although most scholars who have investigated the nature of romantic love acknowledge that there are different—and sometimes exclusive—types or styles of love, these scholars have generally held that this is the result of different combinations of a very small number of constructs. Lee (1973) and Sternberg (1986), for example, both reduce the different types of love to sets of three basic constructs. We believe a clearer understanding of love entails the recognition that the experience of love may be constructed from a far wider range of perceptions and meanings. This is especially true when we consider that love encompasses at least three major realms of experience: cognition, affect, and behavior.

The fourth theoretical assumption follows not so much from a view of love as holistic, as from a view of love as a fundamentally subjective experience; namely, that love is best conceived as an existential construct. There is no preceding nature or essence to love that gives it definition or value. Indeed, the primary definition and value of love is the experience itself—for love is nothing more than the interactive sum of thoughts, feelings, and actions that individuals experience while in love (for an overview of an existentialist view of human emotions, see Sartre, 1957). Thus, romantic love is whatever lovers *experience* as love. Accordingly, love is a phenomenon that is not well suited to strict, a priori theoretical definition, but rather, one that requires that lovers serve as the primary basis for both data and validity in the construction of theories of love.

The final theoretical assumption underlying our conception of love is that although romantic love is a subjective experience, it is also a relational phenomenon, and as such, it is constituted through and maintained by communication. As many theorists have noted, relationships emerge out of communication and, reciprocally, frame the communication within the relationship (see Crosby, 1985; Stephen, 1986; Wood, 1982). Thus, although love may be communicated through a wide variety of behaviors and messages, communication per se is an important component of all loving relationships (Crosby, 1985). Although communication may be treated tangentially by other approaches to love, it is central to the approach advanced here.

In our research we have interviewed and surveyed over 260 individuals with open-ended questions concerning their loveships. These individuals are spread geographically across the country and across the adult life span. Thus far, we have focused on the dominant U.S. culture which is largely derived from heterosexual, European Americans. In both the interviews and surveys, we asked questions such as "How do you define love?," "How does love make you feel?," "How do you communicate love to your partner?," and "How does your partner communicate love to you?" Category systems were developed for coding responses to each of the questions. Coded responses were then cluster analyzed, in accordance with our view of love as a holistic, relational gestalt.

Our analyses of the interview and survey data reveal seven common "love ways," five of which have been confirmed in a subsequent, quantitative study (Hecht, Marston, & Larkey, in press). *Collaborative love* is associated with feelings of increased energy and intensified emotions and is communicated through mutual support and negotiation. *Active love* is experienced through feelings of strength and confidence and through doing things with the other. *Intuitive love* is associated with a variety of physiological responses (such as feelings of warmth or nervousness) and is communicated nonverbally, through facial expressions, sex, and physical contact. *Committed love* is experienced through feelings of togetherness and connectedness and is communicated by making a commitment, discussing the future, and by spending time together. *Secure love* is characterized by feelings of security and is communicated through the discussion of intimate topics. Secure lovers also associated love with the feeling that the other needs them. *Expressive love* is identified by modes of communicating love: doing things for the other as well as saying "I love you." Finally, *traditional romantic love* is associated with feelings of being beautiful and healthy and is communicated through togetherness and commitment.

These love ways are not conceived as exhaustive or mutually exclusive. Lovers may experience hybrid ways of loving, and other ways of loving may remain to be discovered. Nonetheless, these seven love ways reveal several salient gestalts that account for the experiences of a wide variety of actual lovers. Indeed, we found that over 90% of the lovers we talked to could satisfactorily place their love experience in one or more of the love ways (Marston et al., 1987).

It is important to note that the love ways just described corroborate many of the findings of previous research on romantic love in that these love ways include a variety of constructs similar to those derived in other studies (e.g., commitment, intimacy, physiological arousal, expressiveness, etc.). However, within the present theoretical framework, these constructs have been reconceptualized as polyvalent meanings, feelings, and behaviors that may exist in a wide variety of combinations in the subjective experience of particular lovers. Indeed, one of the advantages of a conception of love as a gestalt of polyvalent perceptions and meanings is that it allows us to admit and study the salience of previous conceptions without affirming the necessary superiority of one over another.

Love Ways and the Maintenance of Love

Given that love is a relational phenomenon, it is clear that the love ways of relational partners are interrelated. The behaviors exhibited by one partner—particularly their communication behaviors—are influenced by his or her way of loving and, in turn, affect the perceptions and behaviors of the other. To the extent that these affected perceptions and behaviors are part of the other's love gestalt, we have interdependence between the partners' love ways.

Thus, the simplest model of a loveship, from this perspective, would be two subjective gestalts that may have overlapping elements. Such a model is overly simplistic in that elements that do not overlap may still be interdependent. Let us consider a hypothetical example of a relationship between an expressive lover and a secure lover. The expressive lover may view favors he does for his partner as a central element of his way of loving. His partner, on the other hand, may not view favors per se as central to her love experience, but may feel secure as a result of her partner's attentiveness.

For this reason, we view the maintenance of love not as a product of simple symmetry or convergence in attitudes or behaviors, but rather, as a more complex process of enmeshment. The various elements of two partners' love gestalts may combine in a variety of different ways, resulting in a relational *plexus* of perceptions and behaviors. Some of the elements in this plexus may be common to both lovers, others may be unique to each partner; some elements may be directly related to others, others may be more or less independent. From our perspective, maintaining a successful loveship requires that this relational enmeshment be satisfying to both partners.

At this point, we will describe the various connections that may exist
between the individual elements of any two partners' love ways, grouping these connections into three general categories. These categories are
(1) correspondence relations, (2) functional relations, and (3) structural relations.

Correspondence Relations

Correspondence relations are the most basic, conceptual connections between elements of lovers' love ways, and include symmetry, complementarity,
and asymmetry. They are called correspondence relations because they are
the traditional basis for characterizing a given couple as a good "match" or
"fit," and in this sense, answer the question "How does my way of loving
correspond to my partner's?"

Symmetry, especially in attitude and belief structures, has been widely studied as a contributing factor in relational satisfaction and stability (Byrne &
Murnen, 1988; Cattell & Nesselroade, 1967; Dymond, 1954; Hill, Rubin, &
Peplau, 1976). Two companionate lovers, for example, may share the belief
that love is togetherness and sharing. However, from the love ways perspective, symmetry may extend into the affective and behavioral aspects of love as
well. Two intuitive lovers would both likely communicate their love through
nonverbal expressions such as touch or sex. Two secure lovers may experience
feelings of security in their relationship. In each case, these elements correspond symmetrically. Of course, two lovers need not be symmetrical in their
general love ways in order for there to be symmetrical relationships between
particular elements of their love experiences. For example, a committed lover
and a traditional romantic lover may express their love to one another by
making a commitment.

Whereas symmetrical correspondence refers to the ways in which lovers'
experiences of love "match" each other, *complementary correspondence* or complementarity refers to the ways in which these experiences "fit" together. To
give the simplest possible example, if an individual sends love to her partner
through touch and her partner sends love to her through touch, this is a
symmetrical correspondence; on the other hand, if she *sends* loves through
touch and her partner *receives* love through touch, this is a complementary
correspondence. In the former case, the elements in question "match"; in the
latter case, they "fit."

Although this example illustrates complementarity in relation to loving
behaviors, attitudinal complementarity is also possible. A collaborative lover
who believes that love is supporting or caring for the other may find comple-

mentary attitudinal compatibility with a secure lover, who may believe that love is *being* cared for. Again, we find not a "match," but a "fit" in these particular elements of the individuals' love gestalts. Of course, such attitudinal complementarity will likely coincide with behavioral complementarity, as lovers generally demonstrate consistency and coherence across the cognitive and behavioral elements in their ways of loving (Marston et al., 1987).

This conception of complementarity is, of course, very different from that traditionally found in studies of relational maintenance or satisfaction. The more traditional view of complementarity is captured in the adage "opposites attract" and has received little empirical support (Byrne & Murnen, 1988; Cattell & Nesselroade, 1967; Hatfield & Rapson, 1992). We reject this traditional view for two reasons. First, in the model we are proposing here, we are concerned with symmetry and complementarity of elements *within* the love experiences of relational partners. The traditional view, on the other hand, has typically extended complementarity to encompass attitudes and personality traits that are largely external to the experience of love (e.g., dominance, intelligence, sensitivity, etc.). Second, the range of "opposites" that have been studied in traditional studies of relational complementarity are rarely "complements" in the ordinary sense of the term. Although a submissive behavior might be said to complement a dominant behavior, it is difficult to see how an unintelligent behavior complements an intelligent behavior, or how an insensitive behavior complements a sensitive behavior: they are simply different, not complementary. Certainly, if one lover receives love through gentle touch and her partner sends love through aggressive sex, we would hardly call such an opposition "complementary." In this sense, we suspect the traditional research has investigated the adage "opposites attract" more fully than the notion of complementarity itself.

If elements of lovers' love ways are neither symmetrical nor complementary, they are *asymmetrical.* For example, a collaborative lover may believe that love is doing things together, whereas her partner, if he is a secure lover, might believe that love means that his partner needs him. Even two intuitive lovers may have asymmetrical elements in their ways of loving: one might associate love with feelings of warmth, whereas the other might associate love with nervousness or loss of appetite.

It may seem odd to describe this sort of asymmetry as a correspondence relation when, in a sense, it designates a lack of correspondence. Our purpose is to emphasize that in the enmeshment of love ways in romantic relationships, it is important to consider not only those elements that "match" or "fit" (i.e., are symmetrical or complementary), but also those elements that do not correspond in these basic conceptual ways. Further, as we will see in the subsequent section, even asymmetrical elements in lovers' love ways may be connected by functional relations.

Functional Relations

The elements of lovers' love ways may also share functional relations. These relations may best be described on a continuum ranging from causality to independence. Certain behaviors exhibited by one lover may cause perceptions or behaviors in the other that are part of the other's love gestalt. Such causal relations may occur with symmetrical, complementary, or asymmetrical elements. *Causal symmetry* occurs when a behavior one lover associates with love elicits a symmetrical behavior the other also associates with love; for example, when one lover offers a relational commitment and this offer causes the other to reciprocate. *Causal complementarity* occurs when one lover "learns" to receive love in the way his or her partner sends it; for example, when a sexually inexperienced lover learns to receive love sexually after a series of sexual experiences with a partner who sends love sexually. *Causal asymmetry* occurs when a behavior one lover associates with love elicits an asymmetrical behavior or perception the other associates with love; for example, when an expressive lover's declarations of love cause a secure lover to feel safe and secure in the relationship.

At the other end of the spectrum, elements of lovers' love ways may be *independent*. An intuitive lover's feelings of nervousness may not be associated with any particular behaviors exhibited by his partner or even with any global impression of his partner. There are at least two explanations for such independent elements in an individual's way of loving. First, although the love ways are not conceived as personality traits, there may be consistent elements in the love gestalts of particular lovers. A lover, for example, may express her love through touch and sex in all of her relationships, independently of the love ways of her partners. Such an independent element may be part of a personality trait (e.g., sensation-seeking) or it may be a result of parental attachment styles (see Hazan & Shaver, 1987).

Second, independent elements in lovers' love ways may be reactions to recent past relationships. For example, a lover's perceived need to receive love through a commitment may be a result of having stayed in a long-term relationship without such a commitment and ultimately losing the relationship. In this example, the particular independent element is caused not by the current partner, but by factors in a past relationship.

We would like to emphasize that we view causal and independent elements as the anchors of a continuum. It would certainly be difficult to demonstrate total causality (or, given the highly interdependent nature of romantic relationships, total independence) between elements of partners' love ways. Yet, it is clear that the functional relationships between such elements are more or less causal or more or less independent. We react to and learn from our partners, but our ways of loving are not *just* reactions and conditioned responses—they are a combination of elements that are related to the behaviors of our partners in different ways and to varying degrees.

Structural Relations

Finally, the elements of lovers' love ways are also connected by structural relations. These relations may also be described on a continuum ranging from simple to complex. To this point, the examples we have given of the preceding correspondence and functional relations have compared one element of an individual's way of loving with one element of his or her partner's. Yet, love is a gestalt experience and the structural relations among the elements of lovers' love ways may be more complex: that is, elements may not always be connected in one-to-one relations, and in fact, we should expect such relations to be typically more complex.

Here are two examples of how the elements of lovers' love ways may share more complex structural relations. First, one element of one partner's way of loving may share correspondence and functional relations with several elements of his or her partner's way of loving. For example, a committed lover's discussion of the future may cause her partner to reciprocate (causal symmetry), may give rise to feelings of security and warmth (causal assymetry), and may fit with in his typical mode of receiving love (independent complementarity). Second, two or more elements of one partner's way of loving may be jointly related to elements of his or her partner. For example, it may be the interaction of a secure lover's discussion of intimate topics and performance of favors that causes his partner to feel secure or to reciprocate these loving behaviors.

Given this model of the interdependence of lovers' ways of loving, there are four implications we can draw about the nature and process of relational maintenance in romantic relationships. First, the maintenance of loveships is fundamentally a process of maintaining a mutual love experience. Certainly, relationships may continue if one or both partners "falls out" of love, but our concern in presenting this model is the maintenance of *loveships*, and when love founders, so does the loveship. From this perspective, lovers (and scholars examining romantic relationships) should focus their attention on the love experience. Although it is true that satisfaction, communication competence, interpersonal trust, and solidarity may all be related to successful loving relationships, the present model seeks to reassert the centrality of the love experience to the maintenance of such relationships.

Second, the maintenance of loveships is effected by communication. As our discussion of the foregoing model demonstrates, the elements of lovers' love ways become interdependent through *behavior*. A belief, attitude, or emotion that one lover associates with love cannot interpenetrate the love way of the other unless it somehow becomes manifest in behavior. This requires a very broad view of communication—one that includes intentional and unintentional messages, verbal and nonverbal behaviors, and both particular behaviors and more general modes or "styles" of behaviors (as in "the way she treats me"). In each case, however, the fundamental link between two partners' subjective experiences of love is their behavior toward each other.

Third, the maintenance of love is a highly dynamic process. Changes in one area of a lover's way of loving can affect any number of other areas in both the individual's love experience and the experience of his or her partner. Such changes may be experienced as growth and may make the loveship more interesting and attractive. However, such changes may also disrupt the mutual love experience and lead to relational dissatisfaction or termination. The present model provides a framework for discussing not only the enmeshment of lovers' ways of loving, but also the *dynamics* of maintaining love in romantic relationships, for these dynamics are situated within the larger relational plexus. If changes in one or both partners' love ways are to be accommodated within a loveship, such accommodation must occur within the context of the mutual love experience.

Finally, given these first three implications, the work of maintenance lies in *love problematics*. We use this expression to refer to elements of lovers' love ways that do not "mesh," that may conflict or even contradict within the relational plexus. When the elements of a couple's ways of loving mesh naturally (or unconsciously), love maintenance is not "work." However, as lovers become aware that some elements in their ways of loving do not mesh, maintenance is likely to become a conscious, effortful (although not necessarily bilateral) process. We will discuss some of the ways in which lovers may effectively address love problematics in the next section of this chapter.

Before we move on to this discussion, however, we need to note two limitations of the model just outlined. First, as noted, this model accounts more for the maintenance of love than the maintenance of relationships per se. There are any number of factors outside the subjective experience of love that may affect the stability of relationships: changes in employment status or schedule, the dissolution of supportive adjunct relationships (familial and social), health problems or injuries, and changes in cultural norms and expectations, to name only a few. Although our model does not account for such factors, we believe the value of its specific focus on the maintenance of love outweighs this weakness in scope (for a model of love contextualized within a couple's larger lifestyle, see Williams & Barnes, 1988; for a discussion of the interface between couples and culture, see Montgomery, 1992).

Second, although this model accommodates a dynamic view of love and the maintenance of loveships, it is not in itself a developmental model. This model applies equally well to new loveships as it does to those that are more established. We are, however, currently engaged in a study of turning points in the development of loveships and their relationship to the various love ways. Such a study should shed light on the developmental features of the maintenance of loveships.

The Management of Love Problematics

In this final section, we discuss how our conception of love ways and the corresponding model of loveships may be useful to particular lovers in their relationships. This discussion will be organized as a set of four guidelines or recommendations for the successful maintenance of love in romantic relationships. We would also like to note that each of these guidelines suggests an avenue for future research, to determine whether or not such guidelines are empirically related to relational maintenance, satisfaction, or stability. Accordingly, these guidelines are qualified until such research is done.

First, of course, lovers would likely benefit from recognizing the multiplicity of ways of experiencing love. It is perhaps normal to project our own subjective experiences on others, but the assumption that our way of loving is *the* way of loving can be damaging to relationships. Such projection may lead us to overvalue symmetry in our loveship: we look to our partners not only for compatibility, but also for confirmation or validation of our own subjective experience of love. By virtue of its existential character, however, love is an experience that really needs no confirmation. Because there is likely to be at least some divergence between our love way and that of our partner, this may lead to disappointment and dissatisfaction and further, may prevent us from enjoying (and maintaining) otherwise satisfying loveships (see Planalp, Rutherford, & Honeycutt, 1988, for a discussion of how relational differences and uncertainty can be positive in certain stages of relational development).

Second, lovers should avoid overvaluing particular elements of their love ways within the total experience of love. Overvaluing can occur both with elements that do not mesh with our partner's love way and with those elements that do mesh. One lover may say to another, "If you really loved me, you'd commit to me," or "If you really loved me, you'd be more sexually active with me." Such comments reflect the globalization of a certain element of one's way of loving until it is virtually a "test" of love. In other situations, lovers will say "As long as we're open and honest with each other, everything else will work itself out." This, too, reflects the overestimation of one element of the love experience, and, in turn, may mask significant and real problems in the relationship.

Lovers may benefit from the perspective that love is a gestalt of a number of perceptions, feelings, and behaviors; it is not any *one* of these constituent elements. Maintaining a successful loveship requires us to give each element of our love experience, and the experience of our partners, its appropriate place in the whole relationship and avoid the overestimation of any particular element.

Third, when discussing or working through love problematics, it appears that lovers should focus on the particular problematic elements in their ways of loving as well as their love ways as a whole. As we have maintained throughout this chapter, love is a complex—although holistic—experience. Thus, the maintenance of love requires dialectical judgments that move between the particular elements of love experience and the holistic experience itself. When a couple is working through a problem, there may be temptation to undervalue either the particular element that is problematic or to globalize the problem to the entire relationship. The model proposed here recommends an approach that seeks to balance the various elements of the love experience and the experience as a whole.

Fourth, lovers may need to remember that the elements of one's love way vary in importance or centrality in the love experience. From a strictly experiential view, this is what is meant by describing such elements as polyvalent. However, from in the more active process of actually working through problems in a loveship, a better term might be *prioritized*. Lovers may need to not only acknowledge, but also accept a lack of compatibility in elements that are less important to their experience of love, as it is unlikely that one will find absolute compatibility with any given partner, especially as experiences of love change over time. Of course, decisions as to what priorities should be maintained are the prerogative of particular lovers. The notion that maintaining a loveship may require choices, however, is a general principle that all lovers should recognize (see Williams & Barnes, 1988, p. 312).

Avenues for Future Research

In closing, we would like to note two general avenues for future research suggested by the model of loveships presented here. First, there is the issue of whether or not certain combinations of love ways facilitate relational maintenance or lead to more satisfying loveships. If we view the mutual love experience as a plexus of perceptions and behaviors the relational partners associate with love, this leads naturally to the question: Are some plexus more successful or satisfying than others? Second, there is the issue of whether or not the model accounts for the communication processes associated with relational maintenance: that is, do the messages lovers use when discussing or working out problems in their relationships reflect the various correspondence, functional, and structural relationships we have described?

Maintaining a successful loveship is often a challenge, and so is understanding such maintenance from a research perspective. As the foregoing discussion demonstrates, there are a formidable number of factors affecting the experience and maintenance of love. It is hoped that the conception of love and the model of loveships presented here will provide a basic theoretical and conceptual framework for both researchers and lovers who are interested in better understanding the dynamic processes underlying the maintenance of romantic relationships.

Acknowledgments

The authors would like to acknowledge the assistance of John R. Baldwin, Karyl Kicenski, and Karen Swett in the preparation of this chapter.

References

Berscheid, E., & Walster, E. (1978). *Interpersonal attraction* (2nd. ed.). Reading, MA: Addison-Wesley.

Byrne, D., & Murnen, S. K. (1988). Maintaining loving relationships. In R. J. Sternberg & M. J. Barnes (Eds.), *The psychology of love* (pp. 293–310). New Haven, CT: Yale University Press.

Cattell, R. B., & Nesselroade, J. R. (1967). Likeness and completeness theories examined by sixteen personality factor measures on stably and unstably married couples. *Journal of Personality and Social Psychology, 7,* 351–361.

Crosby, F. R. (1985). *Illusion and disillusion: The self in love and marriage.* Belmont, CA: Wadsworth.

Dymond, M. (1954) Interpersonal perception and marital happiness. *Canadian Journal of Psychology, 8,* 164–171.

Hatfield, E., & Rapson, R. L. (1992). Similarity and attraction in close relationships. *Communication Monographs, 59,* 209–212.

Hazan, C., & Shaver, P. (1987). Romantic love conceptualized as an attachment process. *Journal of Personality and Social Psychology, 52,* 511–524.

Hecht, M. L., Marston, P. J., & Larkey, L. K. (in press). Love ways and relationship quality. *Journal of Social and Personal Relationships.*

Hendrick, C., & Hendrick, S. (1986). A theory and method of love. *Journal of Personality and Social Psychology, 50,* 392–402.

Hendrick, C., & Hendrick, S. (1987). Love and sexual attitudes, self-disclosure and sensation seeking. *Journal of Social and Personal Relationships, 4,* 281–298.

Hendrick, C., & Hendrick, S. (1988). Lovers wear rose colored glasses. *Journal of Social and Personal Relationships, 5,* 161–183.

Hill, C. T., Rubin, Z., & Peplau, L. A. (1976). Breakups before marriage: The end of 103 affairs. *Journal of Social Issues, 32,* 147–148.

Lee, J. L. (1973). *Colours of love: An exploration of the ways of loving.* Toronto: New Press.

Marston, P. J., & Hecht, M. L. (1989). Love and commitment. In R. Burnett (Ed.), *Intimacy* (pp. 48–53). Oxford, UK: Oxford-Andromeda Press.

Marston, P. J., Hecht, M. L., & Robers, T. (1987). "True love ways": The subjective experience and communication of romantic love. *Journal of Social and Personal Relationships, 4,* 387–407.

Montgomery, B. M. (1992). Communication as the interface between couples and culture. In S. A. Deetz (Ed.), *Communication yearbook 15* (pp. 475–507). Newbury Park, CA: Sage.

Planalp, S., Rutherford, D. K., & Honeycutt, J. M. (1988). Events that increase uncertainty in personal relationships: II. Replication and extension. *Human Communication Research, 14,* 516–547.

Rubin, Z. (1973). *Liking and loving: An invitation to social psychology.* New York: Holt, Rinehart, & Winston.

Sartre, J. (1957). *Existentialism and human emotions.* New York: The Philosophical Library.

Stephen, T. (1986). Communication and interdependence in geographically separated relationships. *Human Communication Research, 13,* 191–210.

Sternberg, R. J. (1986). A triangular theory of love. *Psychological Review, 93,* 119–135.

Swensen, C. H. (1972). The behavior of love. In H. A. Otto (Ed.), *Love today* (pp. 86–101). New York: Association Press.

Williams, W., & Barnes, M. J. (1988). Love within life. In R. J. Sternberg & M. J. Barnes (Eds.), *The psychology of love* (pp. 311–329). New Haven, CT: Yale University Press.

Wood, J. T. (1982). Communication and relational culture: Bases for the study of human communication. *Communication Quarterly, 30,* 75–85.

Why Can't Men and Women Get Along?

Developmental Roots and Marital Inequities

John M. Gottman

Department of Psychology
University of Washington
Seattle, Washington

Sybil Carrère

Department of Psychology
University of Puget Sound
Tacoma, Washington

Introduction

Marriage is ubiquitous; about 90% of all people marry and marriage is generally the central and primary relationship in a person's life. However, today, separation and divorce are also ubiquitous phenomena. Separation appears to be a trustworthy road to divorce rather than reconciliation. When couples separate, about 75% of these separations will end in divorce (Bloom, Hodges, Caldwell, Systra, & Cedrone, 1977). Current estimates are that in the United States, the probability that a marriage will end in divorce is somewhere between .50 (Cherlin, 1981) and a startling .67 (Martin & Bumpass, 1989). The divorce rate for second marriages is projected to be about 10% higher than for first marriages (Glick, 1984).

Not only has marital dissolution in the United States reached epidemic proportions, but in most cases the disruption of marriages has large negative effects. Separation and divorce have strong negative and diffuse consequences for the mental and physical health of both spouses. These negative effects include increased risk for psychopathology, increased rates of automobile accidents including fatalities, increased incidence of physical illness, suicide, violence, homicide, and mortality from diseases (for a review see Bloom, Asher, & White, 1978). Also, there is now convincing evidence to suggest that marital distress, conflict, and disruption are associated with a wide range of deleterious effects on children, including depression, withdrawal, poor social competence, health problems, poor academic performance, and a variety of conduct-related difficulties (e.g., Easterbrooks, 1987; Easterbrooks & Emde, 1988; Emery, 1988; Emery & O'Leary, 1982; Forehand, Brody, Long, Slotkin, & Fauber, 1986; Gottman & Katz, 1989; Hetherington, Cox, & Cox, 1978, 1982; Howes & Markman, 1989; Katz and Gottman, 1991a, 1991b).

This chapter explores the potential developmental root causes for the failure of close relationships between men and women. Can we identify differences in the ways that boys and girls are socialized that may be related to difficulties that the sexes have in getting along? We will propose a set of hypotheses that suggest these roots exist. We will also analyze the results of a longitudinal study of marriage to see if there are any recommendations that can be made from the correlates of martial stability and marital happiness.

The Sex Segregation Effect in Childhood

Interestingly enough, in most cultures courtship follows a long period of segregation of the sexes. The explanation for this sex segregation, the causes of which are poorly understood, may potentially generate hypotheses about the trouble that many men and women will eventually have in their marriages. Maccoby (1990) reviewed evidence that showed that the sex segregation effect is cross-culturally universal. She noted that the same-sex playmate preference is widespread, and that its roots can be observed as early as preschool and that it grows stronger over time. The sexes do not begin life avoiding one another. Gottman (1986) reported an unpublished study by Rickelman (1981) that found that although about 36% of mutual friendship choices in preschool (ages 3–4) were cross-sex, this rate dropped to 23% for 5- to 6-year-olds and was nonexistent for 7- to 8-year-olds, and the effect held. This indicates that the sex segregation effect is weakest in young children, grows toward middle-childhood, and reaches its zenith by age 7.

Surprisingly, the evidence for a same-sex preference of some sort has roots that considerably precede the preschool period. Lewis and Brooks (1975) reported that 12-month-old infants prefer to look more at a slide of a same-sex child than cross-sex child. Aitken (1977) obtained similar effects even when the children in the slides were dressed to look like their opposite gender (boy models were dressed in frilly dresses and shown holding a doll and girl models were dressed in dark-colored dungarees and shown banging a drum). Bower (1989) reported the effects of movement when the models were babies. There was a clear same-sex preference for the full-color films of these models. Bower then did a clever experiment. Lights were attached to the joints of the children, so that in the film of the models' movements nothing was visible but 12 lights. This was less information than that provided by an animated stick figure and in a still frame, the lights were not even recognizable as a human. Bower (1989) wrote:

> Nevertheless, when the films were set in motion, babies had little trouble in identifying the gender of the babies who had modeled the display; twelve-month-old boy babies looked more at the pattern generated by the baby boy, girl babies more at the pattern generated by the baby girl. (pp. 34–36)

Furthermore, the light pattern produced better discrimination by boy and girl baby viewers than the full-color film. This study demonstrates a remarkable ability of babies to detect same-sex movement patterns, and it also demonstrates a preference for these movement patterns. These effects are not understood, but they suggest a biological basis for the same-sex preference effect. Regardless, the question remains: Why are the sexes segregated for so long and are then suddenly expected to be able to form and maintain intimate life-long liaisons?

Possible Explanations of the Sex Segregation Effect

There are really two phenomena that need to be explained. The first is a same-sex preference, and the second is an increasing sex segregation effect. We will discuss only the second phenomenon here. Maccoby (1990; cf. Maccoby & Jacklin, 1974) reviewed evidence for two factors that she suggested may account for the early segregation of the genders. The first factor is the preference of boys for rough-and-tumble play and for play that involves competition and dominance. The second factor is that girls find it difficult to influence boys. For example, Sarbin, Sprafkin, Elman, and Doyle (1984) reported that the developmental increase in influence attempts by girls involves increases in polite suggestions, whereas for boys it involves increases in direct demands. The influence styles of girls were effective with other girls and adapted for teachers and other adults. Maccoby noted that these factors would account for why girls would avoid boys, but not for why boys would avoid girls (see also Jacklin & Maccoby, 1978).

Maccoby (1990) also suggested that child and adult male social interaction can be described as constricting, whereas female interaction can be described as enabling (constructs she credited to Hauser et al., 1987). Maccoby wrote:

> A restrictive style is one that tends to derail the interaction—to inhibit the partner or cause the partner to withdraw, thus shortening the interaction or bringing it to an end. Examples are threatening a partner, directly contradicting or interrupting, topping the partner's story, boasting, or engaging in other forms of self-display. Enabling or facilitative styles are those, such as acknowledging another's comment or expressing agreement, that support whatever the partner is doing and tend to keep the interaction going. *I want to suggest that it is because women and girls use more enabling styles that they are able to form more intimate and more integrated relationships* [italics added]. (p. 517)

How true is this negative view of males? There is indeed some truth to her contention. For example, males, even at a very young age, are more aggressive than females (e.g., see Hoyenga and Hoyenga, 1979; for a review see Patterson, 1982). However, there is also evidence that this aggressiveness is part of a cluster of behaviors that have to do with males having less ability than females to recover from strong negative emotions; for example, an early study by Goodenough (1931) showed that boys exceeded girls in the frequency of temper tantrums and anger outbursts and that this sex difference persisted up through age 7.

However, this view of young males must be qualified by data that show that young males make and maintain different kinds of peer social relationships than do young girls. There is evidence that elementary school boys are more likely to choose activities that involve unrestrained movement or pretend assault (e.g., cops and robbers) more often than girls (Sutton-Smith, Rosenberg, and Morgan, 1963). Girls tend to choose activities that involve restrained movement (e.g., dolls, dressing up, house, school, and hopscotch). Thorne (1986) also noted that during recess, boys prefer run and chase games that require larger spaces and more children, whereas girls tend to play in smaller groups closer to the school building. Lever (1976) reported that there were sex differences in children's play, and she concluded that boys more often play outdoors, in larger groups, and that their games last longer than girls' games. Gilligan (1982), reviewing this work, wrote:

> Boys' games appeared to last longer not only because they required a higher level of skill and were thus less likely to become boring, but also because, when disputes arose in the course of a game, boys were able to resolve the disputes more effectively than girls: "During the course of this study, boys were seen quarreling all the time, but not once was a game terminated because of a quarrel and no game was interrupted for more than seven minutes. In the gravest of debates, the final word was always, to 'repeat the play,' generally followed by a chorus of 'cheater's proof'" (p. 482). In fact, it seemed as if the boys enjoyed the legal debates as much as they do the game itself, and even marginal players of lesser size or skill participated equally in these recurrent squabbles. In contrast, the eruption of disputes among girls tended to end the game. (p. 9)

Now, recall the relative deficit that boys appear to have in regulating their negative emotions. In the context of this deficit, we suggest that the goal of the games that boys play in large groups is figuratively to keep the ball in play, that is, to keep the game moving. For boys, the game is the object of the play, as is a fascination with negotiating the rules of the game as it is played. The first author (J. Gottman) has noticed on school playgrounds that an emotional event (e.g., one boy's crying) that threatens to disrupt a large group of boys' game is dealt with quickly by the boys, in a perfunctory fashion. Emotion may be displayed but it cannot be disruptive: The game must continue. So, in a sense, boys are working at containing their emotions by using the outside structure of the rules of the game in which emotions are subordinated to another, more important goal, namely, the game.

In contrast, we suggest that for girls, emotions are the substance of the interaction and the relationship is the context for bringing up, exploring, expressing, and understanding emotions. When conflict occurs that the girls cannot handle, they discontinue the play because the object in a game like hopscotch is not hopscotch but the relationship the girls have when playing hopscotch. Hopscotch is an excuse for talking, feeling, and interacting. The relationship is the thing, not the game, and emotions are the substance of the relationship. Thorne's (1986) anthropological observations of different gender group play on playgrounds supports such a view.

These are complex differences between boys and girls because they involve both differences in the size of the group and the nature of the play. Gilligan (1982) takes this evidence and suggests that boys do not learn how to relate in smaller, more intimate groups such as the best friend dyad, which is more likely to foster role-taking and empathy rather than competition. However, this may not be the case. Although boys play in larger groups than girls on playgrounds, a great deal of the play of both boys and girls occurs in groups of two, with best friends, and usually at home. However, even in the dyadic context there are some striking sex differences that can reliably be observed.

Further Exploration of Sex Segregation Causes

Gottman (1986) reported the results of research comparing the dyadic conversations of boy–boy, girl–girl, and cross-sex best friends among preschool children. In that report it was noted that young boys played in ways that were very different from the play of young girls, and these differences concerned emotion. The boys tended to introduce danger and fear into their play and then to use mastery or humor to deal with their fears. In contrast, the girls tended to avoid introducing danger into their fantasy play, and when fear arose they would discuss the feelings and comfort one another in a parental manner. In cross-sex friendships, this difference was quite dramatic.

In one tape of a pair of cross-sex best friends, the girl wanted to play with a doll, pretending that the two children were a married couple with a new baby whom they were taking around to show to their friends. After a period of this domestic play, the boy suddenly observed that the baby was dead and had to be rushed to the hospital in a very fast ambulance which he pretended to drive, and then at the hospital, he turned into the surgeon who operated on the baby and brought the baby back to life. The girl protested that he was driving the pretend ambulance too fast and that she was afraid. He said not to worry, that it was OK and that they would soon be at the hospital. This type of interaction difference was typical of the conversations of these young best friends.

Furthermore, it was not the case that the conversations of the boys could be described as "constricting," whereas those of the girls could be described as "enabling." For example, here are some excerpts from the conversation of two boys who were best friends, Billy and Jonathan (4 and 3 years old, respectively). They started out playing with water and then ended up talking about what they used to believe about soap when they were babies then discussing all the things that can kill. Discussions of dangerous things is a common theme in conversations surrounding all young children's best-friend play.

> *B.* We'll go wash our hands, OK? Let's pretend we go wash our hands, Jonathan.
> *J.* OK.
> *B.* 'Cause I like it that way.
> *J.* Why do you?
> *B.* I just, well, because, I thought of soapy when I was a baby; then I started to like it.
> *J.* You know what I thought when I was a baby?
> *B.* What?
> *J.* That it was poison.
> *B.* Yes, and it was.

This last suggestion about soap being poison is rapidly taken up by Billy because the word "poison" for children has a delightfully dangerous and forbidden quality and they know it is tinged with great danger.

> *J.* I did not want to have any [soap] when I was a baby.
> *B.* Yeah, like kryptonite hurts Superman? And that's poison.
> *J.* Yeah.

This leads to a discussion of all the things that can kill. Boys are quite eager to engage in an extensive discussion of these things, whereas girls are much less likely to extend such discussions in their play. Billy and Jonathan also become quite excited and worked up emotionally as they talk about these dangerous things.

B. And rattlesnakes are poison.
J. Ark!
B. Yes, they are.
J. No, they rattle their tail before they bite people.
B. Yeah, that makes them sick.
J. Or a person shot the snake. The snake would hurt.
B. Yeah, 'cause I hate snakes.
J. Ycch!

In the fever pitch of this excitement they pick what they consider the ultimate fearful object, the shark. They then employ a strategy of dealing with the evoked pretend fear that is characteristic of boys—they either pretend to be the terrifying object, or they devour it (they kill it and conquer it).

B. And I hate sharks. But I love to eat sardines.
J. I love to eat SHARK.
B. Yeah, but they're so big!
J. But we can cut their tail.

They continue exploring the great power of the shark, realizing that they have imagined a terrible opponent, one that will require special efforts to subdue.

B. Yeah, what happens if we cut them to two?
J. It would bite us, it would swim, and we would have to run. Run very fast, run to our homes.
B. Yeah, but umm . . .
J. By the trees. Mr. Shark bited the door down and we would have to run away into the forest.
B. Yeah, but . . . but if he bited all the trees down . . .
J. And then we would have to shoot him. Yeah, and the shark is poison.
B. But pink is. Red is, yellow is.
B. Yeah, but people are too. What happened if the shark ate us?
J. We would have to bite him, on his tongue.
B. Yeah, what happened if we bite him so far that we made his tongue metal?
J. Yeah.
B. Then he couldn't have breaked out of metal.
J. He can eat metal open. Sharks are so strong they can even bite metal.

B. Yes.

J. How about concrete? Concrete could make it.

Here is the ultimate means of resolving the fear. The creature is capable of nearly infinite metamorphosis—capable of moving from sea to land, capable of biting down trees in a forest so that no one can hide, capable of turning into metal or biting through metal obstacles. But concrete finally will subdue it, they decide.

When young girls introduce the discussion of dangerous things into their play with best friends they cope with the fears generated in entirely different ways than boys. They encourage the direct expression of these fears and then take a parental, comforting role, empathizing with the fear, and then soothing it away with words of comfort, love, loyalty, and affection. Again, the boys have dealt with the emotion indirectly and by subduing and conquering it (humor is another favorite indirect young male strategy). The emotion is dealt with externally and its direct expression is not encouraged; in Billy and Jonathan's conversation, instead of the fear of the shark being discussed, Mr. Shark's qualities and how to defeat him are discussed. Hence, these differences in dealing with emotion in the dyadic context appear to be consistent with the differences in group play previously discussed.

Summary

What do these selected findings suggest about gender differences related to sex segregation? First, the dyadic conversation of boys is clearly not describable by a "constricting" code, as Maccoby suggested. Boys' interaction is facilitative, but it is facilitative of a high energy and adventurous kind of exploration—an exploration that avoids emotions. Boys are learning to employ external exploration to deal with their relative inability to calm themselves in the context of negative emotions. They are learning to suppress emotion and make it unimportant, to consider it disruptive to productive play, adventure, mastery, and exploration. Billy and Jonathan do not express their fear of the shark directly. Instead, they figure out how to kill the shark. We are suggesting that the style of young boys' interaction downplays the direct expression and exploration of emotion, whereas this is not true for young girls. There is evidence from the work of Buck (1976) that boys between 4 and 6 years old are learning to inhibit the facial expression of emotion, whereas this is not true for girls. Buck used a procedure in which mothers (looking at a closed-circuit video of their children's faces) had to guess which slides their children were viewing. Mothers of 4-year-old boys and mothers of 4-year-old girls did equally well on this task; mothers of 6-year-old girls also did well, but mothers of 6-year-old boys did significantly worse than the other three groups. We have direct data that corroborates this result; from both posed and spontaneously elicited facial expressions of 5--year-old girls and boys, girls produced more and more varied facial expressions under both conditions than boys.

Why would boys be socialized to inhibit the expression of emotion and to deal with emotion indirectly through structures that encourage mastery? The hypothesis we suggest, then, is that because young boys are far worse than young girls at regulating their own negative emotions, and because young boys' greater aggression is part of a greater interest in danger and adventure than girls, boys become socialized to suppress their own emotionality in the service of an external goal, which usually involves exciting play, combat, and competitiveness. Maccoby (1990) has suggested reasons for why girls would avoid boys. We suggest that because the play of girls does not afford the opportunities boys need for suppression of emotional expression, for high levels of excitement in pretend adventure, and for a mastery approach to fear, and because girls prefer the direct expression of emotion, boys also avoid girls. If this is true, young girls find young boys quite annoying, and young boys find girls quite dull.

What are the implications of these hypotheses for later cross-sex interaction? The same-sex preference does not suddenly end with the emergence of adolescence; it continues well into young adulthood. If our hypothesis is correct, this avoidance over a period of about 14 years (from age 7 to 21) will have serious consequences when love relationships bloom and become serious in young adulthood.

In Public Women Defer but in Marriages They Confront

Throughout life, boys are encouraged to explore wide physical spaces (Thorne, 1986) to have looser ties with the family than is the case for girls, who are kept close to the family and encouraged to make close social ties with kin (e.g., see Elder, 1984). As a result, it may be the case that initial differences in social behavior in childhood are amplified by socialization. There is evidence that the social behavior of women in stranger groups is tentative, polite, and subordinate (Aries, 1976). Adult women clearly differ from men in social influence, dominance, and power in stranger-group interaction. They are also more emotionally expressive than men and far more competent with close social–emotional relationships than men.

Interestingly enough, in close personal relationships, these gender differences have a surprising effect. Women have been socialized to be experts in close personal relationships. Hence, it should come as no surprise that women's public tentativeness and deference, the acceptance of a subordinate role, and politeness in stranger groups does not hold in marriages. In the research literature on marital interaction that has used observational methods, women's marital interaction, in fact, has been consistently described as more confronting, demanding, coercive, and highly emotional (both positive and negative emotions) than the interaction of their husbands (e.g., Gottman, 1979; Raush, Barry, Hertel, & Swain, 1974; Schaap, 1982). The evidence also suggests that women in marriages have considerable influence (Gottman, 1979; Raush et al., 1974; Revenstorf, Vogel, Wegener, Halweg, & Schindler, 1980; Schaap, 1982; Schaap, Buunk, & Kerkstra, 1988). Men, on the other hand, have been described as conflict avoiding, withdrawing, placating, logical and avoiding emotions (Kelly et al., 1978; Raush et al., 1974).

There is consistent evidence tracing back to the earliest studies on marriage that despite societal changes in sex roles, men are perceived by their wives as emotionally withdrawn in unhappy marriages, whereas women are perceived by their husbands as complaining and conflict engaging. Gottman and Levenson (1988) suggested that men and women differ in their responses to negative affect in marriage and other close relationships. Gottman and Levenson examined the earliest studies on marriage and found evidence for sex differences in what husbands and wives complain about. In Terman, Buttenweiser, Ferguson, Johnson, and Wilson's (1938) report, the affectively oriented grievances of husbands concerned their wives' complaining, criticizing, and escalating emotions ("criticizes me," "wife is nervous or emotional," "quick tempered," "wife's feelings too easily hurt," "wife nags me"), whereas wives' grievances concerned their husbands' emotional withdrawal ("does not talk things over," "does not show affection") or aggressiveness ("husband is argumentative," "quick tempered"). Similarly, Locke (1951) found that divorced men complained of constant bickering more than did divorced women. He also suggested that in unhappy marriages it is men and not women who withdraw in terms of the demonstration of affection: "Women tend to place a higher value on talking things over than do men . . . moreover, divorced women reported much more frequently than divorced men that they and their spouses almost 'never' talked things over together" (p. 251).

Research suggests that in the climate of negative affect that pervades unhappy marriages, men withdraw emotionally whereas women do not. Gottman and Levenson (1988) hypothesized that this gender difference is based, in part, on a biological difference between the sexes. The hypothesis is that men are in some ways more reactive to stress than women. There is some evidence to suggest that this difference is found physiologically (autonomic nervous system and endocrine responses) and in emotion-related behaviors. Because of the aversive nature of autonomic arousal, men may attempt to avoid negative affect in close relationships because it is more physiologically punishing for them than it is for women. Gender differences in marital grievances, in interactive style, and in health were evaluated in terms of this hypothesis. Recently Gottman and Levenson (unpublished) found evidence for the contention that men are more likely to withdraw from marital interaction in response to intense negative affect and accompanying physiological arousal.

Christensen identified a common pattern of marital interaction as the "demand–withdraw pattern." Christensen (1988) studied husband and wife ratings of the demand–withdraw pattern and found that husbands are more likely to be withdrawing and wives are more likely to be demanding. Recent work by Christensen and Heavey (1990) examined naive observers' ratings of a demand–withdraw pattern when, in discussion, a child-rearing issue was raised by the husband or by the wife. Husbands were significantly more likely to be rated as withdrawing from the interaction than wives when discussing the wife's issue; there were no significant differences on withdrawing when they discussed the husband's issue (see also Christensen & Heavey, in press). In addition, in unhappy marriages, men are more likely to use other tactics to minimize the intensity of their partner's emotional confrontations. These tactics may be dysfunctional for the stability of the marriage.

Although Women Confront in Marriage, Inequity Exists

Despite the preceding review about women not being passive in marriages, the evidence also suggests that there are great limits to the amount of influence that women actually have in marriages.

Gender and Inequities in Power

Bernard's (1982) work suggested that there are two marriages in any marriage, his and hers, and that marriages benefit men more than they benefit women. Bernard's proposals have received some support; however, the truth seems to be that both sexes benefit from a healthy marriage, but that women are at greater risk than men (e.g., health risk) in an ailing marriage. Nonetheless, in ailing marriages it is the inequities in power that tend to be associated with women's depression (Mirowsky, 1985; Vanfossen, 1981).

An important index of women's lack of power in many marriages is the gender inequity in performing household and child-care tasks. For women there is a connection between the amount of husbands' participation in household tasks and their marital satisfaction (Staines & Libby, 1986). Wives who feel overworked as mothers also tend to evaluate their husbands more critically (Barnett & Baruch, 1987). There are no analogous results for men. In fact, men resist sharing household and parenting chores, and rate their marriage as happier when they perceive their wives as demanding less change (Harrell, 1986).

Even when women work, it does not lessen the demand that they continue to carry the major burden of household chores. Although over one-half of the men interviewed in one study perceived their working wives expected more help (Pleck, 1985), Crosby's (1991) review of the literature shows that men do not help significantly more when wives work. For example, one astounding result in this literature is that men with employed wives spent 4 minutes more per day on household tasks than other men (Berk, 1985).

How can these two facts about gender differences in marriage be combined? On the one hand, women are more confronting and men more avoidant of conflict than women. On the other hand, there is evidence that women put up with vast inequities in marriages and that they tend not to confront these inequities; that is, women in marriages behave to some degree like the passive (toward boys) 33-month-old girls in Jacklin and Maccoby's (1978) study.

Summary

What can we conclude so far from this discussion? Initial individual differences between the sexes, the gender segregation of childhood and the continued different socialization of the sexes appear to lead clearly to divergent accelerating trajectories. These divergent trajectories, then, come together in courtship and marriage. It seems clear that in general, a man has married a person who is used to having considerably less dominance and power than he has had, except with other women. She is also a person who is much more comfortable and competent with emotion and the regulation of her own emotions than he is. She is also considerably more perceptive about nonverbal and emotional events than he (Hall, 1984). On the other hand, he is more used to getting his way, to having influence by authority not derived from competence with an emotional world, but on the basis of knowledge of rules and structures and patterns of behavior that emphasize mastery over the exploration and direct experience of emotion. He thus has a highly developed ability to control emotions and to avoid them by using external social structures, and to push away the expression and exploration of feelings in the service of getting things accomplished (figuratively keeping the ball in play). If this picture is true, one could not ask for a greater preparation for disaster in marriages than this sex segregation and differential socialization of the sexes.

Can research with marriages suggest a prescription with respect to the gender differences reviewed here that would contribute to the long-term stability and happiness of marriages? To address these questions, we turn now to the recent results from an 8-year longitudinal study of marriage.

Prediction of Separation
and Divorce over an 8-Year Period

In 1983, R. Levenson and J. Gottman began a longitudinal study of 79 married couples. This study combined collecting behavioral data, self-report data, and physiological measures while a couple discussed an area of continuing conflict in their marriage and as they watched the videotape of their interaction. The methods of this study are described in Gottman and Levenson (1992) and Gottman (in press), as well as the results from the 4-year follow-up. Gottman, Carrère, and Levenson have just completed the results of an 8-year longitudinal study of divorce and separation with this sample. This section presents the initial results of this follow-up.

Brief Description of Methods

Couples were recruited in 1983 in Bloomington, Indiana using newspaper advertisements. The approximately 200 couples who responded to these advertisements were administered a demographic questionnaire and two measures of marital satisfaction (Burgess, Locke, & Thomes, 1971; Locke & Wallace, 1959) for which they were paid $5. From this sample, a smaller group of 85 couples was invited to participate in the laboratory assessments and to complete a number of additional questionnaires (including measures of health). The goal of this two-stage sampling was to obtain a distribution of marital satisfaction in which all parts of the distribution would be equally represented. Due to equipment problems, physiological data from six couples were incomplete, leaving a sample of 79 couples, who in 1983 had the following mean characteristics: (1) husband age = 31.8 (standard deviation = 9.5); (2) wife age = 29.0 (standard deviation = 6.8); (3) years married = 5.2 (standard deviation = 6.3); (4) husband marital satisfaction (average of two marital satisfaction scales) = 96.80 (standard deviation = 22.16); and (5) wife marital satisfaction = 98.56 (standard deviation = 20.70).

Procedure

Interaction Session
The procedures employed in this experiment were modeled after those described in Levenson and Gottman (1983). Couples came to the laboratory after having not spoken for at least 8 hours. After recording devices for obtaining physiological measures were attached, couples engaged in three conversational interactions: (1) discussing the events of the day, (2) discussing

a problem area of continuing disagreement in their marriage, and (3) discussing a mutually agreed on pleasant topic. Each conversation lasted for 15 min, preceded by a 5-min silent period. During the silent periods and discussions, a broad sample of physiological measures was obtained and a video recording was made of the interaction.

Prior to initiating the problem area discussion, couples completed the Couple's Problem Inventory (Gottman, Markman, & Notarius, 1977), in which they rated the perceived severity (on a scale of 0 to 100) of a standard set of marital issues such as money, in-laws, and sex. The experimenter, a graduate student in counseling psychology, then helped the couples select an issue that both spouses rated as being of high severity to use as the topic for the problem area discussion. The Couple's Problem Inventory also provided an index of each spouse's ratings of the severity of problems in the relationship (alpha = .79 [husbands]; alpha = .75 [wives]). For this chapter, only data from the problem area discussion were used. This decision was based on our previous research, in which data from the problem area discussion were the best longitudinal predictors of change in marital satisfaction (Levenson & Gottman, 1985), and on our plan to use marital interaction coding systems which primarily code problem-solving behavior.

Recall Session

Several days later, spouses separately returned to the laboratory to view the video recording of their interaction while the same physiological measures were obtained and synchronized with those obtained in the interaction session. As they watched their videotaped interactions, spouses used a rating dial to provide a continuous self-report of affect. The dial traversed a 180° path, with the dial pointer moving over a 9-point scale anchored by the legends *extremely negative* and *extremely positive* with *neutral* in the middle. Participants were instructed to adjust the dial continuously so that it always represented how they were feeling when they were in the interaction. Data supporting the validity of this procedure for obtaining continuous self-reported affect ratings have been presented in Gottman and Levenson (1985).

1987 Follow-Up

In 1987, 4 years after the initial assessment, the original participants were recontacted and at least one spouse (70 husbands, 72 wives) from 73 of the original 79 couples (92.4%) agreed to participate in the follow-up. These 73 participants represented 69 couples in which both spouses participated, one couple in which only the husband participated, and three couples in which only the wife participated. Data from the nonparticipating partner in these four couples were treated as missing data. For the follow-up, spouses completed the two marital satisfaction questionnaires, a measure of physical illness (the Cornell Medical Index3), and several items relevant to other stages of the hypothesized cascade model (i.e., during the 4-year period had the spouses considered separation or divorce, had they actually separated or divorced, and the length of any separation).

1991 Follow-Up

In 1991, 69 subjects were recontacted and asked to fill out a packet of questionnaires. This packet included the Cowan Who Does What Scale, a modified version of the Cowan Parental Responsibilities Scale (modified to fit the older age of children in the present study's families), and Carrère's Marital Maintenance Scale. Typical items on the Who Does What scale concern planning and preparing meals, cleaning after meals, and repairs around the home; typical items on the Parental Responsibilities scale are staying home when a child is ill, helping children with homework, and talking to a teacher about the child's progress in school; typical items on the Marital Maintenance scale are planning a date or evening out, saying "I love you," and initiating sexual intimacy. Subjects were paid $15 for their participation.

Apparatus

Physiological

Five physiological measures were obtained using a system consisting of two Lafayette Instruments six-channel polygraphs and a DEC LSI 11/73 microcomputer.[1] This set of physiological measures was selected to (1) sample broadly from major organ systems (cardiac, vascular, electrodermal, somatic muscle), (2) allow for continuous measurement, (3) be as unobtrusive as

---

[1] These apparatus were (1) cardiac interbeat interval (IBI)—Beckman miniature electrodes with Redux paste were placed in a bipolar configuration on opposite sides of the subject's chest and the interval between R-waves of the electrocardiogram (EKG) was measured in msec; shorter IBIs indicate faster heart rate, which is typically interpreted as indicating a state of higher cardiovascular arousal. (2) Skin conductance level—a constant voltage device passed a small voltage between Beckman regular electrodes attached to the palmar surface of the middle phalanges of the first and third fingers of the nondominant hand using an electrolyte of sodium chloride in Unibase; increasing skin conductance indexes greater autonomic (sympathetic) activation. (3) General somatic activity—an electromechanical transducer attached to a platform under the subject's chair generated an electrical signal proportional to the amount of body movement in any direction. (4) Pulse transmission time to the finger—a UFI photoplethysmograph was attached to the second finger of the nondominant hand. The interval was measured between the R-wave of the EKG and the upstroke of the finger pulse; shorter pulse transmission times are indicative of greater autonomic (sympathetic) activation. (5) Finger pulse amplitude (FPA)—the trough-to-peak amplitude of the finger pulse was measured, finger pulse amplitude measures the amount of blood in the periphery; reduced FPA often indicates greater vasoconstriction, which is associated with greater autonomic (sympathetic) activation.

possible, and (4) include measures used in our previous studies (Levenson & Gottman, 1983). The computer was programmed to process the physiological data on-line and to compute second-by-second averages for each physiological measure for each spouse. Later, averages were determined for each measure for the entire 15-min interaction period and for the 5-min preinteraction period.

Nonphysiological

Two remotely controlled, high resolution video cameras that were partially concealed behind darkened glass were used to obtain frontal views of each spouse's face and upper torso. These images were combined into a single split-screen image using a video special effects generator and were recorded on a VHS video recorder. Two lavaliere microphones were used to record the spouses' conversations. The DEC computer enabled synchronization between video and physiological data by controlling the operation of a device that imposed the elapsed time on the video recording.

Observational Coding

The coding of the videotapes of the problem area interaction was achieved using two observational coding systems: the Rapid Couples Interaction Scoring System (RCISS), which classified couples' problem-solving ability, and the Specific Affect Coding System (SPAFF), which classified couples' emotional behavior.

Rapid Couples Interaction Scoring System

The Rapid Couples Interaction Scoring System (RCISS; Krokoff, Gottman, & Hass, 1989) employs a checklist of 13 behaviors that are scored for the speaker and 9 behaviors that are scored for the listener on each turn at speech. A *turn at speech* is defined as all utterances by one speaker until that speaker yields the floor to vocalizations by the other spouse (vocalizations that are merely backchannels such as "mm-hmm" are not considered as demarcating a turn). In the present study, only codes assigned to speakers were used to classify couples. These codes consisted of five positive codes (neutral or positive problem description, task-oriented relationship information, assent, humor–laugh, other positive) and eight negative codes (complain, criticize, negative relationship issue problem talk, yes–but, defensive, put down, escalate negative affect, other negative). We also computed the average number of positive and negative speaker codes per turn of speech, and the average of positive minus negative speaker codes per turn. Tapes were coded by a team of coders using verbatim transcripts. Using Cohen's kappa, reliability for all RCISS subcodes taken together was .72. For the individual speaker codes, kappas ranged from .70 to .81.

Specific Affect Coding System

To provide information on specific affects, SPAFF (Gottman & Krokoff, 1989) was employed by an independent team of coders. The Specific Affect Coding System is a cultural informant coding system in which coders consider an informational gestalt consisting of verbal content, voice tone, context, facial expression, gestures, and body movement. For present purposes, only the speaker's affect was coded. Coders classified each turn at speech as affectively neutral, as one of five negative affects (anger, disgust/contempt, sadness, fear, whining), or as one of four positive affects (affection, humor, interest, joy). The kappa coefficient of reliability was equal to .75 for the entire SPAFF coding. Kappas for individual codes ranged between .63 and .76. We coded the conflict discussion with two observational systems, one designed to examine problem solving and one designed to examine emotional behavior.

Results of the 8-Year Follow-Up

Of the 69 (of 79) couples we were able to recontact in 1991, 21 had divorced (30.4%, or 4.25% of the sample per year). Table 1 presents the correlations of the Time-1 physiology, behavioral, and self-report variables with whether or not the couple divorced in 8 years. The only significant difference in physiology between the two groups was the wife's interbeat interval (time between R-spikes of the electrocardiogram), suggesting a slower heart rate both during baseline and during the conflict discussion for the wives who remained married after 8 years. The baseline mean for the stable group was 781.73 ms, and the mean for the unstable group was 710.82 ms, $t(77) = 2.13$, $p < .05$. The interaction mean for the stable group was 775.13 ms, and the mean for the unstable group was 705.35, $t(77) = 2.17$, $p < .05$.

Behavioral differences were that couples who divorced in 8 years were initially different from stable couples in that husbands were more defensive, stonewalled more, were less likely to state their complaints in a positive manner, and were less positive listeners, wives laughed less, were more contemptuous and disgusted, and were sadder. These results show that the male approach of avoiding interaction by stonewalling and by responding to complaints with defensiveness is harmful to the long-term stability of the marriage. Also, the results show that what is most destructive in what wives do in a conflict discussion involves the expression of contempt and disgust. These patterns in unstable marriages are consistent with a female style of intense and provocative confrontation and a male style of avoiding and warding off intense negative emotion.

Table 1
**Correlations between Time-1 Marital Satisfaction,
Physiology, Self-Report, and Behavior with
Divorce or Stability 8 Years Later**

Measures	Husband	Wife
Physiological data		
Baseline physiology		
Interbeat Interval (IB)	.12	−.24*
Activity (AC)	.05	.11
Skin Conductance (SC)	.01	−.07
Pulse Transit Time (PT)	.09	−.17
Finger Pulse Amplitude (FA)	−.06	−.10
Interaction physiology		
IB	.14	−.24*
AC	.02	.05
SC	.02	−.07
PT	.15	−.13
FA	−.13	−.07
Behavior		
RCISS		
Complaint	.03	.13
Defensiveness	.23*	.21a
Contempt	.04	.17
Stonewalling	.32**	.19
Pos Agenda	−.26*	−.12
Assent	.13	−.05
Humor	−.12	−.27
Pos List	−.18	−.18
Global RCISS scales		
SPK POS	−.24*	−.22a
SPK NEG	.14	.20a
SPK	−.20	−.23
LIST POS	−.18	−.18
LIST	−.27*	−.20
SPAFF proportions		
PNEUTRAL	.09	−.01
PHUMOR	−.14	−.16
PAFFECTION	.05	−.13
PINTEREST	.00	−.19
PJOY	−.08	−.03
PANGER	−.08	.06
PCONTEMPT	−.12	.28*
PWHINING	.03	.02
PSAD	.16	.35**
PFEAR	−.06	−.09

(*continues*)

Table 1   (*Continued*)

Measures	Husband	Wife
Self-Report data		
Time-1 Marital Sat.	−.14	−.17
Dial	.01	−.08
Severity of Probs.	.00	.21a
Time-2 Serious Consid. of Dissolution	.55***	

*p < .05.   **p < .01.   ***p < .001.

There were no self-report differences, either on the questionnaires or on the video recall rating dial. Marital satisfaction in 1983 did not significantly predict divorce. However, serious considerations of separation and divorce when couples were asked in 1987 (the 4-year follow-up) was a significant predictor of divorce in 1991. This provides validation for the questions we asked in 1987 about whether the couple had seriously considered dissolving their marriage.

Table 2 summarizes the correlations between marital satisfaction in 1991 with who does what in the general areas of housework, parenting, and the initiation and maintenance of intimacy. As can be seen, the husband's dissatisfaction with the family tasks (housework, etc.) is significantly negatively related to both his and his wife's marital satisfaction (see also Vangelisti & Huston, this volume). The husband's dissatisfaction with task division for

Table 2
Correlates of Marital Happiness Based on Three
Domains: Housework, Parenting, and Initiation
of Intimate Contact

Variables (dissatisfaction with who does what)	Husband's marital satisfaction	Wife's marital satisfaction
Husband in home	−.53***	−.48**
Husband out	−.14	−.16
Wife in home	−.19	−.51***
Wife out	−.39*	−.35*
Husband parenting	−.02	−.22
Wife parenting	−.40*	−.65***
Husband maintenance	−.60***	−.52***
Wife maintenance	−.54***	−.57***

*p < .05.   **p < .01.   ***p < .001.

work outside the family was unrelated to either the husband's or the wife's marital satisfaction, but the wife's dissatisfaction with task division for work outside the family is significantly related to both the husband's and the wife's marital satisfaction. The husband's dissatisfaction with how parenting tasks are allocated was unrelated to either his own or his wife's marital satisfaction, but the wife's dissatisfaction with how parenting tasks are allocated was significantly related to both her own and her husband's marital satisfaction. Both the husband's and the wife's dissatisfaction with the initiation and maintenance of intimacy was significantly related to both the husband's and the wife's marital satisfaction.

What are the correlates of these dissatisfactions in terms of perceived equity in the marriage? For these analyses, each scale that asked about who does what was analyzed item-by-item, splitting at the median on husband and wife marital satisfaction. A mean less than 5.0 suggested that the wives tended to do most of this task, whereas a mean greater than 5.0 suggested that the husband did most of this task. Table 3 summarizes these analyses. Splitting on the husband's marital satisfaction, there were no significant differences between happily and unhappily married husbands on any item. However, for the wives, there were significant differences. Dissatisfied wives reported doing more cleaning after meals, more housework, and marginally more contacts with family and friends, looking after the car, and yard work.

In the area of parental responsibilities, dissatisfied husbands differed from satisfied husbands in reporting doing more of the following: helping children with their homework, talking to teachers, supervising children in their household chores, and, marginally, staying home when a child is ill and teaching the children skills. Interestingly, these patterns also held for the wives. Dissatisfied wives reported doing more taking children to weekend activities, talking to teachers, and marginally helping the children with their homework. In one reversal, satisfied wives reported arranging for babysitters more than dissatisfied wives.

In the area of initiating intimate contact, dissatisfied husbands differed marginally from satisfied husbands in doing less remembering of a wedding anniversary, and more planning of surprises. Dissatisfied wives were more likely to take on extra household tasks when their husband was under stress.

Summary and Prescriptions

There are clearly gender differences in responses to strong negative emotions. Usually, wives were the ones who raised the complaints that stood in

Table 3
**Specific Item Analyses Splitting on Husband
and Wife Marital Satisfaction**

Variable	Dissatisfied mean	Satisfied mean	t	df	p
	Who does what?				
Husband					
Preparing meals	3.19	2.48	1.16	42	ns
Cleaning meals	3.38	4.22	−1.65	42	ns
Home repairs	7.90	7.87	.12	42	ns
House cleaning	3.67	3.04	1.18	42	ns
Garbage	6.38	5.57	1.18	42	ns
Groceries	3.81	3.39	.76	42	ns
Bills	4.86	3.35	1.55	42	ns
Laundry	2.90	2.43	.87	42	ns
Calls to friends	3.81	4.21	−.61	42	ns
Car	8.10	7.91	.52	42	ns
Income	6.19	6.78	−1.14	42	ns
Yard	6.29	5.39	1.62	42	ns
Work	6.33	6.27	.11	42	ns
Wife					
Preparing meals	2.39	2.52	−.24	46	ns
Cleaning meals	2.48	3.56	−2.07	46	.044
Home repairs	7.00	7.44	−.97	46	ns
House cleaning	2.35	3.52	−2.65	46	.011
Garbage	5.70	5.54	.18	46	ns
Groceries	3.00	2.79	.40	46	ns
Bills	4.13	4.12	.01	46	ns
Laundry	2.39	2.16	.48	46	ns
Calls to friends	3.04	4.12	−1.83	46	.074
Car	6.43	7.56	−1.96	46	.056
Income	6.61	6.80	−.36	46	ns
Yard	6.04	5.08	1.97	32	.057
Work	6.18	6.25	−.13	46	ns
	Parental responsibilities				
Husband					
Child ill	3.00	1.92	1.89	29	.069
Weekend	4.39	4.08	.49	28	ns
Homework	5.27	3.27	2.73	24	.012
Teachers	4.69	3.08	2.76	26	.011
Clothes	2.28	1.77	1.06	29	ns
Chores	4.56	3.33	2.26	28	.032
Skills	4.88	4.23	1.72	29	.096
Discipline	4.78	4.46	.47	29	ns
Spending time	4.72	4.62	.19	29	ns
Babysitters	2.47	2.25	.36	27	ns

(continues)

Table 3 (*Continued*)

Variable	Dissatisfied mean	Satisfied mean	t	df	p
Wife					
Child ill	2.50	2.82	−.51	35	ns
Weekend	3.45	4.59	−2.21	35	.033
Homework	3.53	4.73	−1.71	30	.098
Teachers	3.00	4.87	−2.95	30	.006
Clothes	2.05	1.58	.85	35	ns
Chores	2.79	3.63	−1.61	33	ns
Skills	3.85	4.41	−1.15	35	ns
Discipline	4.25	4.18	.15	35	ns
Spending time	4.60	5.12	−.96	35	ns
Babysitters	1.79	1.23	−2.73	31	.010
Initiating intimate contact					
Husband					
Plan date	4.80	4.82	−.06	41	ns
Anniversary	4.24	5.00	−1.88	23	.072
I love you	4.95	5.17	−.59	41	ns
Extra chores	5.43	4.83	1.54	42	ns
Affection	5.67	5.57	.20	42	ns
Initiating sex	5.86	6.39	−1.09	42	ns
Surprises	5.45	4.61	1.92	41	.062
Wife					
Plan date	4.17	4.68	−1.02	46	ns
Anniversary	4.78	4.64	.44	46	ns
I love you	4.65	5.00	−1.01	46	ns
Extra chores	4.04	5.04	−2.55	46	.014
Affection	4.70	5.28	−1.21	46	ns
Initiating sex	5.36	6.04	−1.28	45	ns
Surprises	4.26	4.89	−1.34	46	ns

*$p < .05$.   **$p < .01$.   ***$p < .001$.

the way of intimacy between spouses. However, these negative emotions do not arise from out of nowhere. These data show that there are clear and consistent gender inequities in a marriage that have profound consequences for the happiness of women. These effects suggest several prescriptions for both men and women.

Prescription 1: Stating complaints. Women need to be aware of the gender differences in responses to intense negative affect and confrontations. We have found that the greater tendency of men to withdraw is related to feeling flooded by their wives' negative affect (see Gottman, in press), and that men are flooded by less intense negativity than women (for men, flooding can be predicted from just criticism, for women it needs to be at least contempt). It is important for the future health of the marriage for women to confront the differences between them and their partners (Gottman and Krokoff, 1989). However, it appears that although this confrontation can involve complaint, anger, and disagreement, it ought not to involve criticism, contempt, and disgust. This latter statement is a prescription for both genders.

Prescription 2: Responding to complaints. For the future stability of the marriage, men in particular need to be better listeners, and they specifically need to be engaged listeners rather than withdrawn and disapproving listeners. They also need to respond nondefensively to their partner's complaints. This may also mean avoiding feeling flooded by their wife's complaints. Perhaps the strong negative emotion that often accompanies a complaint could be viewed by men as an "underliner" that expresses the importance of the feeling, that is, an attention-getter. Whatever device they use, men need to avoid withdrawing from their wives' expressions of intense negative emotions.

Prescription 3: Equalizing allocation of family work. Men need to do more housework, child care, and affectional maintenance if they wish to have a happy wife. It is clear from the analyses presented in this chapter that women suffer greatly from these inequities. Furthermore, women engage in a kind of conflict avoidance of their own, rather than confront their husbands with their complaints about these inequities, women tend to suppress their own frustration, and perhaps feel some guilt about their resentments as well. Thompson and Walker (1982), in a review of sociological studies, have shown that whereas women are happier in egalitarian marriages, women do not generally demand such marriages from their partners. Hochschild and Machung (1989) found that far more married women were equalitarian than were husbands, but that women generally accommodated to their husbands' traditional views by doing the "second shift" alone, with a resultant high level of resentment.

It appears that it is the husbands' beliefs about allocation of family work that determines the level of sharing (Hiller & Philliber, 1986). Although higher earnings by wives seem to buy them more decision making at home (Blumstein & Schwartz, 1983), it does not seem to result in more housework or child care by husbands. Despite the connection for women between the degree of sharing family work and their own marital satisfaction, women may be ambivalent about asking men to do housework or child care. Perhaps women are aware that men view their wives' working as something they give to themselves (not to the family; Weiss, 1987) or that husbands' view wives' careers as causing more family stress than their own careers (Baruch & Barnett, 1986). Women may be well aware of unfairness in the division of home labor, but feel helpless to change the situation. The attempts to share bring more conflict (Benin & Agostinelli, 1988; Russell & Radin, 1983) and lower levels of husbands' marital happiness (Crouter et. al., 1987), and may result in women giving in. Barrett and McIntosh (1982) demonstrated men's tendency to ask for multiple directions and to give help of a quality not acceptable to many wives. Feree (1987) suggested that men do so little family work that it is not worth it to women to jeopardize their domestic control just to get a little relief.

It is clear that this chapter's suggestions about the effects of childhood sex segregation and its possible root causes continue to have reverberations in marriages that are related to women's marital unhappiness and to the longitudinal instability of marriages. We are probably living through a period of adjustment of major inequities in cross-sex relationships, in which men need to learn about the areas of competence with emotions that the women they married have. Men also need to learn how to truly share power with women within families if they are interested in their wives' happiness and in the longitudinal stability of their marriages. It may also be the case that our society needs to take a proactive look at how the genders are separately socialized with respect to emotion, and how they are segregated by sex. Perhaps a passive attitude toward these separate socialization phenomena are part of the root causes for why men and women have such difficulty relating to and understanding one another. Although these phenomena may be part of our heritage and may have had some functional value at one time, their current value is unclear, particularly if we want families to survive.

References

Aitken, S. (1977). *Gender preference in infancy.* Master's thesis, University of Edinburgh. Cited in Bower (1989).

Aries, E. (1976). Interaction patterns and themes of male, female, and mixed groups. *Small Group Behavior, 7,* 7–18.

Barnett, R., & Baruch, G. (1987). Mother's participation in child care: Patterns and consequences. In F. Crosby (Ed.), *Spouse, parent, worker: On gender and multiple roles.* New Haven, CT: Yale University Press.

Barrett, M., & McIntosh, M. (1982). *The anti-social family.* London: Verso.

Baruch, G., & Barnett, R. (1986). Consequence of fathers' participation in family work: Parents' role strain and well-being. *Journal of Personality and Social Psychology, 51,* 983–992.

Benin, M., & Agostinelli, J. (1988). Husbands' and wives' satisfaction with the division of labor. *Journal of Marriage and the Family, 50,* 349–361.

Berk, S. (1985). *The gender factory: The apportionment of work in American households.* New York: Plenum.

Bernard, J. (1982) *The future of marriage.* New Haven, CT: Yale University Press.

Bloom, B., Asher, S., & White, S. (1978). Marital disruption as a stressor: A review and analysis. *Psychological Bulletin, 85,* 867–894.

Bloom, B., Hodges, W. F., Caldwell, R. A., Systra, L., & Cedrone, A. R. (1977). Marital separation: A community survey. *Journal of Divorce, 1,* 7–19.

Blumstein, P., & Schwartz, P. (1983). *American couples.* New York: William and Morrow.
Bower, T. G. R. (1989). *The rational infant: Learning in infancy.* New York: W. H. Freeman.
Buck, R. (1975). Nonverbal communication of affect in children. *Journal of Personality and Social Psychology, 31,* 644–653.
Burgess, E. W., Locke, H. J., & Thomes, M. M. (1971). *The family from institution to companionship.* New York: American Book.
Cherlin, A. (1981). *Marriage, divorce, remarriage.* Cambridge, MA: Harvard University Press.
Christensen, A. (1988). Dysfunctional interaction patterns in couples. In P. Noller & M. A. Fitzpatrick (Eds.), *Perspectives on marital interaction* (pp. 31–52). Philadelphia: Multilingual Matters.
Christensen, A. (1991, October). *The demand withdraw pattern in marital interaction.* Paper presented at the annual meeting of the Association for the Advancement of Behavior Therapy, New York City.
Christensen, A., & Heavey, C. L. (1990). Situation versus personality in marital conflict. *Journal of Personality and Social Psychology, 59,* 73–81.
Crosby, F. (1991). *Juggling: The unexpected advantages of balancing career and home for women and their families.* New York: Free Press.
Crouter, A., Perry-Jenkins, T., Huston, T., & McHale, S. (1987). Processes underlying father involvement in dual-career and single-earner families. *Developmental Psychology, 23,* 431–440.
Easterbrooks, M. A. (1987, April). *Early family development: Longitudinal impact of marital quality.* Paper presented at the Meeting of the Society for Research in Child Development. Baltimore, MD.
Easterbrooks, M. A., & Emde, R. A. (1988). Marital and parent-child relationships: The role of affect in the family system. In R. A. Hinde & J. Stevenson-Hinde (Eds.), *Relationships within families: Mutual influence.* Oxford: Clarenden Press.
Elder, G. H., Jr. (1984). *Children of the great depression.* Chicago: University of Chicago Press.
Emery, R. E. (1988). *Marriage, divorce, and children's adjustment.* Newbury Park, CA: Sage.
Emery, R. E., & O'Leary, K. D. (1982). Children's perceptions of marital discord and behavior problems of boys and girls. *Journal of Abnormal Child Psychology, 10,* 11–24.
Feree, M. (1976). The view from below: Women's employment and gender equality in working-class families. In B. Hess & M. Sussman (Eds.), *Women and the family: Two decades of change.* New York: Haworth Press.
Forehand, R., Brody, G., Long, N., Slotkin, J., & Fauber, R. (1986). Divorce/divorce potential and interparental conflict: The relationship to early adolescent social and cognitive functioning. *Journal of Adolescent Research, 1,* 389–397.
Gilligan, C. (1982). *In a different voice: Psychological theory and women's development.* Cambridge, MA: Harvard University Press.
Glick, P. C. (1984). How American families are changing. *American Demographics, 6,* 20–27.
Goodenough, F. L. (1931). *Anger in young children.* Minneapolis: University of Minnesota Press.
Gottman, J. M. (1979). *Marital interaction: Experimental investigations.* New York: Academic Press.
Gottman, J. M. (1986). The world of coordinated play: Same and cross-sex friendship in young children. In J. Gottman and J. Parker (Eds.), *Conversations of friends.* New York: Cambridge University Press.
Gottman, J. M. (in press). *What predicts divorce?* Hillsdale, NJ: Lawrence Erlbaum.
Gottman, J. M., & Katz, L. (1989). Effects of marital discord on young children's peer interaction and health. *Developmental Psychology, 25,* 373–381.
Gottman, J. M., & Krokoff, L. J. (1989). The relationship between marital interaction and marital satisfaction: A longitudinal view. *Journal of Consulting and Clinical Psychology, 57,* 47–52.

Gottman, J. M., & Levenson, R. W. (1985). A valid procedure for obtaining self-report of affect in marital interaction. *Journal of Consulting and Clinical Psychology, 53,* 151–160.

Gottman, J. M., & Levenson, R. W. (1988). The social psychophysiology of marriage. In P. Noller & M. A. Fitzpatrick (Eds.), *Perspectives on marital interaction* (pp. 182–200). Clevedon, England: Multilingual Matters.

Gottman, J. M., & Levenson, R. W. (1992). Marital processes predictive of later dissolution: Behavior, physiology, and health. *Journal of Personality and Social Psychology, 63,* 221–233.

Gottman, J. M., Markman, J., & Notarius, C. (1977). The topography of marital conflict: A sequential analysis of verbal and nonverbal behavior. *Journal of Marriage and the Family, 39,* 461–477.

Hall, J. A. (1984). *Nonverbal sex differences.* Baltimore: Johns Hopkins University Press.

Harrell, A. (1986). Do liberated women drive their husbands to drink? The impact of masculine orientation, status inconsistency, and family life satisfaction on male liquor consumption. *International Journal of the Addictions, 21,* 385–391.

Hauser, S. T., Powers, S. I., Weiss-Perry, B., Follansbee, D. J., Rajapark, D., & Greene, W. M. (1987). *The constraining and enabling coding system.* Unpublished manuscript.

Hetherington, E. M., Cox, M., & Cox, R. (1978). The aftermath of divorce. In J. H. Stevens, Jr. & M. Matthews (Eds.), *Mother–child, father–child relations.* Washington, D.C.: National Association for the Education of Young Children.

Hetherington, E. M., Cox, M., & Cox, R. (1982). *Effects of divorce on parents and children.* In M. Lamb (Ed.), *Nontraditional families* (pp. 233–288). Hillsdale, NJ: Lawrence Erlbaum.

Hiller, D., & Philliber, W. (1986). The division of labor in contemporary marriage: Expectations, perceptions, and performance. *Social Problems, 33,* 191–201.

Hochschild, A., & Machung, A. (1989). *The second shift: Working parents and the revolution at home.* New York: Viking.

Howes, P., & Markman, H. J. (1989). Marital quality and child functioning: A longitudinal investigation. *Child Development, 60,* 1044–1051.

Hoyenga, K. B., & Hoyenga, K. T. (1979). *The question of sex differences.* Boston: Little Brown and Co.

Jacklin, C. N., & Maccoby, E. E. (1978). Social behavior at 33 months in same-sex and mixed-sex dyads. *Child Development, 49,* 557–569.

Katz, L. F., & Gottman, J. M. (1991a). Marital discord and child outcomes: A social psychophysiological approach. In K. Dodge & J. Garber (Eds.), *The development of emotion regulation and disregulation.* New York: Cambridge University Press.

Katz, L. F. & Gottman, J. M. (1991b, April). *Marital interaction processes and preschool children's peer interactions and emotional development.* Paper presented at the meeting of the Society for Research in Child Development. Seattle, WA.

Kelley, H. H., Cunningham, J. D., Chrisham, J. A., Lefebvre, L. M., Sink, C. R., & Yablon, J. (1978). Sex differences in comments made during conflict within close heterosexual pairs. *Sex Roles, 4* (August), 473–492.

Krokoff, L. J., Gottman, J. M., & Haas, S. D. (1989). Validation of a rapid couples interaction scoring system. *Behavioral Assessment, 11,* 65–79.

Lewis, M., & Brooks, J. (1975). Infants' social perception: A constructivist view. In L. B. Cohen and P. Salapatek (Eds.), *Infant perception: From sensation to cognition* (Vol. 2). New York: Academic Press.

Levenson, R. W., & Gottman, J. M. (1983). Marital interaction: Physiological linkage and affective exchange. *Journal of Personality and Social Psychology, 45,* 587–597.

Levenson, R. W., & Gottman, J. M. (1985). Physiological and affective predictors of change in relationship satisfaction. *Journal of Personality of Social Psychology, 49,* 85–94.

Lever, J. (1976). Sex differences in the games children play. *Social Problems, 23,* 478–487.

Locke, H. J. (1951). *Predicting adjustments in marriage: A comparison of a divorced and a happily married group.* New York: Henry Holt.

Locke, H. J., & Wallace, K. M. (1959). Short marital adjustment and prediction tests: Their reliability and validity. *Marriage and Family Living, 21,* 251–255.

Maccoby, E. E. (1990). Gender and relationships: A developmental account. *American Psychologist, 45,* 513–520.

Maccoby, E. E., & Jacklin, C. N. (1974). *The psychology of sex differences.* Stanford, CA: Standford University Press.

Martin, T. C., & Bumpass, L. L. (1989). Recent trends in marital disruption. *Demography, 26,* 37–51.

Mirowsky, J. (1985). Depression and marital power: An equity model. *American Journal of Sociology, 91,* 557–591.

Patterson, G. R. (1982). *Coercive family process.* Eugene, OR: Castalia.

Pleck, J. (1985). *Working wives/working husbands.* Beverly Hills, CA: Sage.

Raush, H. L., Barry, W. A., Hertel, R. K., & Swain, M. A. (1974). *Communication, conflict, and marriage.* San Francisco: Jossey-Bass.

Revenstorf, D., Vogel, B., Wegener, R., Halweg, K., & Schindler, L. (1980). Escalation phenomena in interaction sequences: An empirical comparison of distressed and nondistressed couples. *Behavior Analysis and Modification, 2,* 97–116.

Rickelman, K. E. (1981). *Childhood cross-sex friendships: An investigation of trends and possible explanatory theories.* Unpublished honors thesis, University of Illinois, Champaign.

Russell, G., & Radin, N. (1983). Increased paternal participation: The father's perspective. In M. E. Lamb & A. Sagi (Eds.), *Fatherhood and family policy.* Hillsdale, NJ: Lawrence Erlbaum.

Sarbin, L. A., Sprafkin, C., Elman, M., & Doyle, A. (1984). The early development of sex differentiated patterns of social influence. *Canadian Journal of Social Science, 14,* 350–363.

Schaap, C. (1982). *Communication and adjustment in marriage.* The Netherlands: Swets and Feitlinger.

Schaap, C., Buunk, B., & Kerkstra, A. (1988). Marital conflict resolution. In P. Noller & M. A. Fitzpatrick (Eds.), *Perspectives on marital interaction* (pp. 203–244). Philadelphia: Multilingual Matters.

Staines, G., & Libby, P. (1986). Men and women in role relationships. In R. Ashmore & F. DelBocca (Eds.), *The social psychology of female–male relationships: A critical analysis of central concepts.* New York: Academic Press.

Sutton-Smith, B., Rosenberg, G. G., & Morgan, E. (1963). The development of sex differences in play choices during preadolescence. *Child Development, 34,* 119–126.

Terman, L. M., Buttenweiser, P., Ferguson, L. W., Johnson, W. B., & Wilson, D. P. (1938). *Psychological factors in marital happiness.* New York: McGraw-Hill.

Thompson, L., & Walker, A. J. (1982). The dyad as the unit of analysis. Conceptual and methodological issues. *Journal of Marriage and the Family, 44,* 889–900.

Thorne, B. (1986). Boys and girls together . . . But mostly apart: Gender arrangements in elementary schools. In W. W. Hartup & Z. Rubin (Eds.), *Relationships and development* (pp. 167–184). Hillsdale, NJ: Lawrence Erlbaum.

VanFossen, B. (1981). Sex differences in the mental health effects of spouse support and equity. *Journal of Health and Social Behavior, 22,* 130–143.

Weiss, R. (1987). Men and their wives' work. In F. J. Crosby (Ed.), *Spouse, parent, worker: On gender and multiple roles* (pp. 22–47). New Haven, CT: Yale Univ. Press.

Dialectical Approaches

A Dialogic Approach
to Relationship Maintenance

Leslie A. Baxter

Department of Rhetoric and Communication
University of California, Davis
Davis, California

Introduction

The central assumption of this chapter is that personal relationships are indeterminate processes of ongoing flux. Dialogism, a particular variant of dialectical theory associated with the social theorist and literary critic Mikhail Bakhtin, grounds this assumption of indeterminacy. Relational maintenance, conceived dialogically, is the process of coping with the ceaseless change that results from the struggle of contradictory tendencies inherent in relating. Dialogical maintenance thus fits neither maintenance nor repair concepts as these are typically defined in existing research and scholarship on personal relationships. *Maintenance*, typically conceived as preventive efforts to preserve or sustain a relationship's current state (Ayres, 1983; Bell, Daly & Gonzalez, 1987; Canary & Stafford, 1992, 1993; Dindia, 1989; Dindia & Baxter, 1987; Shea & Pearson, 1986; Stafford & Canary, 1991), presupposes that a condition of stability is both possible and desirable for personal relationships. *Repair*, typically conceived as problem-solving efforts to restore or return a relationship to a former state (e.g., Dindia & Baxter, 1987), presupposes that it is possible and desirable for a relationship to go back to a former state. From a dialogic perspective, these conceptions of maintenance and repair are neither possible nor desirable; a healthy relationship is a changing relationship in which a stable state is nonexistent.

Because parties maintain their relationship dynamically by responding to the dialectical exigencies of the relational moment, some might be tempted to position dialogic maintenance as a subset of the repair domain. However, the problems addressed in the repair literature are typically incidental and idiosyncratic from one relationship to another. Further, repair-oriented problems potentially can be resolved permanently by the relationship parties. By contrast, dialectical problems are inherent to relating and ongoing within the normal boundaries of healthy relationship functioning.

One additional difference between dialogic maintenance and nondialogic maintenance/repair warrants mention. As typically conceived, maintenance and repair are temporally positioned in the *middle passage* of a relationship's history, marking the period between *development* and *termination*. Dialogic maintenance disallows such temporal placement, because dialectical pressures are present in some form throughout the entire history of a relationship's existence.

The remainder of this chapter provides an elaboration of the concept of "dialogic maintenance." The first section summarizes key elements of Bakhtin's theory of dialogism which hold relevance for understanding relational maintenance. The second section discusses six contradictions that constitute important relational sites where ongoing dialectical change occurs. The third section discusses directions for future maintenance research from a dialogic perspective.

"Dialogue," Dialogism, and Dialectics

Bakhtin, who produced the majority of his work during the 1920s and 1930s in the Soviet Union, has been hailed by some as one of the foremost intellectual forces of the twentieth century (e.g., Holquist, 1990; Morson & Emerson, 1990; Todorov, 1984). Along the continuum of theory from "narrow" to "middle-range" to "grand" (Skinner, 1985), Bakhtin's diverse theoretical writings about art, literature, religion, culture, and language are best regarded as "grand theory." It is probably fair to say that Bakhtin's dialogism is best known in the academy among literary critics, but his work is receiving growing attention among social scientists as well (e.g., Heath, 1992). Bakhtin did not write on the topic of human relationships, although dialogism can easily be extended to this domain (Baxter, 1993, in press).

The "dialogue" is the centerpiece of dialogism. To Bakhtin, the essential quality of a dialogue was its simultaneous fusion or unity of multiple voices at the same time that each voice retained its differentiated uniqueness. This dynamic tension between fusion-with and differentiation-from the Other served for Bakhtin (1981, p. 272) as a general metaphor for all social processes which he characterized as "a contradiction-ridden, tension-filled unity of two embattled tendencies": the centripetal (i.e., centralizing, unifying forces) and the centrifugal (i.e., decentralizing, differentiating forces). In contrast to the centripetal monologue, which is a static and closed system, the centripetal–centrifugal dialogue is an indeterminate process in which meaning and order are in a perpetual state of becoming as a consequence of the struggle of contradiction. At the level of lived experience, sociality in its many forms is characterized by moment-to-moment disorder and flux. Thus, a view of relational maintenance as the period of stability after a relationship has been constructed and before its demise is fundamentally nondialogic in conception.

In addition to its role as the central metaphor of the social world, dialogue in its literal sense also occupies a central role in dialogism. Bakhtin's life-long intellectual project was that of understanding the everyday dynamics of centripetal and centrifugal forces in human interaction, a project which Morson and Emerson (1990) aptly labeled "the creation of a prosaics." As Bakhtin (1981, p. 272) stated, "The processes of centralization and decentralization, of unification and disunification, intersect in the utterance." A dialogic approach to relational maintenance thus looks to the communication practices of relationship parties as the primary arena where contradictions are revealed.

Focus on Contradiction

Dialogism is clearly dialectical in the centrality it accords to contradiction. However, Bakhtin (1986, p. 147) was critical of the Hegelian and Marxist dialectical thinking of his time and differentiated his dialogic view on two counts. The first distinction that Bakhtin made between dialogism and dialectics was his emphasis on the process of contradicting rather than on specific contradictions. Bakhtin's emphasis on the contradicting process is useful given the frequency with which dialectical contradiction is mistaken for static, structural duality (Giddens, 1979). In contrast to a duality in which opposites are constituted in parallel, noninteractive structures, the opposing tendencies of contradiction struggle with and against one another for dominance (Cornforth, 1968). The result of such dynamic struggle is that the relation between opposing tendencies is in constant motion.

Bakhtin accomplished his process orientation by granting primacy to the centripetal–centrifugal contradiction as the key organizing feature of social life. The privileging of this abstract contradiction may seem ironic given

Bakhtin's (1986, p. 147) criticism that dialectics reduced contradiction to an abstract concept stripped of complexity and fluidity. However, Bakhtin argued that each pole of the centripetal–centrifugal contradiction is constituted in the contextual, interactive moment and thus is characterized by fluidity. The centripetal pole consists of whatever phenomenon occupies the center or dominant position, for example, normative conventions, the discourse of the majority political party, and so forth. By contrast, the centrifugal pole consists of whatever phenomena are subordinate or peripheral, for example, nonconventionalized behavior, the discourse of the minority political party, and so on. A phenomenon that is characterized as centrifugal at one moment may be characterized as centripetal at another, thereby disallowing a fixed or static conception of the centripetal and centrifugal poles of a contradiction.

The concept of the "dialectical moment" is useful in capturing the relation that exists between the two dialectical poles of a given contradiction at a particular point in time. For ease of discussion, let A and B represent the two dialectical poles of a contradiction. The *Pole A-Dominant Moment* refers to a circumstance in which Pole A dominates Pole B; that is, Pole A successfully negates, undermines, or minimizes the second pole. For example, if A and B stand for interdependence and independence, respectively, this moment would probably be experienced by the relationship parties as excessive interdependence between them at the expense of each party's individual autonomy. The *Pole-B-Dominant Moment* captures a similar circumstance of dominance–subordination, but with Pole B now dominant. For example, the relationship parties would feel as if they are excessively independent from one another at the expense of the relationship's interdependence. A third dialectical moment that seems useful to identify is the *Double-Negation Moment;* this moment captures a complex circumstance in which each pole is successfully negating the other but with neither pole in the position of clear dominance over the other. For example, relationship parties would feel that neither the need for interdependence nor the need for independence was being met adequately because efforts directed at one pole undermined efforts directed at the other pole. Last, it is useful to distinguish a *Moment of Equilibrium* in which neither pole successfully negates or undermines the other. Equilibrium, like all dialectical moments, is not a permanent, stable outcome but can emerge as a temporary interval in the ongoing motion between dialectical poles (Cornforth, 1968). Of course, this fourfold typology of dialectical moments is a gross oversimplification. For example, I assumed that A and B poles vary only quantitatively from one moment to another, ignoring the dialectical possibility that the qualitative essences of both A and B are transformed through the struggle of opposition. Nonetheless, the concept of dialectical moments allows us to capture concretely some of the dialectical snapshots in the ongoing motion of contradiction.

Baxter (1988, 1990) has identified several dialectical coping strategies that are likely to be associated with these four kinds of dialectical moments. Pole A Disequilibrium and Pole B Disequilibrium are likely to correlate with the strategies of Cyclic Alternation and Segmentation. *Cyclic Alternation* involves pendulumlike efforts by the parties to enhance the particular dialectical pole that is subordinate at the moment, followed at a later point in time by efforts to enhance the other dialectical pole once it has become subordinate. *Segmentation* involves efforts by the parties to establish separate domains of their relationship for the fulfillment of each dialectical pole; parties shift from one domain to another in an effort to restore the particular subordinated dialectical pole of the moment. The Double-Negation Moment is probably correlated with Baxter's strategy of Moderation. *Moderation* involves compromise efforts in which neither dialectical pole is fulfilled completely; fulfillment of one pole is sacrificed to some extent in order to partially fulfill the opposing pole, and vice versa. The Moment of Equilibrium is probably correlated with the coping strategies of Disqualification and Reframing. *Disqualification* involves semantic "slippage" through intentional ambiguity or equivocation in order to allow both dialectical poles to be fulfilled. *Reframing* involves a reconceptualization of a contradiction such that the parties no longer perceive the two dialectical poles as opposed to one another, thereby allowing both poles to be fulfilled.

The Concept of Change

The second point of departure from dialectical theory that Bakhtin claimed for dialogism was rejection of the thesis–antithesis–synthesis conception of change in which the struggle of two opposing tendencies is ultimately resolved in a qualitative synthesis. According to Bakhtin, the struggle of centripetal and centrifugal forces is an ongoing dynamic, not a systematic, evolutionary process that necessarily culminates in a state of transcendence to some higher order of development. Although the conception of change as transcendent synthesis is not inherent to dialectical thinking (Rychlak, 1976), transcendent synthesis nonetheless is popularly equated with dialectical thought largely because of the influence of Hegel. In aligning myself with the dialogic variant of the dialectical family, I am rejecting the presumption of a linear, evolutionary path of relational change in which parties necessarily reach some higher, transcendent state where the centripetal–centrifugal contradictions have been resolved.

Dialectical change can take many forms, but two underlying dimensions are important to an understanding of dialogic maintenance in personal relationships. The first dimension captures whether or not the struggle of opposing tendencies is manifested in interpersonal conflict between two relationship parties (Giddens, 1979). If two parties align their respective interests with different poles of a given contradiction (e.g., one party wants more interdependence and the other party wants more autonomy), then the contradiction is likely to involve interpersonal conflict between them. Dialectical theorists refer to this type of contradiction as *antagonistic* (Mao, 1965). Among current dialectical researchers in the area of personal relationships, Conville (1991) and Altman, Vinsel, and Brown (1981) most clearly address antagonistic contradictions. For example, the antagonistic variant of the Openness–Closedness contradiction would be a circumstance in which one party wants more openness between the partners, whereas the other party wants more privacy between them. By contrast, *nonantagonistic* contradictions (Mao, 1965) represent those in which the parties do not align with separate poles. Baxter (1988, 1990, 1992b; Baxter & Widenmann, 1993; Baxter & Simon, 1993; Bridge & Baxter, 1992) and Rawlins (1983a, 1983b, 1989, 1992) most clearly focus on this type of contradiction by examining the dilemmas that both parties experience intrapersonally in fulfilling the two poles of a given contradiction. With respect to the Openness-Closedness contradiction, the nonantagonistic variant would involve a circumstance in which each party is torn between a desire to be open and a desire to be closed in interacting with one another. The catalyst for change differs for antagonistic as opposed to nonantagonistic contradictions. Change occurs in antagonistic contradictions through the interpersonal conflict between the two parties. Change occurs in nonantagonistic contradiction through the internal struggle that each party experiences.

In addition to the distinction between antagonistic and nonantagonistic change, it is useful to distinguish so-called momentous change from nonmomentous change. The distinction I am making between these two types of change corresponds to that made by many dialectical theorists between quantitative and qualitative change (e.g., Cornforth, 1968) and shows similarity, as well, to the distinction between first-order and second-order change in the literature on personal relationships (Conville, 1983). Nonmomentous change refers to tiny, incremental shifts in the dominance–subordination relation of two dialectical poles with no fundamental change in the relationship's dialectical moment. For example, if both parties feel that there is too much autonomy and too little interdependence in their relationship, they might spontaneously decide to go out to dinner one night in order to spend some more time together. The overall effect of a single dinner out is insufficient to transform the fundamental dominance of autonomy over interdependence. By contrast, momentous change refers to a major change in the dominance–subordination relation of the two poles with a transformation of the relationship to a different dialectical moment. Momentous changes appear to be experienced retrospectively by relationship parties as turning points or points of crisis or epiphany in the relationship (Baxter, 1988; Conville, 1991). The couple just described, who spontaneously decided to go out to dinner one night, would likely experience increasingly intensified pressure for more interdependence until a crisis point would be reached. The pair might manage this crisis by fundamentally reorganizing their lives to enable more systematic forms of connection, thereby altering the fundamental balance between autonomy and interdependence.

Consistent with a dialogic world view, I have suggested in this section that relationship maintenance is fundamentally about processes of change rather than stability. Using dialogism's emphasis on the contradicting process as a foundation, I have articulated two underlying dimensions of dialogic maintenance in this section: (1) antagonistic change versus nonantagonistic change, and (2) momentous versus nonmomentous change. Four variants of dialogic maintenance result in the intersection of these two dimensions. Because the focus of dialogism is on the general process of contradicting, context-specific contradictions are understandably outside its scope. However, in the interests of developing a dialogic theory of personal relationships, specific contradictions need explication, and this becomes the task in the next section of this chapter. Bakhtin's emphasis on the contradicting process and the special significance of communication practices in that process constitute an important theoretical backdrop.

The Primary Sites of Dialogic Maintenance

Giddens (1984, p. 198) refers to contradictions as "fault lines," a metaphor which I find useful in framing the six contradictions described in this section. These dialectical tensions do not represent all of the fault lines of relationships, but rather only those of San Andreas magnitude that can be identified from existing scholarship in personal relationships. Fault lines are never static, as any resident of California can quickly testify; similarly, the relational fault lines discussed in this section need to be thought of not as static, structural relations but as dynamic tensions in ongoing flux.

Dialectics and Contradictions

Dialectical flux in personal relationships occurs at three primary sites, which I refer to elsewhere as the Dialectics of Integration–Separation, Stability–Change, and Expression–Privacy (Baxter, 1993). The *Dialectic of Integration–Separation* in its general sense captures the basic tension between social integration and social division; the *Dialectic of Stability–Change* refers to the fundamental opposition between continuity and discontinuity; and last, the *Dialectic of Expression–Privacy* captures a basic oppositional tension between what is said and what is left unsaid.

Each of these basic dialectics is manifested in two forms—internal and external. *Internal contradictions* are constituted within the social unit under study, whereas *external contradictions* are constituted between the social unit and the larger system within which the unit is embedded (Ball, 1979; Riegel, 1976). With respect to personal relationships, an internal contradiction is inherent within the relationship and refers to opposing tendencies, both of which are necessary for intimacy. An external contradiction is inherent between the relationship and the broader social order and refers to opposing tendencies, both of which are necessary to sustain the social order and the relationship's place in it. The following table summarizes the various internal and external manifestations of the three dialectics.

	Dialectic of Integration–Separation	Dialectic of Stability–Change	Dialectic of Expression–Privacy
Internal Manifestations	Connection–Autonomy	Predictability–Novelty	Openness–Closedness
External Manifestations	Inclusion–Seclusion	Conventionality–Uniqueness	Revelation–Concealment

In its internal manifestation, the Dialectic of Integration–Separation refers to the tension between integration and separation of the two relationship parties, that is, the *Connection–Autonomy contradiction*. In its external manifestation, the *Inclusion–Seclusion contradiction*, Integration–Separation takes the form of an oppositional tension between a pair's involvement with their social network versus the isolation of the pair from others. The Dialectic of Stability–Change is manifested internally in the *Predictability–Novelty contradiction*, that is, the basic opposition between a relationship pair's simultaneous needs for predictability, certainty, and routinization, on the one hand, and novelty, stimulation, and spontaneity, on the other hand, as the partners interact with one another. The external manifestation of the Dialectic of Stability–Change is one I label the *Conventionality–Uniqueness contradiction*. On the one hand, the social order is reproduced through the enactment of conventionalized ways of relating from one relationship to another; in complying with such conventions, a pair constructs a public identity for the relationship that is familiar and easily legitimated by others. On the other hand, however, a highly conventionalized relationship denies the parties a sense of their pair uniqueness, a quality which is central to intimacy. Last, the Dialectic of Expression–Privacy in its internal manifestation, the *Openness–Closedness contradiction*, captures the dilemma of candor and discretion faced by the relationship parties in their interactions with one another. In its external manifestation, the *Revelation–Concealment contradiction*, the parties face the dilemma of what to make known about their relationship to outside third parties versus what to keep private between just the two relationship partners. The remainder of this section will summarize existing research for these six contradictions, beginning with the internal contradictions.

Supporting Research

An intimate relationship necessitates that the two parties forsake some of their autonomy in order to construct an interdependent bond; yet too much connection between partners paradoxically can jeopardize that bond because the parties have lost their individual identities. Thus, woven into the very construction of intimacy is the Connection–Autonomy contradiction. Research with friendships and with romantic and marital relationships documents the salience of this contradiction in the everyday lives of relationship partners (Baxter, 1988, 1990; Baxter & Simon, 1993; Bridge & Baxter, 1992; Conville, 1991; Cupach & Metts, 1988; Goldsmith, 1990; Rawlins, 1983a, 1989, 1992). The fact that couples are sometimes unable to manage the Connection–Autonomy contradiction is evident in the research on complaints and breakup accounts among romantic and marital relationships. The inability to meet interdependence needs is evident in such complaints and reasons for breakup as insufficient time together, a lack of partner loyalty and commitment, and disparate relationship needs (Baxter, 1986; Cody, 1982; Cupach & Metts, 1986; Harvey, Wells, & Alvarez, 1978; Hill, Rubin, & Peplau, 1976; Kelley, 1979; Orvis, Kelley, & Butler, 1976; Riessman, 1990). The inability to fulfill autonomy needs is apparent in such expressed complaints and reasons for breakup as the desire for freedom and independence and a feeling of entrapment by the relationship (Baxter, 1986; Cody, 1982; Harvey et al., 1978; Hill et al., 1976; Kelley, 1979; Riessman, 1990).

The Predictability–Novelty contradiction also appears integral to personal relationships. On the one hand, as research under the rubric of uncertainty reduction theory has well documented (Berger & Gudykunst, 1991), conditions of intimacy are facilitated when the parties have certainty and predictability about one another, their interactions together, and the state of their relationship. However, research also documents that parties need the stimulation of spontaneity and novelty to prevent an emotional deadening of affections (e.g., Byrne & Murnen, 1988; Livingston, 1980). Although this contradiction has been studied less extensively than the Autonomy–Connection contradiction, research consistently has found this tension present among romantic and marital relationship parties (Baxter, 1990; Baxter & Simon, 1993; Cupach & Metts, 1988). Both excessive predictability (e.g., Baxter, 1986; Cody, 1982; Cupach & Metts, 1986; Hill et al., 1976) and excessive novelty (e.g., Kelley, 1979; Planalp, Rutherford, & Honeycutt, 1988) have been reported as sources of complaint and breakup by relationship parties.

The last internal contradiction, Openness–Closedness, captures the dilemma that relationship parties face with respect to candor and discretion. A bond of intimacy necessitates open self-disclosure between the relationship parties (e.g., Altman & Taylor, 1973), yet parties have need of individual privacy, as well (e.g., Altman et al., 1981; Petronio, 1991). The Openness–Closedness tension appears to be salient in self-reports by friends, romantic partners, and marital partners (Baxter, 1990; Baxter & Simon, 1993; Bridge & Baxter, 1992; Cupach & Metts, 1988; Rawlins, 1983b, 1989, 1992). Many pairs are unable to manage this contradiction successfully, as evidenced in the reports of communication-based problems in the research on complaints and accounts of breakup (e.g., Baxter, 1986; Cupach & Metts, 1986; Kelley, 1979; Kitson & Sussman, 1982; Riessman, 1990).

Although these three contradictions appear to be pervasive in relating, some research suggests that the salience of a given contradiction will vary systematically by relationship type. Sillars, Weisberg, Burggraf, and Wilson (1987), for instance, have reported that couples who vary with respect to Fitzpatrick's (1988) Martial Types differ in the likelihood that themes of togetherness and separateness surface in their conflict-based conversations. The Sillars et al. study was not framed within the dialectics tradition, but it nonetheless is suggestive of probable differences in how the Autonomy–Connection contradiction is experienced and managed. I suspect that different relationships vary with respect to the other contradictions, as well.

Two studies have systematically examined how each of these three internal contradictions is managed by relationship parties. In the first study (Baxter, 1990), I conducted in-depth, qualitative interviews with 106 respondents who were involved in romantic relationships of at least a 1-month duration. Respondents were asked to divide the natural history of their relationship into as many or as few stages as they thought meaningful and then to discuss their experiences related to each of the three internal contradictions for each stage. Responses were coded using the typology of contradiction-management strategies derived deductively in prior work (Baxter, 1988). The most frequent way of managing the Connection–Autonomy contradiction was Cyclic Alternation, that is, autonomy-enhancing efforts alternating with connection-enhancing efforts in a pendulumlike manner. The most frequent way of coping with both the Predictability–Novelty and Openness–Closedness contradictions was Segmentation, that is, the designation of certain topics or domains as arenas for dominance by one pole of a given contradiction and the designation of other topics and domains as arenas for dominance by the other pole. Both Cyclic Alternation and Segmentation are based on functional specialization, with efforts targeted in a specialized way toward one pole or the other of a given contradiction.

The typology employed in the 1990 study was cast at an abstract level and ignored the concrete behaviors that constitute functional specialization. Further, the typology was developed independent of the research in the strategies of relationship maintenance. In order to examine the maintenance strategies involved in the management of internal contradictions, a colleague and I (Baxter & Simon, 1993) recently asked the 324 partners from romantic and marital relationships to report their current satisfaction with the relationship and their perceptions of the partner's relationship maintenance strategies. These respondents also completed a series of Likert-type items that allowed us to divide respondents into Pole A-dominant and Pole B-dominant dialectical-moment groups for each of the internal contradictions. Perceived partner efforts to increase contact were more strongly correlated with participant satisfaction for respondents in the autonomy-dominant moment than for respondents in the connection-dominant moment. Partner efforts to increase contact clearly functioned to enhance connection, a desirable outcome under circumstances of excessive autonomy. Perceived partner romantic efforts were more strongly correlated with participant satisfaction for respondents in the predictability-dominant moment in contrast to respondents in the novelty-dominant moment. Romantic efforts typically involved such spontaneous and creative actions as surprising one's partner with a candlelight dinner; understandably, such efforts served to alleviate the boredom that is characteristic of the predictability-dominant moment. Last, perceived partner avoidance of communication about relational problems was reacted to more negatively by respondents in the closedness-dominant moment in contrast to respondents in the openness-dominant moment. For respondents already experiencing insufficient openness, evidence of further avoidance of communication by the partner understandably evoked a negative reaction. Overall, these findings support the notion of functional specialization previously discussed; relationship maintenance strategies appear to function in specialized ways that are targeted toward one of the two dialectical poles of a given contradiction.

Personal relationships are embedded in webs of sociality, yet simultaneously they are isolated havens of privacy for the two parties. The Inclusion–Seclusion contradiction thus is built into the very fabric of relating. On the one hand, a relationship requires legitimation and support from others (Parks & Eggert, 1991), and such legitimation is obtained, in part,

.through the everyday integration of the relationship pair into social networks of family and friends (Lewis, 1973). By responding to a relationship pair as a single social unit, others grant social recognition and support to the relationship; reciprocally, in interacting as a single unit with others, relationship parties affirm to themselves, as well as to others, their relationship identity. In addition, because excessive predictability can become problematic for long-term married relationships (Baxter & Simon, 1993), pair integration with others can potentially provide an important source of stimulation and novelty for a couple. On the other hand, however, relationship partners need social isolation and privacy from others in order to construct and sustain their dyadic culture (Baxter, 1987; Lewis, 1972; McCall, 1970). Couples experience difficulty in fulfilling the demands of both inclusion and seclusion, as evidenced in the literature on complaints and breakups. In expressing such complaints as "not enough social life" and "no sense of family" (Kitson & Sussman, 1982), former spouses testify to the difficulties associated with pair seclusion. By contrast, the problems posed by integration are evident in complaints such as excessive time spent as a couple with extended kin (Riessman, 1990) or accounts by remarried spouses of efforts by stepchildren to undermine the solidarity of their marriage (Cissna, Cox, & Bochner, 1990).

Although relationship parties need to manage the simultaneous demands for both inclusion and seclusion, our understanding of the maintenance strategies by which this is executed is relatively limited. Nevertheless, existing research in the social networks tradition provides us with a general profile of the pattern of inclusion and seclusion for developing romantic relationships. A romantic pair tends to develop an overlapping social network as their relationship develops (Kim & Stiff, 1991; Parks & Eggert, 1991), providing the parties with structural opportunities to interact jointly with others who know them as a couple. When relationship parties do spend time with social network members, such interaction increasingly takes the form of joint appearances with the partner as relationship closeness intensifies (Baxter & Widenmann, 1993). However, the amount of leisure time spent with social network members, as opposed to time spent alone with the partner, appears to decline overall with relationship development (Surra, 1985). Such withdrawal from integration may account for Stafford and Canary's (1991) finding that married couples more so than dating couples reported inclusion with the joint network as maintenance effort directed toward the relationship's well-being. Overall, the relationship maintenance strategies of withdrawal from the network and romantic efforts appear to be reported more for respondents experiencing excessive inclusion as opposed to excessive seclusion (Baxter, 1992b).

The external contradiction of Conventionality–Uniqueness has been variously referred to among relationship dialectical theorists as the Communality–

Identity contradiction (Altman & Gauvain, 1981), the contextual dialectics of Public–Private and Ideal–Real (Rawlins, 1989, 1992), and the Connection–Autonomy contradiction (Montgomery, 1992). Despite this profusion of labels, the fundamental tension is that of conformity to conventionalized ways of relating versus construction of a unique relationship identity. From a macro perspective, the society reproduces itself to the extent that each relationship adopts conventional forms and practices of relating; yet conventionality dampens exploration of alternative ways of relating, which could prove adaptive for the society in the long run (Montgomery, 1992). From the perspective of a given relationship pair, conformity to social expectations increases the likelihood that they will be understood and legitimated by others, yet at the same time, intimacy is based in part on a pair's sense of themselves as totally unique from all other relationships (Baxter, 1987; Mc-Call, 1970; Owen, 1984).

The Conventionality–Uniqueness contradiction is likely to be particularly salient for parties whose personal relationship has a role-based component, for example, family members who are business associates, spouses who are co-workers, and so forth. The pair is constrained not only by the conventions for personal relationships, but it additionally faces the expectations associated with the role relationship, and these two sets of expectations are often incompatible with one another. A colleague and I (Bridge & Baxter, 1992) recently examined a relationship type in which we correctly anticipated that the Conventionality–Uniqueness contradiction would be particularly salient, that is, close friends who simultaneously are work associates. The most frequent contradiction experienced by our sample of 162 adults was that of Impartiality–Favoritism, a variant of Conventionality–Uniqueness. On the one hand, the conventions of the workplace involved expectations that work associates would treat one another with impartiality and with the absence of favoritism (i.e., an expectation of non-Uniqueness). Yet, on the other hand, the expectations of close friendship also involved the belief that friends should recognize one another's unique needs and circumstances. Friends allowed their personal relationship to show on the job when they felt their immediate work group was cohesive; otherwise, and particularly if the pair occupied a superior–subordinate work relationship, the conventions associated with the work relationship prevailed in the workplace despite the perception that the friendship was potentially beneficial to work performance.

The Conventionality–Uniqueness contradiction is probably the most amenable of all of the external contradictions to a coping strategy of integrative Reframing, that is, a transformation in which the two poles are no longer regarded as oppositional to one another (Baxter, 1988, 1990). For example, pair uniqueness would be regarded as a conventionalized norm of relating. The basis of this transformation lies with the central role which selfhood plays in the perception of relationship uniqueness. A number of cultural analysts (e.g., Carbaugh, 1988; Katriel & Philipsen, 1981) have recently observed that contemporary American conventions for personal relationships celebrate individual selfhood. Thus, relationship parties can conform to these conventions in celebrating one another's individual selves and thereby construct the basis of their uniqueness as a relationship pair.

Of the three external contradictions, the most research has been done with respect to the Revelation–Concealment contradiction. On the one hand, the bond of intimacy necessitates a norm of confidentiality between the two relationship parties (e.g., Krain, 1977). On the other hand, relationships are social entities that benefit from the legitimation and support provided by others, and others are positioned to provide such affirmation only if they have knowledge of the relationship's existence and status. Four studies (Baxter & Widenmann, 1993; Goldsmith, 1988; Goldsmith & Parks, 1990; Holland & Eisenhart, 1990) have examined the reasons people identify for revealing and concealing relational information to friends and family.

Consistently, results indicate that the oppositional tension between revelation and concealment is salient to relationship parties. First, parties are predisposed to inform others in order to gain their emotional or material support. Research tends to support the wisdom of this motive in documenting the benefits which relationships reap from social network support (e.g., Parks & Eggert, 1991). On the other hand, relationship parties are apprehensive about revealing their relationship because of anticipated nonsupport from others. This apprehension appears well founded given the research on perceived network interference (e.g., Johnson & Milardo, 1984; Leslie, Huston, & Johnson, 1986). Second, relationship parties are motivated to reveal their relationship out of sheer catharsis or joy of expression, yet they are also fearful of losing control over relational information once it becomes gossip among social network members. Because the relationships of fellow network members appear to be a frequent topic of discussion among friends (see, e.g., Holland & Eisenhart, 1990), this apprehension seems well founded. Third, parties are motivated to reveal relational information because they think it is expected of or desirable for their relationship with the recipient of the information; at the same time, parties are motivated to conceal information because they anticipate that revelation would be inappropriate or would otherwise hurt the recipient or the relationship with the recipient. Finally, parties are motivated to reveal their relationship because they think that "going public" is expected of, or desirable for, the relationship with their partner; yet, at the same time, parties are hesitant to reveal relational information because they think it could violate the confidentiality established between the two partners.

Although relationship parties unwittingly reveal the status of their relationship to observant third parties through a variety of verbal and nonverbal leakages (Goffman, 1971), we know substantially less about how relationship parties strategically manage the information that is available to others. In a questionnaire study in which married and nonmarried respondents were asked to report on their relationship maintenance strategies and their perceptions of the state of their relationship with respect to the three external contradictions, Baxter (1992b) found that respondents experiencing excessive revelation were less likely than respondents experiencing excessive privacy to report disclosure to third parties and more likely to withdraw from couple-based interactions with third parties. These results suggest dialectical management of the Revelation–Concealment contradiction through the overarching strategy of Cyclic Alternation, with use of efforts which alternate between revelation-enhancing and concealment-enhancing functions depending on the particular dialectical moment.

In a qualitatively based study, a colleague and I (Baxter & Widenmann, 1993) conducted in-depth interviews with romantically involved respondents in order to determine what, how, and to whom relational information was revealed and concealed. In general, we found a differentiated pattern of information management that bears resemblance to the Segmentation strategy previously discussed; respondents established some target recipients and some topics as more appropriate for revelation and other targets and topics as less appropriate. In particular, we found that parents were the targets of proportionately more acts of concealment than were other social network members, whereas close friends were the targets of proportionately fewer acts of concealment. At least in part, this difference was attributable to an expectation of less support from parents than from friends. With respect to kind of information, two topics differed in their likelihood of revelation as opposed to concealment. Not surprisingly, sexual activity was more likely to be concealed than revealed. Information about the partner's background, personality, and other attributes was also more likely to be revealed than concealed, a finding which suggests that parties regard themselves in the business of promoting their partner, not defending his or her character weaknesses. The results of this study are consistent with other research (Goldsmith & Parks, 1990; Leslie et al., 1986) in pointing to the varied communication repertoire available to relationship parties in managing the strategic revelation and concealment of information. In particular, respondents controlled information availability through the following six communicative tactics: (1) verbal description (e.g., disclosures of relationship information), (2) co-presence (e.g., joint appearances as a "couple" at various public events), (3) use of conventionalized relationship labels (e.g., introducing the partner as one's "boyfriend" or "girlfriend"), (4) overt verbal and nonverbal display of affection (e.g., use of affectionate nicknames or hand holding), (5) display of material objects that were associated with the partner (e.g., wearing a ring), and (6) manipulation of the situation in order to use third parties as information conduits (e.g., telling third-party gossips some relationship information with the expectation that they would transmit the information to others).

Summary

In this section, I have moved toward the articulation of a dialogic theory of personal relationships in presenting three sites where dialogic maintenance occurs: Dialectics of Integration–Separation, Stability–Change, and Expression–Privacy. Each of these dialectics is manifested in both internal and external contradictions. The bulk of research efforts to date have been devoted to the descriptive task of documenting that these six contradictions are experienced in people's relational lives, with some secondary attention to how these contradictions are managed. The last section of this chapter addresses possible directions for future research.

What Next?

The most obvious direction for future research in this dialogic perspective on maintenance is linking the process-oriented issues discussed in the first section with the six dialectical contradictions presented in the second section. The struggle of a given contradiction could be momentous or nonmomentous at a given point in a relationship's history and thus might involve different maintenance practices. I suspect, for example, that the maintenance strategies of increasing contact and romantic efforts might suffice for dialectical struggles of a nonmomentous nature but might be inadequate for dialectical tensions that are of crisis proportions for the couple. Similarly, antagonistic and nonantagonistic forms of dialectical flux might necessitate different maintenance efforts by the relationship parties. On its face, for example, it strikes me as a qualitatively different matter when both parties are experiencing excessive connection as opposed to a circumstance in which one party desires more autonomy and the other party is satisfied with the current state of interdependence.

Although dialogic maintenance is posited as an ongoing dynamic throughout a relationship's history, researchers need to examine the extent to which parties cope differently over time with a given contradiction. In finding that the two poles of the Connection–Autonomy contradiction do not mean the same thing to romantic partners at different developmental stages, Goldsmith (1990) usefully demonstrated that indeterminacy in a contradiction can take qualitative form. As a consequence of ongoing dialectical struggle, the two poles of a different contradiction become altered not only quantitatively in their dominance–subordination relation, but qualitatively as well. Research needs to examine the indeterminacy of the constituent poles of the other contradictions, exploring variations in their meanings and how such variations are related to maintenance efforts by the relationship parties.

Relationships and individuals are likely to vary systematically in how dialectical flux is experienced and managed. As previously discussed, some research is already suggestive of relationship-type differences with respect to the internal contradiction of Connection–Autonomy. Future research needs to address systematically possible relationship differences in both internal and external contradictions. I suspect, for example, that relationships which are characterized by different trajectories of development (e.g., Surra, 1985) might experience and manage dialectical flux in systematically different ways. In addition, a variety of individual-differences variables are likely to be relevant to how dialectical flux is experienced and managed, for example, attachment style, tolerance for ambiguity, and cognitive complexity.

Dialectically oriented scholars in the personal relationships field have focused the majority of their attention to date on the internal manifestations of the Dialectics of Integration–Separation, Stability–Change, and Expression–Privacy. Such a focus is not surprising given the general tendency for researchers to ignore context factors that affect relationships in favor of studying factors internal to the dyad itself (Parks & Eggert, 1991). Future research obviously needs to redress this imbalance.

Future research also needs to move closer toward achieving the dialectical principle of "totality," that is, the assumption that a given contradiction does not function in isolation but is dynamically interdependent with other contradictions (Rawlins, 1989). Existing dialectical research tends to focus on contradictions as they function independently of one another. The three internal contradictions are likely to be interdependent with one another (e.g., Baxter, 1988), just as the three external contradictions are likely to be interdependent with one another (e.g., Baxter, 1992b, 1993). Further, internal and external contradictions probably function in highly interdependent ways. For example, I have suggested that insufficient inclusion with others is likely to correlate with excessive predictability between relational partners.

The six contradictions discussed in the second section of this chapter should not be interpreted as exhaustive. Although my own dialectical work tends to focus in an a priori manner on these contradictions, other dialectical researchers such as Conville (1991) and Rawlins (1992) have productively identified additional dialectical tensions that are important in dialogic maintenance, for example, time-related oppositions such as the past versus the present, or affect-based oppositions such as positivity–negativity or judgment–acceptance.

In addition to these theoretically substantive concerns, three methodological issues need research attention from a dialogic perspective. As part of the broader effort to understand the efficacy of maintenance strategies under different moments of dialectical flux, researchers could benefit from reexamining the corpus of maintenance strategies that are often employed in maintenance research. Maintenance strategies research (e.g., Baxter & Dindia, 1990; Canary & Stafford, 1992, 1993; Dindia, 1989; Dindia & Baxter, 1987; Stafford & Canary, 1991) has developed a set of strategies that were elicited by asking romantic and marital parties what they do in general to maintain their relationships. Such an elicitation procedure may be systematically biased against localized strategies which are effective in response to very particular dialectical exigencies. As a result, existing maintenance research may be tapping only a portion of the strategy repertoire available to relationship parties.

A second methodological issue is the need for longitudinal research. Both dialectical researchers and maintenance researchers have relied, to date, on cross-sectional or retrospective approaches. If the ongoing flux of dialogic maintenance is to be fully understood, then longitudinal research must become a top priority in future research. Unlike some theoretical approaches for which longitudinal data are useful but not essential, a process-oriented perspective such as dialogism requires nonstatic approaches to data collection.

The third methodological issue involves the need for multimethod research. Dialectical research has largely been dominated by qualitative or interpretive research methods, and, like any theoretical perspective, it could benefit from the application of complementary methods. However, efforts to employ traditional psychometric scaling procedures will need to abandon the logic of bipolarity that has guided item construction and interpretation. The semantic differential, for example, presupposes that the two poles of a scale exist in a fixed, zero-sum relation to one another such that an X placed near one bipolar adjective automatically negates the other pole. Although the domination of one pole may negate the subordinate pole, dialectical flux can also result in temporary equilibrium or temporary double negation, neither of which can be captured in the zero-sum logic of bipolarity. Similarly, such bipolar logic leads researchers to interpret a "strongly disagree" response to a Likert-type statement such as "Our relationship is characterized by autonomy and independence of action" as evidence of high interdependence in the relationship. From a dialogic perspective, it is possible that the respondent could also mark "strongly disagree" if presented with a statement about interdependence. In short, the logic of bipolarity that has guided traditional scale construction functions to preclude some of the ways in which contradictory poles can dynamically interact. Alternative scaling methods, such as multidimensional scaling in which dialectical poles are represented as separate stimuli whose proximity can vary in a space of changing dimensionality, might be more suitable to a dialogic perspective.

My purpose in this chapter has been the presentation of an alternative conception of relational maintenance, one which conceives of maintenance as rooted in dialectical change. I have emphasized six contradictions that I posit as key sites of dialectical change in personal relationships, but I would like to end this chapter by returning to Bakhtin's emphasis on the contradicting process more generally. Fundamentally, a researcher who thinks dialogically seeks out the centripetal–centrifugal dynamic in all facets of communicative practice. For every dominant theme or modal pattern that is identified in research, the dialogic thinker asks, "What is occurring with the centrifugal opposite?" This core question is a useful heuristic by which to transform nondialogic research into dialogic research for any substantive domain, including relational maintenance.

References

Altman, I., & Gauvain, M. (1981). A cross-cultural and dialectic analysis of homes. In L. Liben, A. Patterson, & N. Newcombe (Eds.), *Spatial representation and behavior across the life span* (pp. 283–320). New York: Academic Press.

Altman, I., & Taylor, D. A. (1973). *Social penetration: The development of interpersonal relationships.* New York: Holt, Rinehart, & Winston.

Altman, I., Vinsel, A., & Brown, B. (1981). Dialectical conceptions in social psychology: An application to social penetration and privacy regulation. In L. Berkowitz (Ed.), *Advances in experimental social psychology* (Vol. 14, pp. 107–160). New York: Academic Press.

Ayres, J. (1983). Strategies to maintain relationships: Their identification and perceived usage. *Communication Quarterly, 31,* 62–67.

Bakhtin, M. M. (1981). *The dialogic imagination: Four essays by M. M. Bakhtin.* M. Holquist (Ed.), C. Emerson & M. Holquist (Trans.). Austin, TX: University of Texas Press.

Bakhtin, M. M. (1986). *Speech genres and other late essays.* C. Emerson & M. Holquist (Eds.), V. McGee (Trans.). Austin, TX: University of Texas Press.

Ball, R. (1979). The dialectical method: Its application to social theory. *Social Forces, 57,* 785–798.

Baxter, L. A. (1986). Gender differences in the heterosexual relationship rules embedded in breakup accounts. *Journal of Social and Personal Relationships, 3,* 289–306.

Baxter, L. A. (1987). Symbols of relationship identity in relationship cultures. *Journal of Social and Personal Relationships, 4,* 261–280.

Baxter, L. A. (1988). A dialectical perspective on communication strategies in relationship development. In S. Duck (Ed.), *Handbook of personal relationships* (pp. 257–273). New York: Wiley.

Baxter, L. A. (1990). Dialectical contradictions in relationship development. *Journal of Social and Personal Relationships, 7,* 69–88.

Baxter, L. A. (1992a). Interpersonal communication as dialogue: A response to the "Social Approaches Forum." *Communication Theory, 2,* 330–337.

Baxter, L. A. (1992b). *Self-reported relationship maintenance strategies and three external contradictions of relating.* Unpublished manuscript, University of California, Davis.

Baxter, L. A. (1993). The social side of personal relationships: A dialectical perspective. In S. Duck (Ed.), *Understanding relationship processes* (Vol. 3 pp. 139–165). Newbury Park, CA: Sage.

Baxter, L. A. (in press). Thinking dialogically about communication in personal relationships. In R. Conville (Ed.), *Structure in communication study.* New York: Praeger.

Baxter, L. A., & Dindia, K. (1990). Marital partners' perceptions of marital maintenance strategies. *Journal of Social and Personal Relationships, 7,* 187–208.

Baxter, L. A., & Simon, E. P. (1993). Relationship maintenance strategies and dialectical contradiction in personal relationships. *Journal of Social and Personal Relationships, 10,* 225–242.

Baxter, L. A., & Widenmann, S. (1993). Revealing and not revealing the status of romantic relationships to social networks. *Journal of Social and Personal Relationships, 10,* 321–338.

Bell, R. A., Daly, J., & Gonzalez, C. (1987). Affinity-maintenance in marriage and its relationship to women's marital satisfaction. *Journal of Marriage and the Family, 49,* 445–454.

Berger, C. R., & Gudykunst, W. (1991). Uncertainty and communication. In B. Dervin & M. Voigt (Eds.), *Progress in communication sciences* (Vol. 10, pp. 21–66). Norwood, NJ: Ablex.

Bridge, K., & Baxter, L. A. (1992). Blended friendships: Friends as work associates. *Western Journal of Communication, 56,* 200–225.

Byrne, D., & Murnen, S. (1988). Maintaining loving relationships. In R. Sternberg & M. Barnes (Eds.), *The psychology of love* (pp. 293–310). New Haven, CT: Yale University Press.

Canary, D., & Stafford, L. (1992). Relational maintenance strategies and equity in marriage. *Communication Monographs, 59,* 243–267.

Canary, D., & Stafford, L. (1993). Preservation of relational characteristics: maintenance strategies, equity, and locus of control. In P. Kalbfleisch (Ed.), *Interpersonal communication: Evolving interpersonal relationships* (pp. 237–259). Hillsdale, NJ: Lawrence Erlbaum.

Carbaugh, D. (1988). *Talking American: Cultural discourses on "Donohue".* Norwood, NJ: Ablex.

Cissna, K. N., Cox, D. E., & Bochner, A. P. (1990). The dialectic of marital and parental relationships within the stepfamily. *Communication Monographs, 57,* 44–61.

Cody, M. (1982). A typology of disengagement strategies and an examination of the role intimacy, reactions to inequity and relational problems play in strategy selection. *Communication Monographs, 49,* 148–170.

Conville, R. L. (1983). Second-order development in interpersonal communication. *Human Communication Research, 9,* 195–207.

Conville, R. L. (1991). *Relational transitions: The evolution of personal relationships.* New York: Praeger.

Cornforth, M. (1968). *Materialism and the dialectical method.* New York: International Publishers.

Cupach, W., & Metts, S. (1986). Accounts of relational dissolution: A comparison of marital and non-marital relationships. *Communication Monographs, 53,* 311–334.

Cupach, W., & Metts, S. (1988, July). *Perceptions of the occurrence and management of dialectics in romantic relationships.* Paper presented at the Fourth International Conference on Personal Relationships, Vancouver.

Dindia, K. (1989, November). *Towards the development of a measure of marital maintenance strategies.* Paper presented at the Speech Communication Association Convention, San Francisco.

Dindia, K., & Baxter, L. A. (1987). Strategies for maintaining and repairing marital relationships. *Journal of Social and Personal Relationships, 4,* 143–158.

Fitzpatrick, M. A., (1988). *Between husbands & wives: Communication in marriage.* Newbury Park, CA: Sage.

Giddens, A. (1979). *Central problems in social theory: Action, structure and contradiction in social analysis.* Berkeley: University of California Press.

Giddens, A. (1984). *The constitution of society.* Berkeley: University of California Press.

Goffman, E. (1971). *Relations in public: Microstudies of the public order.* New York: Harper & Row.

Goldsmith, D. (1988, November). *To talk or not to talk: The flow of information between romantic dyads and networks.* Paper presented at the Speech Communication Association Convention, New Orleans.

Goldsmith, D. (1990). A dialectic perspective on the expression of autonomy and connection in romantic relationships. *Western Journal of Speech Communication, 54,* 537–556.

Goldsmith, D., & Parks, M. (1990). Communicative strategies for managing the risks of seeking social support. In S. Duck (Ed.), *Personal relationships and social support* (pp. 104–121). Newbury Park, CA: Sage.

Harvey, J., Wells, G., & Alvarez, M. (1978). Attribution in the context of conflict and separation in close relationships. In J. Harvey, W. Ickes, & R. Kidd (Eds.), *New directions in attribution research* (Vol. 2, pp. 230–264). Hillsdale, NJ: Lawrence Erlbaum.

Heath, D. (1992). Fashion, anti-fashion, and heteroglossia in urban Senegal. *American Ethnologist, 19,* 19–33.

Hill, C., Rubin, Z., & Peplau, L. (1976). Breakups before marriage: The end of 103 affairs. *Journal of Social Issues, 32,* 147–168.

Holland, D. C., & Eisenhart, M. A. (1990). *Educated in romance: Women, achievement, and college culture.* Chicago: The University of Chicago Press.

Holquist, M. (1990). *Dialogism: Bakhtin and his world.* New York: Routledge.

Johnson, M. P., & Milardo, R. M. (1984). Network interference in pair relationships: A social psychological recasting of Slater's theory of social regression. *Journal of Marriage and the Family, 46,* 893–899.

Katriel, T., & Philipsen, G. (1981). "What we need is communication": "Communication" as a cultural category in some American speech. *Communication Monographs, 48,* 301–317.

Kelley, H. H. (1979). *Personal relationships: Their structures and processes.* Hillsdale, NJ: Lawrence Erlbaum.

Kim, H. J., & Stiff, J. B. (1991). Social networks and the development of close relationships. *Human Communication Research, 18,* 70–91.

Kitson, G. C., & Sussman, M. B. (1983). Marital complaints, demographic characteristics, and symptoms of mental distress in divorce. *Journal of Marriage and the Family, 44,* 87–101.

Krain, M. (1977). A definition of dyadic boundaries and an empirical study of boundary establishment in courtship. *International Journal of Sociology of the Family, 7,* 107–123.

Leslie, L., Huston, T., & Johnson, M. (1986). Parental reactions to dating relationships: Do they make a difference? *Journal of Marriage and the Family, 48,* 57–66.

Lewis, R. A. (1972). A developmental framework for the analysis of premarital dyadic formation. *Family Process, 11,* 17–48.

Lewis, R. A. (1973). Social reaction and the formation of dyads: An interactionist approach to mate selection. *Sociometry, 36,* 409–418.

Livingston, K. (1980). Love as a process of reducing uncertainty—Cognitive theory. In K. Pope et al. (Eds.), *On love and loving* (pp. 133–151). San Francisco: Jossey-Bass.

Mao, T. (1965). *On contradiction.* Beijing: Foreign Languages Press.

McCall, G. (1970). The social organization of relationships. In G. McCall, M. McCall, N. Denzin, & S. Kurth (Eds.), *Social relationships* (pp. 3–34). Chicago: Aldine de Gruyter.

Montgomery, B. M. (1992). Communication as the interface between couples and culture. In S. Deetz (Ed.), *Communication yearbook 15* (pp. 476–508). Newbury Park, CA: Sage.

Morson, G. S., & Emerson, C. (1990). *Mikhail Bakhtin: Creation of a prosaics.* Stanford: Stanford University Press.

Orvis, B. R., Kelley, H. H., Butler, D. (1976). Attributional conflict in young couples. In J. Harvey, W. Ickes, & R. Kidd (Eds.), *New directions in attribution research* (Vol. 1, pp. 353–386). Hillsdale, NJ: Lawrence Erlbaum.

Owen, W. (1984). Interpretive themes in relational communication. *Quarterly Journal of Speech*, *70*, 274–287.

Parks, M. R., & Eggert, L. L. (1991). The role of social context in the dynamics of personal relationships. In W. H. Jones & D. Perlman (Eds.), *Advances in personal relationships* (Vol. 2, pp. 1–34). London: Jessica Kingsley.

Petronio, S. (1991). Communication boundary management: A theoretical model of managing disclosure of private information between married couples. *Communication Theory*, *1*, 311–335.

Planalp, S., Rutherford, D., & Honeycutt, J. (1988). Events that increase uncertainty in personal relationships: II. Replication and extension. *Human Communication Research*, *14*, 516–547.

Rawlins, W. K. (1983a). The dialectic of conjunctive freedoms. *Human Communication Research*, *9*, 255–266.

Rawlins, W. K. (1983b). Openness as problematic in ongoing friendships: Two conversational dilemmas. *Communication Monographs*, *50*, 1–13.

Rawlins, W. K. (1989). A dialectical analysis of the tensions, functions and strategic challenges of communication in young adult friendships. In J. A. Andersen (Ed.), *Communication yearbook 12* (pp. 157–189). Beverly Hills, CA: Sage.

Rawlins, W. K. (1992). *Friendship matters: Communication, dialectics, and the life course.* New York: Aldine de Gruyter.

Riegel, K. (1976). The dialectics of human development. *American Psychologist*, *31*, 689–700.

Riesmann, C. K. (1990). *Divorce talk: Women and men make sense of personal relationships.* New Brunswick, NJ: Rutgers University Press.

Rychlak, J. F. (Ed.) (1976). *Dialectic: Humanistic rationale for behavior and development.* New York: S. Karger.

Shea, B., & Pearson, J. (1986). The effects of relationship type, partner intent, and gender on the selection of relationship maintenance strategies. *Communication Monographs*, *53*, 354–364.

Sillars, A., Weisberg, J., Burggraf, C., & Wilson, E. (1987). Content themes in marital conversations. *Human Communication Research*, *13*, 495–528.

Skinner, Q. (Ed.) (1985). *The return of grand theory in the human sciences.* New York: Cambridge University Press.

Stafford, L., & Canary, D. (1991). Maintenance strategies and romantic relationship type, gender and relational characteristics. *Journal of Social and Personal Relationships*, *8*, 217–242.

Surra, C. A. (1985). Courtship types: Variations in interdependence between partners and social networks. *Journal of Personality and Social Psychology*, *49*, 357–375.

Todorov, T. (1984). *Mikhail Bakhtin: The dialogical principle.* W. Godzich (Trans.). Minneapolis: University of Minnesota Press.

Relationship Rejuvenation

William W. Wilmot
Department of Communication Studies
University of Montana
Missoula, Montana

Introduction

The study of personal relationships used to be limited to issues of initiation and dissolution but is now beginning to focus on the more complex and far-reaching issues of maintenance and rejuvenation (Canary & Stafford, 1992; Wilmot & Stevens, in press). Whether it is labeled *maintenance* (what you do to keep a relationship from going downhill; Dindia & Baxter, 1987), *repair* (when you think the relationship has gone downhill and you want to restore it to its previously healthy state; Dindia & Baxter, 1987), or *rejuvenation* (trying to arrest the decline that occurs in relationships; Wilmot & Stevens, in press), the basic conceptual issue is, How can people improve their relationships or keep them from moving to dissatisfaction and dissolution? Specifically, *relationship rejuvenation* is used in this chapter to refer to the process of improving a relationship that has gone through a period of decline.

This chapter focuses on relationship rejuvenation in response to a decline and highlights both empirical and conceptual issues. Specifically, it (1) casts the discussion firmly within a dialectical framework, (2) investigates partners' reactions to decline, probing the conditions necessary for rejuvenation to occur, (3) looks at the different paths that may be taken to rejuvenate a relationship, (4) highlights some of the basic prototypes underlying the self–other connection in relationships that are manifested in rejuvenation choices, and (5) offers a concluding commentary.

The Dialectical Framework

The dialectical approach presumes there are opposite forces in all relationships that are connected and that affect one another (Wilmot, 1987; Rawlins, 1992). The dialectical opposites in personal relationships have been characterized a number of ways. One set of dialectic poles comprises (1) autonomy–interdependence, (2) expressiveness–protectiveness, and (3) predictability–novelty (Wilmot, 1987). Another specific set of dialectic options that has been tagged to friendship relations comprises (1) private–public, (2) ideal–real, (3) freedom to be independent and freedom to be dependent, (4) affection–instrumentality, and (5) expressiveness–protectiveness (Rawlins, 1992).

Regardless of the chosen labels attached to the dialectical poles, dialectical approaches all share a view of the antagonistic choices relationship partners face. The dialectical perspective highlights the continuing tensions relationship partners face. For example, friends, family members, and romantic partners all struggle with the major dialectic of autonomy–interdependence. If they choose to be completely independent, then their relationships cannot survive. Likewise, choosing to be totally dependent on the other and exercising no autonomy is widely recognized as paralyzing the individual growth of the relationship partners. The dialectical perspective does not try to *solve* these contradictory impulses and needs in relationships, rather, it descriptively recognizes the continuing choices individuals must make to respond to the opposing forces present in all relationships. One formulation (as adapted to personal relationships by Wilmot, 1987) notes that participants struggle with the dialectical tensions by (1) dialectic emphasis, (2) pseudosynthesis, or (3) reaffirmation. Using *dialectic emphasis* means swinging to one pole for an extended period of time. For instance, the young adult who leaves home and does not maintain contact with the family of origin, or the person "giving her all" to a relationship without considering her own needs for independence, *emphasizes* one pole of the dialectic. *Pseudosynthesis* occurs when the two disparate poles are brought together by glossing over the complex, contradictory pulls on the relationship. For example, saying "Oh, we don't have separate needs, what I want is what she wants" is denial of two individual identities. *Reaffirmation* of the dialectic is when an individual recognizes the opposites and believes they are truly contradictory and cannot be easily explained away. Thus, a participant would shift back and forth between the poles as conditions warrant.

Looking at relationship rejuvenation from a dialectical perspective and through the lens of "reaffirmation of the tensions," suggests that the oscillation between "close" and "far" in a relationship is a *normal* process. And the key to relationship rejuvenation seems to be the recognition that "the relationship is going downhill" and making some change to arrest further deterioration. Stated differently, relationships can go into periods of decline or regressive spirals where misunderstanding and discord produce more misunderstanding and discord. But, "unless regressive spirals are arrested, they continue until they lead to the dissolution of the relationship" (Wilmot, 1987, p. 152). The central issue facing both researchers and the relationship participants is How does one go about arresting decline and improving a relationship that is in a regressive spiral?

The decline of a relationship from a dialectical perspective is part and parcel of the drive for improvement or maintenance. Instead of viewing relationships as steady states that are merely maintained through "maintenance," this view of rejuvenation presumes ebb and flow in relationships, seeing them as complex, ever-changing phenomena. The earlier trajectory models characterized by Altman and Taylor's (1973) metaphor of a positively sloped line and Knapp's (1984) staircase analogy are not the only potential models from which to view relationships. Altman, Vinsel, and Brown (1981), Baxter (1988, 1990, this volume), Wilmot (1987), and Rawlins (1992, this volume) have suggested a third alternative for relationship movement based on the dialectical notions. The approach assumes that relationships continually oscillate between opposite poles such as openness and closedness. For example, they assume that a relationship may remain intact but alternate between periods of closeness and periods of distance. This ebbing and flowing between periods of closeness and distance can occur in relationships regardless of *whether or not* they move to dissolution. Stated another way, the dialectical approach suggests that relationships alternate between *regressive* and *progressive* spirals over time even if they maintain a predominate trend (Wilmot, 1987).

Reactions to Relational Decline

Why should people attempt to improve their relationships? Culturally, we often speak of the "growth" of an individual or the "growth" of a relationship, as well as the decay of relationships over time. Rejuvenation only becomes an issue if there is a focus on the *quality* of the relationship, or if a decrease in quality threatens the stability of a relationship. For most people interested in rejuvenation, the question Did this marriage survive? is not the most salient issue, rather, it is the litmus test of quality that emerges as a central issue. If an individual is not troubled with downturns, regressive spirals, or unsatisfactory relationships, then rejuvenation is not a goal to be sought. Rather, that person may choose to go through an ongoing series of relationships, letting the presumably natural decay and downturns slowly overwhelm the positive elements and gradually lead to permanent stagnation or dissolution. Proponents of serial monogamy, for instance, would argue that growth and subsequent decay in relationships are normal and, rather than trying to fix or improve a relationship, one's energy is best spent searching for a new romantic partner, new friend, or family surrogate.

It can be hypothesized that relational rejuvenation efforts do not happen in a vacuum; in fact, they probably occur in response to some decrease in relational satisfaction. When a relationship regresses there are two disparate paths toward downturns and dissatisfaction. Some relationships, whether family, friends, or romantic, tend to become embroiled in escalatory conflict spirals. Such conflicts have only upward and onward trends. They are characterized communicatively by a heavy reliance on overt power moves such as threats, coercion, and deception (Deutsch, 1973). In escalatory spirals, the damaging interactions become self-perpetuating and its attendant features are misunderstanding, discord, and destruction (Hocker & Wilmot, 1991). The relationship participants fight openly, relying on continuing destructive conflict moves to overpower the other, "get even," and gain goals at the other's expense.

A more subtle, but nevertheless more common decline pattern also occurs. A *de-escalatory conflict spiral* is characterized by lessened dependence, withdrawal, avoidance of the relationship issues, and decreased investment in the relationship. The basic dynamics of such de-escalatory spirals are (1) less direct interaction, (2) active avoidance of the other party, (3) reduction of dependence, (4) harboring resentment or disappointment, and (5) complaining to third persons about the other party (Hocker & Wilmot, 1991, p. 36).

We do not know empirically if participants in escalatory spirals either rejuvenate more frequently or in a different form than those in de-escalatory spirals. In fact, the paucity of knowledge about how relationship partners communicatively deal with their downturns while retaining an intact relationship makes it impossible to answer such questions at this time. One recent study, although not linking rejuvenation moves to the type of decline, did highlight the major paths to decline (Wilmot & Stevens, in press). When 116 participants were asked what led to the decline in a relationship, the responses from those in the romantic and friendship relationships were grouped into three categories: (1) relational issues, (2) escalation events, and (3) influences external to the dyad. Of these categories, relational issues were mentioned the most frequently, followed by escalation events, and then by influences external to the dyad.

Relational issues, the most often mentioned type of decline event, centered on the interaction patterns or perceptions of the partner. For example, the most frequently mentioned relational issue was experiencing reduction of interaction or involvement–spending less time together, decreasing communication, and sharing fewer activities. Unequal investment/involvement was the second most mentioned relational issue, comprising different relationship expectations, dissatisfactions, uncertainty about role, unequal affection, and unequal time spent on the relationship. The third most frequent response was undesirable/unacceptable behaviors, with one partner finding the other's behavior unusual, unacceptable, compulsive, deceitful, or abusive. The final relational issue was unequal power or dependence centering on illness, financial dependence, or control issues of dominance/submissiveness. All of these types of relational issues were associated with decline because they changed the quality of the relationship per se.

Escalation events were behaviors by either partner which hastened the decline by threatening or worsening the relationship. For example, respondents increased overt conflict by using threats, crying, and physical fighting. The second most frequently mentioned behavior was using physical separation from one another in direct response to the decline in the relationship. The third avenue for escalation was avoidance of certain topics or limiting themselves to superficial exchanges, and sometimes avoiding all communication. All the escalation events share one common thread—they are acts that directly added to the decline in the relationship.

The third major category, *influences external to the dyad*, took two major forms: interference from a third party and lifestyle changes. Third-party interference took many forms. For example, in the case of romantic relationships, interference usually centered on the partner's involvement with another romantic partner, whereas in family relationships, it was more often the disapproval of the family member's involvement with a friend or romantic partner. Lifestyle changes were influential in relationship decline when, for example, one partner moved, changed jobs, or expected a child. All the influences external to the dyad were exogenous events that brought about a decline in the quality of the dyadic relationship.

These responses give an interesting perspective on the decline of the relationships and illustrate that the events connected to a decline are varied and numerous. On the average, each respondent nominated 3.2 events associated with the decline of their relationship, events that varied from the internal dynamics of the relationships ("we fought all the time") to external attributions ("she fell in love with someone else") or ("he had to take a job in another city"). There were no differences in the type of decline for romantic relationships compared to friendships.

This beginning look at some paths for decline suggests that the most frequent type of decline is de-escalatory spirals, that is, reduction of interaction and involvement, decreasing communication, and spending less time together. If we can presume for the moment that this study can be generalized, it means that the most prominent issue facing a relationship is Will we continue to let the energy drain out of this relationship, let it continue its downward slide, or will we engage in rejuvenation behaviors? Or, stated more simply, *When is it too late?*

It is obviously too late for a relationship when either person is not willing to engage in rejuvenation, or at least participate in "holding actions." Rejuvenation (or maintenance for that matter) necessitates some conditions before it can be accomplished. *At a minimum*, rejuvenation of any type of relationship requires that (1) both parties are committed enough to not leave or dissolve the relationship, (2) both parties are willing to change behavior and/or talk about the relationship, and (3) both parties have the skills necessary to adjust to one another, which may include talking.

Given this set of conditions, it is no wonder that the divorce rate is high, relational turnover is frequent, and we are asking What can people do to rejuvenate their relationships? Any personal deficit or choice can keep the relationship on a downward slide and not allow the participants enough energy and commitment to "turn it around." In romantic relations, the downward slide is often associated with one party's external involvements, whereas in friend relations it may be a slow ebbing away and disinvolvement over a period of months or years (Wilmot, 1987). The challenges are no less daunting in family relations. If one person is unwilling to make changes and is locked into destructive conflict and "holding firm" waiting for the other to move first, such a standoff will keep both parties dissatisfied and the relationship on a downward path.

If we want to help individuals rejuvenate or enrich their relationships, their choice of *avoiding* dealing with relationship difficulties needs examination. The avoidance, in fact, magnifies the negative spirals present, often through continuation of the de-escalatory spiral of neglect. Avoidance is the most common response to difficulties, not the "yell and scream" variety most of us see as synonymous with conflict (Hocker & Wilmot, 1991). With intervention in family and personal disputes, it can be seen that the participants use a variety of attributions to stay locked into destructive cycles (Wilmot & Hocker, in press). If, for example, family members believe "you can't change someone else's personality anyway," then they are unlikely to use collaborative moves to work through the conflict. Even the work on marital enrichment programs bypasses the most frequent problems facing marital couples—they are so disinvested and in such a self-sealing spiral that third party assistance is not sought to help them improve their faltering relationship.

The central question that emerges, then, is Why would relationship parties want to rejuvenate their relationship? Given that our cultural learning about relationships—about one-half of all marriages terminate and most premarital romantic involvements are not going to last forever—it is no wonder that many people choose not to reinvest in their relationship after it faces some of the inevitable forces of decay and decline. Of course, such decision making is never simple, therefore we need to study the decision-making processes individuals use. Whether we look at it through the lens of equity theory and argue that "under-benefited" individuals would be less likely to reinvest in the relationship (Canary & Stafford, 1992), or cast a broader net, we have yet to understand the complexities and perplexities individuals face when deciding to let a relationship slide or make a decision to try to rejuvenate it. Lack of participant interest, skill, knowledge, a loss of faith in the possibilities of change, or simply not having outside help available, any one of these can keep the participants from redirecting the relationship. Because it is so easy *not* to reinvest in a relationship, we need to know how individuals make the decision to rejuvenate a faltering relationship. To date, we do not know the answers to the simplest questions such as what percentage of individuals monitor their relationship and decide to rejuvenate it.

Paths to Rejuvenation

Although not arguing for a rational approach to the decision to rejuvenate, at some point individuals either consciously or intuitively make some decision to improve a relationship. Once that decision is made, communication researchers may begin to piece together some of the typical paths that individuals take toward rejuvenation. Though limited, what we know to date suggests some interesting patterns in the rejuvenation processes. Table 1 summarizes three sets of research bearing on the process of both maintenance and rejuvenation. Following the work of Stafford and Canary (1991), Canary and Stafford (1992) summarized strategies isolated in studies dealing with maintenance; the Dindia and Baxter (1987) work lists strategies for both maintenance and repair (finding little difference in use in the two situations); and the Wilmot and Stevens (in press) research lists rejuvenation strategies.

In examining all three studies, one pattern is abundantly clear—*most* of the strategies used in both maintenance and rejuvenation efforts are behavioral changes, rituals, or other signals used to "tell" the other of a desire to improve the relationship. In other words, participants more often try to signal the other about their increased reinvestment in the relationship through a

Table 1
Maintenance and Rejuvenation Strategies[a]

Canary & Stafford, maintenance	Dindia & Baxter, maintenance/repair	Wilmot & Stevens, rejuvenation
Positivity	Change environment	Change behaviors
Openness*	Communication*	Big relational talk*
Assurances*	Metacommunication*	Gesture of reconciliation
Network	Avoiding metacommunication	Reassess importance of
Tasks	Antisocial	the relationship
	Prosocial	Accept or forgive
	Ceremonies	Seek third party help
	Antirituals/spontaneity	
	Togetherness	
	Seeking/allowing autonomy	
	Seeking outside help	

[a] Strategies with asterisks focus on direct oral communication.

variety of means other than engaging in overt communication about the status of the relationship.

The *implicit relational moves* are meant to inform the lover, friend, or family member that you are trying to improve the relationship. Or, another way of saying it is "Watch what I do and notice that I am trying to help our relationship improve." The Wilmot and Stevens (in press) study also found some relationship-specific generic structures to the rejuvenation attempts. Family members were more apt to "accept and forgive" the other than were friends or lovers in order to turn the relationship toward a more progressive phase. Such cognitive intrapersonal alignments were reported to occur both with and without any changes in overt communication.

Overt communication strategies were used more often by romantic partners than friends or family members (Wilmot & Stevens, in press). Participants in romantic relationships used more "big relationship talk" (communicating with one another about the decline) and third party involvement (seeking counseling for example) than did friends or family members. The romantic bonds are more fragile than family ties, thus, the participants must do more open negotiation and work to clear up declines in a relationship. If the bonds are fragile, then a decline sets off warning signals that some repair is needed. On the contrary, when the bonds are more resilient one can more confidently go though a decline (such as in a family relationship) without overtly addressing it. Talk seems both more permissible and needed in more fragile romantic relationships than in friendships and family.

Two items stand out at this point: (1) much more research is needed on implicit rejuvenation processes, and (2) the role of talking about relationship issues also needs much more comprehensive study. For example, participants seem to say "watch my behavior" more often than "listen to what I say" as a way to signal rejuvenation and reinvestment efforts. The adequacy of those implicit choices to "make it through" to the other, that is, the fidelity of the implicit messages, needs further investigation. Also, the kind of decision making participants go though in deciding on or intuitively trying new patterns of behavior are in need of explanation.

Second, the role of overt talk within the entire process of rejuvenation needs further study. Dindia and Baxter (1987) found that relationship satisfaction was not related to strategy preference for maintenance and repair, yet the folk belief in the importance of communication lingers. Whereas talking *can* lead to rejuvenation, so can the lack of talking. One finding from Wilmot and Stevens (in press) is that whereas 75% of the respondents both talked and used behavior change, fully 90% of those who did not have a relational talk reported behavior change. Although talking and changes co-occur, *more* change occurred without talk. Further, when respondents were asked "What can others do to improve their relationships?" most said "communicate." Yet, such advice to others about communication as a path to rejuvenation was not isomorphic with whether those participants themselves had a relationship talk—people recommend to others to talk more during times of relationship downturn whether they themselves talked or not during their own downturn.

Basically, the two overall paths to rejuvenation can be separated into implicit relational moves and explicit relational talk. The correspondence and disjunction between these two modes obviously need more comprehensive examination.

Self/Other/Relationship: Conceptual Conundrums

An examination of relationship maintenance and rejuvenation could be concluded easily without probing some of the deeper assumptions regarding this entire enterprise. Often, for example, both the outside behavioral scientist and the inside participant speaks about relationship rejuvenation without highlighting some underlying assumptions. This section is an excursion into some common underlying assumptions about self, other, and relationships that underlie both the scientists' findings and the participants' choices in a relationship. It was argued at the outset that the dialectic approach offers a heuristic frame for viewing rejuvenation, maintenance, or any aspect of a relationship. This section will further attempt to specify some of the assumptions about relationships and how self, other, and relationship are dialectically interwoven.

Probably the prevailing view of self/other/relationship in our current culture is what could be characterized as totally individuated selves who just happen to have relationships. This prototype language comes from the work of Wilmot and Baxter (1989) on cognitive schemata as explained in Wilmot and Shellen (1990). The notion of prototypes is intended here to generate lenses for processing the self/other/relationship linkages as seen by both relationship partners and researchers. Each prototype contains assumptions about why people maintain their relationships, for they each have important implications for the values people assign their involvements.

Prototype I: Individual Selves Loosely Connected

Grounded firmly in many of the basic assumptions, this view of how self and other are related presumes the person is the center and an integrated whole in and of him- or herself (Sampson, 1989).[1] As Geertz (1979) notes: "The Western conception of the person as a bounded, unique, more or less integrated motivational and cognitive universe, a dynamic center of awareness, emotion, judgement and action, organized into a distinctive whole and set contrastively against other such wholes" (p. 229).

Such a conception, thoroughly familiar to all of us raised in a Western culture, is "a rather peculiar idea within the context of the world's cultures" (p. 229). Yet, firmly rooted in it we are. Such notions stress that there are Cartesian atomic units "dependent upon nothing outside themselves for their existence" (Wilden, 1980, p. 92). Graphically, such views would be expressed as in Figure 1.

Note the Self and Other are independent units, loosely connected by the relational thread. Prototype I emphasizes the self, de-emphasizes the other, and reduces the relationship to a connecting mechanism. Those who view relationships from such a perspective would be prone to emphasize individual growth, individual responsibility, and want to look inside the envelope of the individual for explanations (Harre, 1989). Further, individual achievement is the goal and so ego identity requires that the person have some control over the process, and anything less than a separated individual identity would be seen as a deficit (Slugoski & Ginsburg, 1989). Such an ideology of individualism necessitates that we specialize in looking at our own reactions, determining if a relationship is worth the effort based on whether we are happy or satisfied. The "bridge" between people is precarious at best and ineffectual at worst. The assumptions of such a view are clearly highlighted by Chodron (1990):

[1]The use of "self" in this section is consistent with the much broader use made popular by Jungian psychology. Normally, there is confusion between "ego" or "persona" and "self." Self, as used here refers to the complete aspects of one, not just the presenting, conscious aspect. For clarification of this use of the term see Stevens (1990).

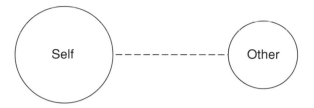

Figure 1

Prototype I.

> We think things exist in a way they don't. We have a wrong conception of who we are, thinking we are a permanent, concrete, findable entity. Then, we cherish this illusory "real self" dearly. The one thought in our minds from morning to night is, "I want happiness and my happiness is the most important." We think and act as if we were the center of the universe, for the thought "my happiness, my suffering" is foremost and ever-present in our minds. Our concern for others comes after our concern for ourselves. (p. 107)

If one can transcend the self-cherishing attitudes of Prototype I, instead of wondering How can this relationship fulfill my needs? we may think What can I give to the other? (Chodron, 1990, p. 43).

It is interesting to note that the entire concept of self arose during the middle ages, when people were, for the first time, seen as having separate rights and obligations (Wilber, 1983). The word *self*, in fact, did not appear until about 1595 (Slugoski and Ginsburg, 1989). Bellah, Madsen, Sullivan, Swindler, and Tipton (1985) note that people use the language of individualism and sound more isolated than their lives really are.

One of the ramifications of Prototype I is that in contemporary Western culture, relationship difficulties (whether between lovers, friends, or family members) can be identified by the degree of *blame of the other*. Because the two persons are loosely connected, if there are difficulties, the first line of defense is to blame the other, taking great care to show how the disturbances traveled down that thin wire of the relationship back to cause the behavior. Paradoxically, in such a self-oriented culture, the self is the last object for analysis for many people in times of relationship difficulty. The person seldom blames self or interconnected communication patterns or other features, but rather defaults to blame of the other. If one subscribes to Prototype I, then, during times of difficulty the first impulse is to take care of one's self at the expense of the other, and during such times the relationship threads are not vital enough to hold the two together.

The potency of Prototype I is displayed in most studies of relationships. For example, the popular social exchange model rests on the assumption that one's self-interest is what is being maximized (Roloff, 1981). Talk of profits, rewards, and costs connotes an image of a banker investing in a separated stock, hoping for a profit. If the payoff is not high enough, rather than reinvesting in the unchangeable stock, a partner switches investments. Such views, of course, set difficult standards for relationship rejuvenation when the prime value is *self rejuvenation*, not enhancement of the relationship. Lay persons who do not subscribe to Prototype I often criticize those who do as "selfish," trying to make the point that there is an overemphasis on self. It is a value question of course, but it may be that our stress on individualism has grown "cancerous" (Bellah et al., 1985).

Scholars who adopt perspectives such as social exchange are merely reflecting a prevailing Prototype I view endemic to our culture. The choice of this perspective is to judge relationships from the standpoint of the viability for individual growth. It is said, "She is finding herself" not "The relationship is finding itself."

Before proceeding to the next prototype, there is a common variation on the Individual Selves Loosely Connected Prototype that is worthy of mention (see Levinger & Shoek, 1978). Although diagrammically the Prototype I variation appears different from Prototype I, it does share the most basic assumption that the locus for understanding relationships is lodged in the separate individuals. Figure 2 illustrates the variation of Prototype I.

The relationship context arises from the mere overlap of the two separate, autonomous selves who just happen to have enough overlap to create a relationship. Such a view, while appearing to give more due to the relationship elements, still rests on the assumption of two discrete selves as the starting point. After all, all the selves have to do is just pull away and the relationship withers to nothing.

Prototype II: The Embedded Self

This fundamental shift in thinking moves from the individual as a separate nonaffected self to a self embedded within relationships. Note in Figure 3 the essential self cannot be described outside a relationship context.

Although an individual might talk about the self, its very definition hinges on the relational context from which it arises. As Senn notes, research conducted from this perspective assumes that

> studying individual members of dating couples does not do justice to the dynamics of their interpersonal relationship. Simply providing a detailed explanation of the structure and function of an individual person will not lead to an adequate account of social behavior and the structure of the social order. (Senn, 1989 p. 46)

Prototype II explains self-esteem by seeing it composed as a system of mutual exchanges, dependent on others for its creation and maintenance,

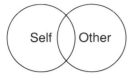

Figure 2

Prototype I variation.

whereas self and other are in a sense created by one another. As Wilber says, "the identity of 'I' is possible solely through the identity of the other who recognizes me, and who in turn is dependent upon my recognition" (Wilber, 1983, p. 272.). In a sense, we spin the self within the relationship web and the relationship web is spun with the other. The self is developed always within the context of the other (Bellah et al., 1985). Or, in the terms of the deconstructionists, there is an *interpenetration* of the society (relationships) and the individual (Sampson, 1989). Such views bring with them a very different research agenda from Prototype I, such as a call for examining "relationship constellations" as a needed step in the understanding of personal relationships (Wilmot & Sillars, 1989).

Prototype II assumes that relationships serve a transcendent function. The relationship itself is treated as an entity, and has even been called the "spiritual child" of the two people (Stewart, 1990, p. 26). Of course, if a relationship becomes destructive for the participants it can become a "demonic child" that devours the parents. Rather than seeing self and other as opposite poles, Prototype II assumes that self and other have permeable boundaries.

Relationship participants who subscribe to some of the variations of this

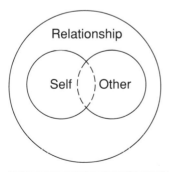

Figure 3

Embedded self.

major Prototype II, would talk about "our relationship" being in trouble, suggesting that the relationship has an entity or even self-esteem. They are also likely to stress collaboration, the interweaving of self and other into ongoing, unfolding complex patterns. When they have faith in the relationship or believe in it, especially if they think it has a future, then they have a relationship (Leatham & Duck, 1990).

Some typical differences in male/female communication could arise from different prototypes of relationships, with males more often relying on a Prototype I position and females using a Prototype II stance. It has been clearly demonstrated that females do value and monitor their relationships more than males do (Baxter & Wilmot, 1983). And, in terms of maintenance or rejuvenation, females more often see the need for proactive relational work and are more motivated to invest energy to maintain the relationship (Dindia and Baxter, 1987).

For participants, when a relationship becomes suffocating or constricting, they are ascribing power to the relationship entity itself, noting its impact on their choices, often explaining how they cannot move or make independent choices. Critics of marriage would also ascribe much power to the relationship itself, thus one should avoid or jettison a marriage because of its power to form the self (Guggenbuhl-Craig, 1977). When participants begin to feel that the relationship can bring lasting happiness and they cling to the relationship, they are assuming that the relationship has a real findable essence (Chodron, 1990).

Prototype II adherents would argue for relationship rejuvenation work, per se, because the relationship has a definable essence of its own that transcends the two individuals, and with relationship improvement comes a different set of forces on the self. Of course, there are some conundrums inherent in this approach. One is that the self is created by all the relationships it has and is in, *and* the relationship(s) literally creates the self; no easy logical jump for those with a Cartesian bent.

Prototype III: Non-Separable Self/Other/Relationship

The third prototype anchors the position opposite of Prototype I. Rather than taking the individual as a sacred entity to be preserved and nurtured at the exclusion of and in isolation from others, it challenges the very notion of an identifiable "I." It sees the self and other as so inextricably tied that to take care of one necessitates taking care of the other. The principle of Dependent Co-Arising can be interpreted as saying, "So we are friends, and our happiness depends on each other. According to that teaching I have to take care of myself and you take care of yourself. That way we take care of each other" (Hanh, 1992). Or, stated even more simply, "I am therefore you are" (Hanh, 1992). Such an approach goes even beyond the dialectic approach noted

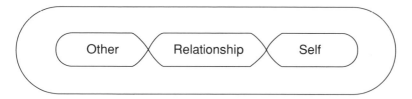

Figure 4

The non-separable self/other/relationship.

earlier and suggests that we cannot stand outside and observe our relationships and that duality itself is an illusion. As Murdock (1990) notes, "it is an illusion to think you can have right without left, good without evil, women without men, the rose without the garbage. . ." (p. 171). And, although we cannot obviously wholly enter into another person's subjective world, neither can we be separate from it (Bugental, 1978). Yet, while rejecting the either/or aspects of how dialectics are usually seen, Prototype III embraces the essence of the interweaving of self/other/relationship. They simply are *not* separable, as Figure 4 attempts to illustrate.

Adherents to Prototype III would find themselves struggling not to default to the "I," but rather seeing self and other as inextricably tied—instead of thinking "How can this relationship fulfill my needs?" think instead, "What can I give the other?" (Chrodron, 1990, p. 43). Relationship work would reflect a fundamental premise that it would not be undertaken to benefit self but would be chosen as a way to enhance relationship, other, and self—all interwoven. Such views, given that they do not align with our current cultural assumptions, necessitate some mental gymnastics. Researchers have yet to probe any of the variations on this theme. For example, it is unclear how, in a culture bent on searching for the independent "I," individuals transcend that dominant perspective.

Research Questions

There are many more unsolved puzzles than answers about relationship rejuvenation. The following research questions may serve to stimulate the examination of many neglected aspects of the entire rejuvenation process.

1. The different rejuvenation processes that are functional in one relationship genre may or may not be the best choice in another.

We need to know which processes are context bound and which are context free.

2. Much more data is needed on family and friendship rejuvenation processes. It is easy to overestimate the importance of romantic relationships in a person's total relationship constellation. Therefore data from other types of personal relationships are needed.
3. Are there behavioral differences in maintenance and rejuvenation strategies yet untapped by researchers who rely on self-reports?
4. What are the prototypes the participants have in mind when they choose to enter or not to enter rejuvenation processes?
5. Can we track the cognitive processes of individuals over time, specifying the choices they make to avoid or to engage in rejuvenation?
6. When is it too late for rejuvenation to occur?
7. What are the precise functions that implicit relational moves and explicit relational talk serve? How and under what conditions do these two function in tandem?
8. Do different fundamental beliefs about the viability of relationships have an impact on the decision to rejuvenate and the strategies used if one chooses to do so?
9. How do partners decode the implicit relational rejuvenation attempts made by the other?
10. Does the perceived "voluntariness" of a relationship have an impact on the rejuvenation processes or lack of them?
11. Do the suggested prototypes actually reflect the conceptual underpinnings of the self/other/relationship conundrums? If so, what impact do the different prototypes have on the choices made during a time of relational decline? And how do individuals frame or make sense out of their and the other's attempts to rejuvenate a relationship?

Conclusion

The processes of rejuvenating a relationship provide a rich context in which to study the intricacies of relationships. After all, what could be a more fundamental question than What can these people do to arrest decline and improve their relationship? This excursion has examined the dialectical view of the inherent tensions in relationships within Western cultures, noting that the oscillation between phases of satisfaction and dissatisfaction is to be expected. The various reactions to relational decline have been charted, asking whether escalatory or de-escalatory spirals bring different rejuvenation patterns. Further, the various paths of the decline have been described, focusing on the question When is it too late for rejuvenation?

It was argued that at a minimum, rejuvenation requires (1) each person wanting the relationship to continue and not dissolve or decline further, (2) participants who are willing to change their communication with one another, and (3) participants who have the skills necessary to infuse new energy into the relationship. It was also noted that most rejuvenation attempts are *implicit relational moves* and not explicit relational talk.

Finally, various prototypes for fundamental beliefs about the interconnection of self/other/relationship were sketched in order to highlight some differing assumptions people make about relationships. The heightened sense of self extant in our culture is only one option for viewing self/other/relationship interconnections. One can, for example, argue that there is no such thing as an independent self, rather, it is co-arising with the other. The different prototypes probably have profound impacts on the rejuvenation views and choices of individuals and are worthy of empirical study to heighten our understanding of such diverse views of self, other, and relationship. Within this broader context, we may begin to more fully understand the rejuvenation process.

References

Altman, I., & Taylor, D. A. (1973). *Social penetration: The development of interpersonal relationships.* New York: Holt, Rinehart, & Winston.

Altman, I., Vinsel, A., & Brown, B. B. (1981). Dialectic conceptions in social psychology: An application to social penetration and privacy regulation. In L. Berkowitz (Ed.), *Advances in experimental social psychology* (Vol 14, pp. 105–160).

Baxter, L. A. (1988). A dialectical perspective on communication strategies in relationship development. In S. Duck (Ed.), *A handbook of personal relationships* (pp. 257–273). New York: Wiley.

Baxter, L. A. (1990). Dialectical contradictions in relationship development. *Journal of Social and Personal Relationships, 7,* 69–88.

Baxter, L. A., & Wilmot, W. W. (1983). Communication characteristics of relationships with differential growth rates. *Communication Monographs, 50,* 264–272.

Bellah, R. N., Madsen, R., Sullivan, W., Swindler, A., & Tipton, S. (1985). *Habits of the heart: Individualism and commitment in American life.* Berkeley: University of California Press.

Bugental, J. F. T. (1987). *The art of the psychotherapist.* New York: Norton.

Canary, D. J., & Stafford, L. (1992). Relational maintenance strategies and equity in marriage. *Communication Monographs, 59,* 243–267.

Cermak, T. L. (1987). *Diagnosing and treating co-dependence: A guide for professionals who work with chemical dependents, their spouses, and children.* Minneapolis, MN: Johnson Institute Books.

Chodron, T. (1990). *Open heart, clear mind.* Ithaca, NY: Snow Lion Publications.

Deutsch, M. (1973). Conflicts: Productive and destructive. In F. E. Jandt (Ed.), *Conflict resolution through communication.* New York: Harper & Row.

Dindia, K., & Baxter, L. A. (1987). Strategies for maintaining and repairing marital relationships. *Journal of Social and Personal Relationships, 4,* 143–158.

Geertz, C. (1979). From the native's point of view: On the nature of anthropological understanding. In P. Rabinow & W. M. Sullivan (Eds.), *Interpretive social science* (pp. 225–241). Berkeley: University of California Press.

Gergen, K. J., & Semin, G. R. (1990). Everyday understanding in science and daily life. In G. R. Semin & K. J. Gergen (Eds.), *Everyday understanding: Social and scientific explanations* (pp. 1–18). London: Sage.

Guggenbuhl-Craig, A. (1977). *Marriage dead or alive.* Murray Stein (Trans.). Dallas, TX: Spring.

Hanh, T. N. (1992). Peaceful heart, peaceful politics. *Lotus, 1* (3) Spring, 28–31.

Harre, R. (1989). Language games and texts of identity. In J. Shotter & K. J. Gergen (Eds.), *Texts of identity* (pp. 20–35). London: Sage.

Hocker, J. L., & Wilmot, W. W. (1991). *Interpersonal conflict.* Dubuque, IA: Wm. C. Brown.

Knapp, M. L. (1984). *Interpersonal communication and human relationships.* Newton, MN: Allyn and Bacon.

Leatham, G., & Duck, S. (1990). Conversations with friends and the dynamics of social support. In S. Duck (Ed.), *Personal relationships and social support* (pp. 1–29). London: Sage.

Levinger, G., & Shoek, J. D. (1978). Attraction in relationships: A new look at interpersonal attraction. In G. Levinger & J. D. Shoek (Eds.), *Attraction in relationships.* Morristown, NJ: General Learning Press.

Murdock, M. (1990). *The heroine's journey.* Boston, MA: Shambhala Publications.

Planalp, S. (1985). Relational schemata: A test of alternative forms of relational knowledge as guides to communication. *Human Communication Research, 12,* 3–29.

Rawlins, W. K. (1992). *Friendship matters: Communication, dialectics, and the life course.* Hawthorne, NY: Aldine de Gruyter.

Roloff, M. E. (1981). *Interpersonal communication: A social exchange approach.* Beverly Hills, CA: Sage.

Sampson, E. E. (1989). The deconstruction of the self. In J. Shotter & K. J. Gergen (Eds.), *Texts of identity* (pp. 1–19). London: Sage.

Senn, D. J. (1989). Myopic social psychology: An overemphasis on individualistic explanations of social behavior. In M. R. Leary (Ed.), *The state of social psychology* (pp. 45–53). Newbury Park, CA: Sage.

Slugoski, B. R., & Ginsburg, G. P. (1989). Ego identity and explanatory speech. In J. Shotter & K. J. Gergen (Eds.), *Texts of identity* (pp. 36–55). London: Sage.

Stafford, L., & Canary, D. J. (1991). Maintenance strategies and romantic relationship type, gender and relational characteristics. *Journal of Social and Personal Relationships, 8,* 217–242.

Stewart, J. (1990). *Bridges not walls: A book about interpersonal communication.* New York: McGraw-Hill.

Stevens, A. (1990). *On Jung.* London: Routledge.

Tannen, D. (1990). *You just don't understand: Women and men in conversation.* New York: William Morrow.

Wilber, K. (1983). *Up from Eden: A transpersonal view of human evolution.* Boulder, CO: Shambhala Press.

Wilden, A. (1980). *System and structure: Essays on communication and exchange* (2nd ed.). London: Tavistock Publications.

Wilmot, W. W. (1987). *Dyadic communication.* New York: Random House.

Wilmot, W. W., & Hocker, J. L. (in press). Couples and change: Intervention through discourse and images. In N. Coupland & J. Nussbaum (Eds.), *Discourse and life span development.* Hillsdale, NJ: Lawrence Erlbaum.

Wilmot, W. W., & Shellen, W. N. (1990). Language in friendships. In H. Giles & W. P. Robinson (Eds.), *Handbook of language and social psychology* (pp. 413–431). New York: Wiley.

Wilmot, W. W., & Sillars, A. L. (1989). Developmental issues in personal relationships. In
    J. Nussbaum (Ed.), *Life-span communication: Normative processes* (pp. 119–135). Hillsdale, NJ:
    Lawrence Erlbaum.
Wilmot, W. W., & Stevens, D. C. (in press). Relationship rejuvenation: Arresting decline in
    personal relationships. In R. Conville (Ed.), *Communication and structure*. Norwood, NJ: Ablex.

Being There
and Growing Apart

Sustaining Friendships during Adulthood

William K. Rawlins
Department of Communication
Purdue University
West Lafayette, Indiana

Introduction

This chapter examines some predicaments and practices of sustaining friendships during adulthood. Although recognizing the difficulty of defining the boundaries of adulthood precisely, I consider middle adult friendships as spanning Neugarten's (1968) time periods of maturity (from 30 to 40 years old) and middle age (from 40 to 65 years old), with later adulthood and old age occurring thereafter. I concentrate on the lived experiences of a group of middle-class, North American men and women in managing physical and emotional separations from friends, occasioned by the demands of their encompassing configurations of roles, relationships, and responsibilities.

I begin by discussing distinctive features of friendship and a dialectical perspective on sustaining friendships during adulthood. Then, I describe the interviewees and the aims of this investigation. Next, I explain and exemplify the social patterning of friendship discontinuities evident in these persons' accounts and their individual and relational practices for handling them. Clearly, the tensions and contradictions generated by the situated nature of friendships produce dialectical demands that routinely affect friends' face-to-face interactions. Elsewhere, I have analyzed the communicative management of these dialectical tensions of friendship across the life course (Rawlins, 1992). My concern here, specifically, is with how friends handle contextually occasioned threats to the very continuity of their friendship as a shared feature of their lives. In the press of multiple involvements, and with the tugs and pulls of time and distance, how do adult friends sustain or subvert a shared definition of their importance to each other as friends? To address this question, this chapter examines individual and relational practices of sustaining friendships. The chapter closes with selected implications of this investigation.

A Focus on Friendship

Friendship is a commonplace category of relationship that has celebrated ideals dating back at least to ancient Greece. Friendship is also an everyday form of connection whose specific expectations and practices, although culturally patterned, are only minimally regulated by social institutions in American culture and can vary as much as the persons who pursue it (Blieszner & Adams, 1992; Brain, 1976). By and large, people choose each other as friends and sustain or relinquish their attachment within normatively constrained circumstances (Rawlins, 1992). Even so, every case develops through the voluntary interaction of particular persons. People may feel compelled by their job or marriage, or may be motivated by civic concerns to enact friendly relations with others, but the caring and commitment of close friendship emerges from within the dyad (Kurth, 1970).

Friendship's contextually negotiated core allows it to assume diverse social forms. Some friendships develop as ends in themselves, aspiring to the classical ideals of shared ethical comportment, good will, and trust (Rawlins, 1991). Transcending institutional guidelines, the behavioral standards of these discretionary bonds arise primarily from ongoing mutual commitments to behaving and interpreting conduct in ways that preserve assumptions of benevolence between the friends (Rawlins, 1992). The enduring character of these friendships derives from jointly defined responsibilities and discursive practices (Rawlins, 1991).

In different cases, friendship may complement or fuse with other relationships, such as marriage, business, or political associations. Here, the ideals of friendship may significantly influence the relational practices of the parties involved. They may regard and treat each other as friends even as they enact the institutional requirements of their affiliation. In contrast, prevailing social conventions may pointedly constrain opportunities to act as friends, and in particularly glib or utilitarian relationships, persons may tactically employ the notion or practices of friendship. Calling someone a "friend" in this case is a strategic maneuver designed to trade on friendship's moral and positive connotations for instrumental gains (Bloch, 1971). The contextually patterned and privately negotiated normative essence of friendship permits such a range of cases.

The combination of ideal attributes, cultural norms, and inconsistent actualities can make friendships ambiguous. Friendship's potentially frustrating bonds are difficult to recognize and manage in daily life, much less to describe conclusively in scholarly work. The situationally negotiated nature of friendships lends a flexibility to them that permits them to course in and out of private and public situations, facilitating personal integration and/or social participation in given cases, a capacity I term *double agency* (Rawlins, 1992). But lacking definitive social moorings, friendship's flexibility in one context is its fragility in another. The nebulous qualities of friendship allow for opportunistic and hurtful moments as well as edifying and joyful ones.

Having acknowledged the varieties of friendship, this chapter focuses primarily on those formed for personal and intrinsic reasons by middle-class, midwestern North American adults. In such dyads, adults want someone to talk to, to depend on, to enjoy spending time with—in essence, someone to care about who cares about them for "who they are." As we will see, for most of the persons interviewed here, sustaining such bonds across the years and changes of middle adulthood is not an easy or uncomplicated matter.

First of all, friendship pairs are highly susceptible to what Simmel (1950) termed *the mortality of the dyad.* When someone exits a social group, the remaining members can maintain their collective identity and shared practices by recruiting other persons. In contrast, when an individual abandons a friendship, the dyad dissolves. Moreover, friendship lacks the legal and/or religious sanctions buttressing marriages, the economic contracts reinforcing partnerships and business associations, and the blood ties linking kin throughout their lives. Given friendship's voluntary, idiosyncratic, and mutually developed practices, seeking another partner is *de facto* searching for another friendship.

Meanwhile, friendships are highly *contingent* relationships for the middle-aged, middle-class American adults who have assumed the typical roles and responsibilities of that life course stage (Rawlins, 1992). The routines and demands of combinations of work, marriage, parenthood, family, neighborhood, and community involvement usually result in an elaborate configuration of ongoing interactions with others. Most friendships are pursued in the contexts of meeting the expectations of these socially sanctioned endeavors. Free-standing friendships, that is, friendships made outside such pursuits, are a luxury (Paine, 1969). Giving voice to friendship's conditional status, Naegele (1958) observed that "the extent and importance of friendship is a measure of the extent and importance of the 'permissive' sphere in the ordering of society" (p. 236). We will now explore how friendships trace the ebb and flow of this permissive sphere within the temporal horizons of middle class adult lives.

A Dialectical Perspective on Sustaining Friendships during Adulthood

---

Dialectical conceptions of interpersonal life share several theoretical commitments (Altman, Vinsel, & Brown, 1981; Baxter, 1988; Rawlins, 1983a, 1989). I thematize these basic elements as totality, contradiction, motion, and praxis. Viewed as a *totality*, communicating in friendships involves the constant interconnection and reciprocal influence of multiple individual, interpersonal, and social factors. Discrete "things," actions, or events are inconceivable from a dialectical perspective; reality is composed of relations and relations among relations. Moreover, dialectical totalities are not static or fixed, but are in constant movement and alternate between contextualizing and being contextualized. Thus, I conceive any component or aspect of friendship as existing in dynamic connection with all of the others of friends embracing life situations.

Contradictions are the antagonistic yet interdependent aspects of communication between friends. Such dialectical tensions are considered inherent features of ongoing friendships because friends' activities and experiences necessarily interweave personal biographies, dyadic practices, social collectivities, and cultural matrices, the demands of which often oppose while presupposing each other. One can examine a given friendship for the contradictions evident within the relationship, and those occurring between the dyad and the external social formations contextualizing it (Bopp & Weeks, 1984; Rawlins, 1989). Two friends experience the former type, for example, when attempting to manage the contradictory requirements of expressive versus protective communication within their relationship (Rawlins, 1983b). By comparison, external contradictions develop when the constraints of marriage or job undermine freedoms negotiated between friends. Animated by such contradictions, social life is characterized by *motion*—activity and change. The present state of any relationship or social formation is considered an incessant achievement.

Elsewhere I have discussed in detail contextual dialectics of the private and the public, and the ideal and the real (Rawlins, 1989, 1992); and interactional dialectics of the freedom to be independent and the freedom to be dependent (Rawlins, 1983a), affection and instrumentality (Rawlins, 1992), judgment and acceptance (Rawlins & Holl, 1988), and expressiveness and protectiveness (Rawlins, 1983b). In diverse interpersonal situations, Baxter (1988, 1990, this volume; Bridge & Baxter, 1992) has examined and empirically documented similar dialectics, as well as a tension between predictability and novelty, across the development of relationships.

Finally, the concept of *praxis* emphasizes the reflexive constitution of human beings and their social worlds. Human communicators are conceived as both ongoing producers and products of their own choices within encompassing and historically conditioned cultural contexts. Persons act with others to produce contexts, which in turn function to produce the subject as an object. The notion of praxis focuses attention on the decisions friends make in the face of objective constraints existing in their temporally and spatially specific social circumstances. But a praxic view also notes that many of these constraints derive from prior choices the individual has made that now manifest themselves as objective and concrete limitations on action. Accordingly, this chapter depicts individuals as conscious, active selectors of possible choices from a field that is partially conceived by them, partially negotiated with others, and partially determined by social and natural factors outside of their control. The choices a person makes throughout life in concrete circumstances simultaneously generate and constrain options.

Informed by a dialectical perspective, I do not consider *maintenance* to be an appropriate comprehensive metaphor for guiding inquiry into the lived experience of sustaining friendships for several reasons.[1] First, the language of maintenance and repair invokes mechanistic and cybernetic imagery, as if baseline specifications exist for relational "performance" to be "maintained." The terms suggest that individuals following specified procedures and/or timetables in their connections with others can preserve the existing state of their relationships from decline or adjust them to a desired setting. Problems (or malfunctions) can be repaired. Although such language expresses optimism and faith in a technological and instrumental ethic for conducting relationships (and echoes of this stance were apparent in some participants' accounts), I consider the maintenance metaphor a potentially disturbing and objectifying rubric.

Perhaps more importantly, I believe the discourse on "maintenance" and "repair" reflects naive and misleading conceptions about enduring connec-

---

[1] While this chapter was in press, Montgomery (1993) published an article arguing similarly for a conception of sustaining relationships versus maintaining them. This is an intriguing example of how a dialectical perspective can sometimes lead scholars to shared insights regarding relational matters.

tions with others, especially friendships. In adulthood much of what makes friendship possible, or problematic, is beyond the friends' direct control. Working from a dialectical view of social life, one sees that both partners are continuously making choices and responding to exigencies inside and outside of their dyad that ramify throughout a broad array of relationships (Rawlins, 1992). Within the limits determined by their place in the social structure, individuals shape and reflect their values and priorities in choosing the relationships and collectivities in which they will participate as well as the extent of their commitment to them. What creates problems between friends during adulthood is often larger than the friendship itself.

Moreover, dyadic relationships are embedded in each partner's encompassing configuration of involvements that is itself part of a larger life story. In emphasizing the dyad and steady state notions, discussions of relationship maintenance risk looking at the ongoing practices of being friends as if they were somehow separate from their sociocultural envelope, as well as each party's embracing life course events (Blieszner & Adams, 1992; Milardo & Wellman, 1992). As considered here, friendships are doubly embedded and therefore doubly contingent. First, there must be times and places for friendship within the press of each person's configuration of social obligations, conceived synchronically as a contemporary personal network (Wellman, 1992). Second, there must be times and places for particular friendships diachronically as one or both persons' social worlds reconfigure themselves over time. These changes may be due to events in the lives of people or contexts indirectly implicated in the friendship. For example, a friend's spouse may take a new job in another town or at a status level that "requires" new friends. One's close friend may marry or divorce. The practices of friends must address both synchronic and diachronic arrangements and lived contingencies.

A dialectical perspective on sustaining friendships recognizes that one individual's choice of interactional strategies has only conditional impact on the overall trajectory of given relationships. We must look at patterns of thoughts and deeds that are *jointly* enacted in composing the relationship's continuity. Moreover, we should note that our choices as relational actors and communicators shape and reflect multiple levels of social constraints and opportunities. To a significant degree, the viability of friendships depends on the continuity of the social configurations within which they occur, for example, remaining in the same community or work network. Sometimes, new social contexts are chosen at the expense of former friendships; sometimes, though probably less often, friendships are developed at the risk of one or both parties' situations. The activities sustaining friendships therefore may need to address persons outside the dyad or factors affecting the embracing organization of one's own life or the friend's life. Throughout adulthood, the continuing connection and dyadic interactions of friends must mesh with multiple contending voices and enveloping conversations.

Adults' Descriptions of Their Friendships

The following discussion is based on open-ended interviews conducted with 56 middle-class, middle-aged women and men living in the midwestern United States. Thirteen pairs of these participants were married to each other. The interviewees ranged in age from 28 to 69 years old. The average age of the women was 45.8 years. Their occupations included: administrative assistant, director of a volunteer bureau, financial advisor, floral designer, graduate teaching assistant, guidance counselor, homemaker, housekeeper, market researcher, part-time waitress, professor, registered nurse, residence hall director, salesperson, secondary school teacher, and secretary. Twenty of these women were married for the first time and three for the second time; three were divorced and two were widowed. All had children, with a mean distribution of 2.3 per woman. The average age of the men was 46.7 years. Their occupations included: accountant, administrative assistant, army officer, assistant manager, building contractor, business executive, college counselor, dentist, electrical engineer, graphic designer, industrial arts instructor, industrial systems manager, investment counselor, professor, purchaser for manufacturing, salesperson, and secondary school administrator. Twenty-three of the men were married, one was divorced, and three were single. Of the men who were or had been married, all but one had children, with an average distribution of 2.4 per man.

Using the "experience-near concepts" of these participants, I examined some of the expectations and meanings they associated with their friendships, and the thoughts and actions they described in trying to sustain them (Geertz, 1976). The approach taken here is phenomenological and interpretive. I attempt to construe each person's statements according to meanings that the actor's situation had for him or her. This approach acknowledges that each participant's account involves interpretation and depiction of a negotiated, lived, and socially constituted context (Taylor, 1977). Identical interview protocols guided the interactions with all of these participants. While each person was asked questions about the meanings, communicative practices, activities, and important events of her or his friendships, specific concerns and emphases were discussed further as they arose.

The Social Patterning of Friendship Discontinuities

This section portrays how these adults' friendships were both supported and undermined by the social networks in which they occurred. First, the intermittent yet restorable character of friendships is contrasted with the socially recognized continuity of relationships such as marriage, kinship, and work bonds. Then, two contradictory themes in these participants' accounts of their friendships are examined. On the one hand, they considered mutual availability, that is, "being there" for each other, as definitive of friendship. However, they also reported having minimal time for friends because other social arrangements and responsibilities interfered with or assumed precedence over them. Consequently, they detailed a variety of social processes occurring outside their friendships that resulted in separations from friends, a trajectory they called "growing apart."

Sigman (1991) has analytically distinguished between "the life history of a social relationship and the interactional co-presence of the relationship partners" (p. 106), arguing that little attention has been paid to how relational partners enact their relationships as persisting in the face of extended periods of physical and interactional non-co-presence. Sigman (1991) states:

> From this perspective, relationship members are not only confronted by the agendas and intentions of their partners but also by more abstract (i.e., socioculturally general) demands. The socio-cultural reality of relationships involves a 'problem' for the co-members: reification of the relationship itself, maintenance of the particular form the reality of the relationship takes both for partners and for other persons, and establishment of the continuity of the tangible existence of the relationship across space and time, that is, both when the co-members are in each other's interactional presence and when they are absent from each other. (p. 107)

Sigman (1991) argues that certain relationships are socio-culturally defined as *continuous* and viewed as persisting despite the partners' non-co-presence. Examples include marriages, kin relationships, and contractually regulated business affiliations. In contrast, there are relationships that are considered *repeatable* and *restorable* (Sigman, 1991). These are connections that may be resumed on an ongoing basis but are not socially recognized as necessarily continuing when the members are not co-present. Of course, restorable relationships vary widely in terms of their mutual obligations and acknowledgment by others. They range from the utterly episodic link between a ticket teller and customer to the ongoing interweaving of lives enacted by close friends or longtime lovers. Certainly, friends and lovers themselves vary in the degree to which they perceive their own relationship as continuous or restorable. Achieving shared perceptions and assumptions about the relationship's capacity to endure separations is one of the challenges facing friends and lovers.

A combination of social patterning and individual initiative decides how, when, and whether friendships are developed and sustained during adulthood. The ongoing accomplishment of friendship must be examined in terms of life course moments, and situated in social and geographical space and time. Some of these adults' friendships were established earlier in the friends' lives when they lived in close proximity and were more easily able to spend a lot of time together. In retrospect, life seemed less serious to them then, with both friends assuming fewer adult responsibilities and having more time for fun. Frequently, images of selves, relationships, and social contexts created during such periods are cherished throughout peoples' lives (Rawlins, 1992). As persons take on more of the tasks and obligations of adult life, their time for friendship often dwindles, while the demands of domestic, community, and occupational domains typically take precedence (Rawlins, 1992). Once-close friends now may be separated by social priorities, and/or time and space. Even so, these friendships may persist through ongoing interaction or intermittent contact, or become memories.

A desire for readily available friends still informed these adults' conceptions of friendship. A chief expectation of a friend was for that person to "be there" to talk to and to help. The following statements are representative of the participants' answers to a question about their expectations of friends:

I would expect that person to be interested in me for who I am, not necessarily what I can do for them. Um, I would expect that person to be there when I needed them. If I am going through a hard time with something, I would expect them to be there for that. (Tim, married, academic counselor, 36 years old)

Uh, someone that is always there. If you want to talk to them, they always have time for you. Even if they're busy, they'll make time for you. (Loretta, married, professor, mother of two, 40 years old)

Mmm, I would expect them to be umm, trustworthy; I would expect them to be there when I need them and umm, to help me out or be a shoulder, or listening and a good ear, a good shoulder to cry on when I need them. (Andrea, married, registered nurse, mother of two, 44 years old)

I don't know, kinda be there I guess if you want to talk, or do, or whatever. They're kind of in a default position. Somebody you keep coming back to for whatever, a situation may arise for fun or for trouble or for advice, or whatever. (Keith, married, purchaser for manufacturing, father of three, 52 years old)

To be there when I need them. To be able to discuss most anything, personal or otherwise. Just themselves being there, not material things. (Alicia, married, homemaker, mother of four, 54 years old)

That they would be there when you need them. True friendship is not the surface kind of friendship that many acquaintances have with one another. But, when you need somebody, whether it be for emotional support or even financial support, although that's not important. But a person that when you need something is there to help you. (Arnold, married, school administrator, father of four, 59 years old)

Having friends who would "be there" was both a comforting thought and a practical achievement. It took time to develop and sustain the kind of friendship that included such mutually held assumptions of availability, time that was typically contingent on other relationships and demands. William, a married, 56-year-old business executive and father of three children, succinctly described what separates such friendships from the rest:

How much you put into it. I mean, I could probably have more close friendships if I really, I mean if I simply put more into it. Simply took the time to put more into it, and tested the friendship and climbed into it. But, I'm a pretty active person; I don't really have a lot of spare time. So, I don't really have enough time to sit down and develop all these interpersonal skills, although I have to have them with my wife and children.

For William, whether or not he develops other close friendships boils down to social priorities, which was a common observation by interviewees.

Friendships were typically pursued as part of encompassing configurations of adult activities and responsibilities, which could facilitate or hinder a wide range of involvements with others, including close friends. Vicki, a married, 41-year-old salesperson and mother of two, observed:

I think your friendships change as situations change. You know, you go through the little fill-the-house type thing with all the little kids babysitting, and taking turns. And that's a kind of friendship and you have something pulling you together that maybe normally that kind of person wouldn't be someone you would maybe normally find yourself drawn to. And some of those will mature into a real friendship and some will just kind of fade away, kind of a convenience type thing.

Andrea described how the passage of time and the appropriate social circumstances shaped a friendship of hers:

I develop rapport immediately because I can usually get people talking, but friendships usually don't happen overnight; it's very unusual when they do. And it's amazing as you grow older, some of those people you thought were just acquaintances, as you get older your lives change, they become friends. At first they were like classmates, like Patty Thompson and I, we weren't that good of friends in school. But now that we're out, we are good friends. 'Course, we lived together and our husbands knew each other, so all those extenuating circumstances. All of a sudden as your life, as you grow older, those kinds of things draw you together.

These persons' experiences of friendship were significantly structured by the challenges and happenstances of coordinating couples' activities, aligning family compositions, synchronizing life stages, pursuing careers, and matching schedules. Although talking and doing things together remained the lifeblood of close friendships, their very possibility noticeably reflected socially constituted constraints.

The social patterning of friendships was especially apparent in the participants' depictions of how friends "grow apart" from each other. There were several related trajectories. First, friends could remain close geographically, but a shift in one or the other's marital or occupational status could result in social or emotional distancing and sharply diminished time spent together. Second, these and other changes in social configurations, such as the gradual development of a different set of friends, could shape and reflect new interests or personal priorities that are not shared with the original friend. Third, any or all of these developments could occur in conjunction with a friend moving a significant distance away. Finally, a person may need to move away for reasons that initially suggest little change in the friendship (for example, to care for a relative), but the separation eventually results in the friends growing apart and losing touch.

I was struck by how pervasively the phrase, "growing apart," was used by these participants in discussing their friendships, and by its double meaning. First, growing apart implies that friends are gradually and "naturally" loosening their connection with each other as their lives unfold. Second and relatedly, the phrase could suggest that the former friends are developing separately as individuals. Even so, these accounts display resignation. These adults had to address the subsequent continuation, dormancy, or dissolution of their friendships in facing the literal and/or figurative distance that now separated them. The following examples show how friendship discontinuities are shaped by other social circumstances, like marital and family status, occupation, emerging interests, and friendship circles. The accounts suggest precious little that interaction between the friends could do to reverse or "repair" these processes.

An extended excerpt from Loretta's interview depicts how tangibly such constraints have affected her friendships. In reading her words, recall her expectation, quoted previously, for her close friends' constant availability.

I noticed when I was in college it seemed like I still, I made new friends, but I was still friends with the same people I knew in high school. . . . But, it's funny now. I don't really see a lot of those people now. They're still in town but I just, it's just kind of like your, the things you do are different. You grow apart, so you just really don't go out with them as much as you did, and do things with them. Now we've lost a, I guess I shouldn't say lost, but um, we don't see them as much anymore because of divorce. So it's kind of awkward, good friends that split up, a lot of times one or both will move out of town.

. . . And then we have a problem with friends who stayed in town, remarried, and we're still friends with the husband *and* the wife, and now they have different spouses, so who do you ask? So there have been a lot of times when there's a large group of people, you'll ask both. But I always tell both of them the other person was invited because to me that would be, I've never been in that situation, but I would feel real awkward if I didn't know the other one was going to be there and they're not friends. So normally what happens is that the girl usually comes and the husband, the ex-husband, doesn't come. And then there's been a lot of times when we'll just go out with the ex-husband and his new wife and a couple of other people and not ask the wife and her new husband.

. . . Divorce plays a part because it makes the friendship awkward. And if one doesn't remarry, or date, um, we've had, like Sheila Wilson, we've asked her to things, but I think she feels funny because she doesn't have, have a date. Yeah, so it's kind of like you lead separate lives if you're married and you're single, I don't know, even if you're the same age.

Wayne, a married, 47-year-old industrial supervisor with two children, described how friends moving disrupted two of his friendships:

Well there have been a couple; but it's only been the case of where we grew apart geographically, where he moved away and then we just never kept up the relationship. I would still consider him a friend, but not a real close friend, because I just haven't seen him in so many years. . . . In both cases I did make attempts to talk to them, but in both cases they had changes in their lives that, umm, were dramatic and they didn't reciprocate, like they grew apart. You know, it happens.

Keith refers to the process as a "gentle parting of the ways":

Friendships and relationships change a little bit over time. Uh, I'm old enough to—people move, people change, their interests change—and it's not that you get angry at somebody or situations like that. It's just kind of a gentle parting of the ways over time, people come and go. . . . I think people will, uh, there's some outside influences that can be rather unexpected, people take job offers and leave and that causes some separation. . . . Changes in interests and I think too there's, uh, let's say an involvement; people are involved in certain social circles. Sometimes you see people moving towards other interests in other groups and you can kind of sense they're going away.

These narratives reflect the ongoing reconfiguring of friendships during middle adulthood evident throughout the interviews. An almost tangible irony permeated these adults' discussions of close or "real" friendship. On the one hand, a premier expectation of such a friend was that he or she would "be there" when needed to talk to or depend on for assistance. Such availability was widely cited as definitive of friendship, and was greatly facilitated by living or working near each other, being part of the same network, facing similar life course challenges, or simply having the time. On the other hand, the interviews were riddled with accounts of how vulnerable their friendships were to altered circumstances—people marrying, divorcing, remaining single, remarrying, shifting schedules, having children, changing jobs, moving away, developing new interests. It felt like valued friendships were continually slipping away from these adults, in most cases due to events that transcended the friendships. However, when the contexts of friendships altered, these persons repeatedly described certain thoughts and actions that they selectively employed in attempting to sustain some of them. We turn now to these practices.

Individual and Relational Practices of Sustaining Friendships

For various reasons these adults experienced extended periods of separation from and/or no contact with their friends. During these junctures, ranging from days to decades, they did not share a "vivid present" and moments of "growing older together" in Schutz's (1970) sense. Several issues shaped friends' experiences of these breaches. For one thing, the friends reflected on the extent to which the breach was due to the time demands of other relational involvements and obligations (such as family, work, and hobbies) or to a personal inclination on their own or the other's part. In cases involving friends who still resided in the same locale, considerable ambiguity existed about the onset of the separation. Several people described themselves as "wondering" if they had done or said something that hurt the other's feelings. For the most part, however, people observed (as in some of the preceding quotations) that their drifting or growing apart was "not anybody's fault," and therefore they "still considered them friends." This view of the other left the door open to continued friendship.

Another concern was the nature of the hiatus itself. What did it signify about the friendship? Did the partners continue to share an active friendship, except with a more relaxed rhythm of encounters and time spent apart? Or was this a dormant friendship, involving an indefinite period of separation and an anticipation of renewal by either party's initiative? Or perhaps no contact was expected and the friendship was now considered a memory. Finally, with increasing time passing since the friends were together and the recollection of possible actions that could have hurt or angered the friend, maybe this was a dissolved friendship? Were these two persons no longer friends?

This is a potentially nettlesome collection of issues for friends to live with for several reasons. First, an individual cannot answer these questions for certain without contacting the other or getting back together again (Rawlins, 1983a). But this situation makes the original quandary about the meaning of their separation both paradoxical and interactive. It is paradoxical because of friendship's essentially voluntary nature. That is, getting back together only answers the question for the moment; once the friends part, the temporal and existential meter of separation begins to tick again. It requires a mutually enacted pattern over time to describe fully the nature of their continued involvement. It is an interactive quandary because without resuming contact, friends do not necessarily know what the other is thinking. If either one assumes apathy or disdain on the other's part, he or she may not contact that person, thereby perpetuating one side of their separation and preventing the testing of the suspicions. It is also an interactive quandary because none of these scenarios may actually be formulated consciously; rather, they are played out while both friends are living through the activities and schedules mapping their days, months, and years. Only one or the other's pause to reflect registers this passage of time in the context of their friendship.

Finally, how discontinuities are interpreted and enacted depends on the mutual definition of the friendship and certain assumptions that have developed over its history. These participants remarked that friends who were tied to limited or specific contexts, such as work, recreation, or community participation, or who shared only a brief period of closeness, often were not expected to preserve their connection indefinitely. Further, closer bonds with more and varied experiences were more likely to have developed some key mutual assumptions. One is the assumption of benevolence, which refers to good friends' tendency to see each other's actions in the best light and to give each other the benefit of the doubt in questionable circumstances (Rawlins, 1991, 1992). Consequently, a common and valued past and the assumption of benevolence may lead a person to excuse a friend's failure to keep in touch for an inordinately long period of time. Both shared history and well wishing enabled friends to assume the restorability if not the continuity of their caring for each other.

Several persons kept the *idea* of their ongoing friendship with others alive through fond thoughts about their friends. Even with minimal contact, they reflected on their friends' continued presence in their lives, emphasizing that the friendship was "still there." Rhonda, a married, 51 year-old marketing supervisor with three children, remarked:

> It doesn't matter how far apart we get or how often we see each other, especially if it's somebody that you don't have a chance to see very often. It's just like you know that they're out there somewhere and they know you're out there somewhere. . . . Maybe some of the friends we only see for dinner a couple of times a year, or we exchange written notes or whatever. But, they're still there and we care about them; it's just that we don't have time to actively nurture the friendship.

Without contacting friends, such thoughts may provide private solace and gratification, but their relational significance appears to be the sustained image of such friendships as eligible for restoration. In answering the question, "How do you know when friendships won't last?" Ellen, a married, 53-year-old financial advisor and mother of three, replied:

> I guess I don't! If it's an acquaintance, maybe an acquaintanceship won't last because it's on a different level than a friendship. But if it's gone past an acquaintanceship and has gotten to a deeper level where you really consider this person a friend—like I said, we have friends that go back twenty-some years. And there's a few female friends that go back to childhood that I will stay in touch with. Now we don't see each other as often. And there's a few yet from college that I don't see them a whole lot; they live in different parts of the country and everything.
> And I don't know if you consider that still a friendship. But to me it's still a friendship because, even though I don't see them, I write to them every once in a while, and occasionally I get a letter back. But, as far as I'm concerned, I still care about them and what's going on in their lives. And if there was ever an opportunity for us to get together, I just think that would be wonderful to revisit all those old times we had together and everything. I guess I don't really think about a friendship not lasting.

Interactionally, the continuation of separated friendships becomes a question of "staying in touch," however predictably or sporadically the mutually acknowledged activities occur. The primary culprit cited for problems with friends and losing touch was a lack of time. Consequently, keeping friendships alive and rekindling them involved "taking," "making," or "finding the time." Having no time could make virtually any physical distance between friends too far to traverse. Still, friends who lived within striking distance of each other found that actually making the friendship a priority and scheduling opportunities to spend or share some time together was essential. Several mentioned, however, that these occasions often were talked about more than they were accomplished.

Closely associated with taking the time was "making the effort" to keep in touch, especially with people who had moved or remained at prior locations. People mentioned telephone calls ("the almighty phone"), letters, greeting cards (especially Christmas cards), as well as visits as important for staying in contact. With telephone calls people share "real time" with each other (Sigman, 1991), and several adults spoke of "telephone friendships," where their primary interaction was over the phone. A number of persons, mostly women, described preserving ties through writing letters and sending Christmas cards, but these endeavors involved their own constraints. Angie, a married, 50-year-old market researcher and mother of two, discussed her attempts to keep in touch with a woman who had moved away 6 years prior to the interview:

> It takes a lot of effort because you have to sit down and write a letter, and we do call each other probably twice a year. And it was wonderful being in Florida with each other for a week because we were right there. But it's harder because you have to sit down and write a letter, and that's hard because it takes time. When I know I'm going to write her, I'm going to write probably 8 or 10 pages. And so you don't just do that in 10 minutes. So it's hard.

Later, she narrated a commonplace trajectory for these adults:

> My best friend from high school, I have probably not seen her probably in thirty years since high school. And we wrote—No, I saw her when I was in college.—But we wrote letters, and we called each other for awhile, then it was just Christmas cards, then all of a sudden it was nothing. And I think, I'm sure that a lot of the reason that friendship ended was because we didn't spend time together, because I think you can only write just so much on a Christmas card.

Clearly, mutual visits, even if few and far between, offered the most expansive opportunities for renewing and sustaining friendships. One of the most celebrated features of enduring bonds was the friends' mutual ability to "pick right up with the friendship" after virtually any duration. By all accounts, whether face-to-face or over the phone, accomplishing this with old friends was a clear case of restoring the friendship, particularly if conversations did not merely replay the past. Sally was a married, 66-year-old director of a volunteer bureau with five children. She recounted how an evening visit with old friends who had "drifted" away condensed the time that had lapsed and reinstated their moments of friendship:

> A few months ago, some friends here in town, we were just really close when we first came and then drifted apart. And we went to visit them, and it just felt so good. It was like we have seen each other. We could walk in and sit down and just feel like a day had hardly passed between the last time we were together. And we sat there, laughed at the same things, and shared together how it feels to get old and talked about retirement, talked some about our families but not a whole lot, mostly shared our feelings. It was just such a warm great evening it really made me think, "We've got to do this more often.

Conclusion

These persons concretely experienced the contingent nature of their friendships at the intersections of individual initiative and social patterning. Becoming friends involved individuals choosing each other to care about and developing practices that both found mutually fulfilling. They expected their close friends to be there for them to talk to, depend on, and enjoy sharing activities. Even so, across the adult years, friendships were negotiated within constantly evolving configurations of social roles and affiliations. Seldom purely dyadic endeavors, their continuation was constrained and/or facilitated by the friends' embracing activities, such as work, marriage, parenthood, family, other friends, and neighborhood and community life. In many cases, friends were separated by social demands and exigencies transcending the dyad, a pattern commonly referred to as "growing apart."

The narratives I examined positioned the primary challenges of sustaining friendships as questions of individual volition in the grips of enveloping and divisive social arrangements. How could friends be there for each other in social configurations that required them to grow apart? How available could friends be for each other in the face of multiple claims on their time, especially when they were dispersed geographically? Some dyads developed patterns of routine contact; others tried to schedule fairly regular visits, recreation, or phone conversations. Still others "touched base" monthly, seasonally, or even less often.

But what is being sustained by these practices? It appeared that a range of stances toward friendships was cultivated, with potential ambiguity about whether both friends viewed their connection or disconnection similarly. These participants' descriptions suggested to me three modes of sustaining friendship: (1) active, (2) dormant, and (3) commemorative. *Active* friendships reflected mutually negotiated habits of ready availability, satisfactory contact, and emotional commitment. Such friends were expected to be there when needed, even if it involved significant travel or phone bills. The interviewees celebrated friends who had "come through" when called on or who had stood "the test of time." *Dormant* friendships shared a valued history and/or maintained sufficient contact to anticipate or remain eligible for a resumption of the friendship at any time. In these dyads there was less of an expectation for such friends to be there and more of an assumption that their friendship continued to exist ("the friendship is there") as a comforting, helpful, or enjoyable potential. Such bonds could be viewed indefinitely by one or both friends as dormant. For a variety of reasons including, for example, the passage of time, lost contact, or attributions of neglect, some friendships were considered merely memories. Such *commemorative* friendships often retained significance, however, as poignant symbols of particular places and moments of the life course or editions of the self-with-others. Reflecting on these friends was a bittersweet activity. Remembering times spent with them captured key feelings, thoughts, and activities from earlier periods in life. Even so, these memories could be tinged with regrets about life's undeniable finitude and the choices that left various friends behind.

In many respects, these adults' descriptions of their friendships expressed ambivalent feelings about middle-class immersion in a striving, competitive social system. Although their opportunities and resources for friendship were structured extensively by their career quests and accomplishments in this system, it continuously goaded them to abandon friendships and communities for "greener pastures," even within the same geographical area. And despite the fact that contemporary communication technologies and means of travel often diminished the salience of physical distance, busy schedules and other priorities preserved time as the deepest chasm, wherein there was often little place for friendship.

In scholarly work and everyday lives it is easy to psychologize or interpersonalize the quandaries of separated friends, and, in fact, most of these participants narratized their restoration in terms of individuals' initiatives. But the relational discontinuities in these accounts were typically not matters of psychological compatibility. Rather, they involved the social contexts and larger life stories in which they were embedded. In this regard, questions about how these adults sustained their friendships transmute into inquiries like, What kinds of social arrangements do we want to live and work together in? and What is the nature of the well-lived life? As Sadler (1970) sagely noted over 20 years ago:

> It is hard to find a place for friendship when one's primary values are: intellectual domination over oneself and the environment; highly successful individual achievement; keeping busy; lucrative productivity; effective manipulation of data, programs, and personnel; having exotic experiences; and finding the security of moral certainty that in our striving we are doing what is right. (p. 196)

Judging together and taking action on these larger issues and contexts have direct implications for our possibilities for friendship (Beiner, 1983).

We need more research about how the social construction of time, identities, and communities shapes and reflects the practices of relationships in general and friendship in particular across the life course. Further understanding is also necessary regarding precisely how relationships are facilitated and disqualified by the requirements and communicative endeavors of embracing networks. How do individuals establish the priorities patterning their involvements with others? How do both parties enact and feel about distinctions among active, dormant, and commemorative friendships? Clearly, demographic and network data have much to offer in describing the distribution of the various activities of multiple participants (Wellman, 1992). Still, they lack the indepth insight of personal narratives depicting how persons have actually experienced and managed these socially constituted exigencies. Moreover, we need more than just a snapshot of relational configurations at one point in time, as this investigation and most network studies provide; we need research that covers the temporal development of focal persons' biographies.

Finally, because we, as scholars of interpersonal life, cannot be separated from the subjects of our work, we also need to reflect continuously on the moral imperatives that guide our collective efforts. Are the contexts, predicaments, or practices we describe the ones that we want to reproduce and share with others?

References

Altman, I., Vinsel, A., & Brown, B. B. (1981). Dialectic conceptions in social psychology: An application to social penetration and privacy regulation. In L. Berkowitz (Ed.), *Advances in experimental social psychology* (Vol. 14, pp. 107–160). London: Academic Press.

Baxter, L. A. (1988). A dialectical perspective on communication strategies in relationship development. In S. W. Duck, D. F. Hay, S. E. Hobfoll, W. Ickes, & B. Montgomery (Eds.), *Handbook of personal relationships* (pp. 257–273). London: Wiley.

Baxter, L. A. (1990). Dialectical contradictions in relationship development. *Journal of Social and Personal Relationships, 7,* 69–88.

Beiner, R. (1983). *Political judgment.* Chicago: The University of Chicago Press.

Blieszner, R., & Adams, R. G. (1992). *Adult friendship*. Newbury Park, CA: Sage.

Bloch, M. (1971). The moral and tactical meaning of kinship terms. *Man, 6*, 79–87.

Bopp, M. J., & Weeks, G. R. (1984). Dialectical metatheory in family therapy. *Family Process, 23*, 49–61.

Brain, R. (1976). *Friends and lovers*. New York: Basic Books.

Bridge, K., & Baxter, L. A. (1992). Blended relationships: Friends as work associates. *Western Journal of Communication, 56*, 200–225.

Geertz, C. (1976). "From the native's point of view": On the nature of anthropological under-standing. In K. H. Basso & H. A. Selby (Eds.), *Meaning in anthropology* (pp. 221–237). Albu-querque: University of New Mexico Press.

Kurth, S. B. (1970). Friendships and friendly relations. In G. J. McCall, M. M. McCall, N. K. Denzin, G. D. Suttles, & S. Kurth (Eds.), *Social relationships* (pp. 136–170). Chicago: Aldine de Gruyter.

Milardo, R. M., & Wellman, B. (1992). The personal is social. *Journal of Social and Personal Relationships, 9*, 339–342.

Montgomery, B. M. (1993). Relationship maintenance versus relationship change: A dialectical dilemma. *Journal of Social and Personal Relationships, 10*, 205–223.

Naegele, K. D. (1958). Friendship and acquaintances: An exploration of some social distinctions. *Harvard Educational Review, 28*, 232–252.

Neugarten, B. L. (Ed.). (1968). *Middle age and aging: A reader in social psychology*. Chicago: University of Chicago Press.

Paine, R. (1969). In search of friendship: An exploratory analysis in "middle-class" culture. *Man, 4*, 505–524.

Rawlins, W. K. (1983a). Negotiating close friendships: The dialectic of conjunctive freedoms. *Human Communication Research, 9*, 255–266.

Rawlins, W. K. (1983b). Openness as problematic in ongoing friendships: Two conversational dilemmas. *Communication Monographs, 50*, 1–13.

Rawlins, W. K. (1989). A dialectical analysis of the tensions, functions and strategic challenges of communication in young adult friendships. In J. A. Anderson (Ed.), *Communication yearbook 12* (pp. 157–189). Newbury Park, CA: Sage.

Rawlins, W. K. (1991). On enacting friendship and interrogating discourse. In K. Tracy (Ed.), *Understanding face-to-face interaction: Issues linking goals and discourse* (pp. 101–115). New York: Lawrence Erlbaum.

Rawlins, W. K. (1992). *Friendship matters: Communication, dialectics, and the life course*. Hawthorne, New York: Aldine de Gruyter.

Rawlins, W. K., & Holl, M. (1988). Adolescents' interactions with parents and friends: Dialectics of temporal perspective and evaluation. *Journal of Social and Personal Relationships, 5*, 27–46.

Sadler, W. A. (1970). The experience of friendship. *Humanitas, 6*, 177–209.

Schutz, A. (1970). Interactional relationships. In H. R. Wagner (Ed.), *Alfred Schutz on phenome-nology and social relations* (pp. 163–199). Chicago: University of Chicago Press.

Sigman, S. J. (1991). Handling the discontinuous aspects of continuing social relationships: Toward research on the persistence of social forms. *Communication Theory, 1*, 106–127.

Simmel, G. (1950). *The sociology of Georg Simmel*. Kurt Wolff (Ed. and Trans.). Glencoe, IL: The Free Press.

Taylor, C. (1977). Interpretation and the sciences of man. In F. R. Dallmayr & T. A. McCarthy (Eds.), *Understanding social inquiry* (pp. 101–131). Notre Dame: University of Notre Dame Press.

Wellman, B. (1992). Men in networks: Private communities, domestic friendships. In P. M. Nardi (Ed.), *Men's Friendships* (pp. 74–114). Newbury Park, CA: Sage.

Epilogue

Tracing the Threads of Spider Webs

Laura Stafford

Department of Communication
Ohio State University
Columbus, Ohio

Introduction

This volume has served as a forum for various views on relational maintenance. And regardless of the orientation taken, the primary focus of all the
chapters, as reflected in the title, has been on communication. Given that
communication is a dynamic and ongoing process, it is not surprising to find
some similarity among these chapters: In one way or another maintenance is
portrayed as part of a process of relating. This general orientation is unequiv-
ocally adopted as opposed to more static approaches of relationship stability
based on some set of characteristics (i.e., demographic, compatibility, or
similarity models; see Cate & Lloyd, 1992). Though this baseline agreement
is apparent throughout, it is equally apparent that there is no one emergent
vision of "maintenance."

Definitional Issues

Understanding what various authors mean when the term *maintenance* is
employed is necessary for conceptual clarity (see also Dindia & Canary,

1993). An important point at which to enter this dialogue is in examining what is meant by "maintenance" and its cohort terms. An ostensibly underlying assumption manifest in most definitions is that maintenance is a temporal state: some midpoint or stage of relational life. As Montgomery (1993) notes "most scholars do agree about when maintenance occurs—namely, just after a relationship has finished beginning and just before it has started to end" (p. 205). This stance also is exemplified in Duck's (this volume) articulation of "relationship maintenance as a point *between* initial development and possible decline; a period of continuous existence" [emphasis added]. In other words, maintenance is generally studied as a "stage" somewhere after "escalation" and before "de-escalation" (see Dindia, this volume). Despite this general consensus, the definition of maintenance is not so neatly packaged. Baxter (this volume) argues that "dialogical maintenance disallows such temporal displacement." Yet for most, it appears given that maintenance only occurs when "stuck in the middle."

The question of the temporal placement of maintenance is only one area in which definitional consensus is lacking. Basic definitions of maintenance are divergent as well. Dindia and Canary (1993) offer four definitions of relational maintenance: "(1) to keep a relationship in existence; (2) to keep a relationship in a specified state or condition; (3) to keep a relationship in satisfactory condition; and (4) to keep a relationship in repair" (p. 163).

Most of the contributors to this volume see maintenance as fundamentally a state of existence. For some, keeping the relationship intact is the primary concern. For example, Roloff and Cloven ask how partners *stay together* in the face of relational transgressions. This is basically a question of relational stability. This is not to imply that staying in the stage of togetherness is stable in the sense that relationships do not change, but rather stable in the sense that they are together. Gottman considers maintenance as partners not divorcing (i.e., being stable). He also discusses marital satisfaction; yet, satisfaction is mostly relevant in that it is predictive of stability.

The mere state of existence is a necessary, but not sufficient, condition for most of the contributors. Maintenance appears to be a state of relational stability with manifest positive relational characteristics. Dindia and Canary (1993) have partialed this into two distinctions: (1) the primary focus on relational satisfaction (by far the most commonly studied variable), and (2) additional relational properties such as liking, love, trust, and so forth.

Authors in this volume who appear to adopt the primary stance of maintenance as existence plus satisfaction include Rusbult, Drigotas, and Verette, and Attridge. Rusbult and colleagues ask "Why do some relationships make it through both good times and bad times whereas others do not?" They note that remaining in a relationship is the minimum requirement for maintenance; additional concern is with the promotion of "healthy functioning."

Attridge also extends the notion of maintenance from mere survival to that of the satisfactory nature of the relationship.

Other authors see maintenance as not only the intact state or global satisfaction, but are concerned with other relational proprieties. Vangelisti and Huston examine satisfaction and love, where maintenance is conceived of as a "relative lack of change in marital satisfaction and love over time." Canary and Stafford are primarily concerned with the preservation of relational characteristics such as liking, control mutuality, trust, and commitment. Dindia also considers characteristics other than satisfaction in referring to maintenance as the period in which *advanced* levels of familiarity, attraction, and connection are sustained.

Some of the authors herein concentrate on repair, or preempting the need for repair. Roloff and Cloven ask "How do partners stay on track in the face of decay and threatening circumstances?" Rejuvenation is also conceivably repair oriented, as seen by Wilmot's interest in "the process of improving a relationship that has gone through a period of decline." Burleson and Samter's emphasis on maintenance as a response to relational exigencies implies a repair-oriented stance.

In summary, in addition to the four definitions noted by Dindia and Canary (1993), one other vision of maintenance emerges: the view of maintenance as a period or stage in relational time in which processes of some sort are used to ensure this period continues. In short, we have the notion of maintenance as an intact relationship, and for many, the ensuring of relational properties and characteristics whether through the prevention of their decline, through their enhancement, or through their reestablishment. In addition, maintenance is portrayed as a temporal point in time versus a process throughout relational history.

As was foreshadowed by the basic juxtaposition of maintenance as a temporal point or continuous phenomenon, this simple synopsis is deceiving. Disentangling definitions of maintenance are actually much more troublesome for several reasons. First, in most (if not all) conceptualizations of maintenance, state and process have been entangled. Second, the term maintenance itself has been deemed problematic by some. The concern with the term and the meaning of stability may lie at the bottom of this quagmire.

Process and State

In regard to the entanglement of stage and state, it becomes apparent that maintenance has been viewed as a state and/or timeframe (stage), and/or the processes used within that state/stage to ensure its continuence. In essence, it seems that much of the concern about the terminology resides in one fundamental confusion: Is maintenance a *state* of existence (or existence plus some relational characteristics) or is maintenance a *process* (the "to keep" part of Dindia and Canary's definitions, i.e., the acts, behaviors, and so forth that function to keep a relationship in whatever state a researcher preferentially defines)? *Or* is maintenance *both*, as Canary and Stafford propose?

It seems that the most representative definition that can arise from this conundrum is that maintenance is the process of maintaining a given state. However, this tautology (as do all tautologies) tells us very little about the state and/or process. More precisely, the two uses of the word maintenance (as a state and as a process) constitute divergent classes and are clearly of different logical types (see Russell, 1951, cited in Watzlawick, Bavelas, and Jackson, 1967). As Watzlawick et al. (1967) note, such a confusion of logical types is not false, but rather "meaningless."

Authors such as Attridge, Canary and Stafford, Duck, Dindia, Gottman, Roloff and Cloven, Rusbult et al., and Vangelisti and Huston seem to adopt the view of maintenance as a state, although they generally study the mechanisms by which partners stay within this state. To illustrate: Attridge proposes maintenance occurs due to the presence and/or increase of barriers; Gottman's maintance occurs via communicative acts such as stating and responding to complaints; Roloff and Cloven see maintenance as approaches such as retribution reformulation; Duck argues maintenace occurs primarily via talk. Vangelisti and Huston note that given both love and satisfaction tend to decline during marriage, the struggle to keep satisfaction and love at relative high levels is an ongoing process. Despite this focus on process, the processes are only important as they serve to meet the goal (or fail to meet the goal) of keeping the relationship in some preferred state.

Alternatively, dialectical views of *maintaining* relationships are generally more reflective of processes as opposed to states. Baxter, Rawlins, and Wilmot stress the management of dialectal tensions. However, these authors also reference some sort of desired relational state. For example Baxter (this volume) envisions management of dialectal tensions within the paramarters of a healthy relationship; and Wilmot (this volume) assumes these processes occur to keep the relationship from deteriorating beyond acceptable boundaries into extinction. Hence, although dialectical views may emphasize process over state, again both process and state are considered.

Of course a process orientation does not require a dialectical framework. Maintenance is also seen from a functional standpoint. For Burleson and Samter, maintenance occurs whenever persons enact beheaviors that service the particular tasks or functions defining a particular relationship. They see maintenance as a dyadic process. Yet they also merge the stability and satisfaction components in emphasizing the "continuation of a healthy relationship" (Burleson & Samter, this volume).

Likewise, Rusbult's investment model (Rusbult et al., this volume), although concerned with satisfaction and commitment, stresses maintenance phenomena as processes: inclinations and tendencies which motivate prorclationship behavior. Marston and Hecht (this volume) are concerned with the "management of love problematics" in order to preserve the loveship. As should be evident, both state-oriented views as well as process ones (whether dialectical or not) in actuality incorporate both concepts of process and state.

The dialectic approach taken by Wilmot provides an excellent example of this intermingling of process and state; he argues that "Maintenance may be viewed as a constant struggle [process] to keep relationships in a state of rejuvenation" Specifically, he asks "How can people improve their relationships or keep them from moving to dissatisfaction *and* dissolution?" [emphasis added]. Though it appears he believes nonetheless that relational tensions are never resolved and maintenance is a constant process of negotiating these tensions. Wilmot explicitly realizes that there is a realm of acceptance within which relationships will survive.

Clearly then, whether one starts with a process-oriented view or a state view, it seems that scholars generally find themselves evolving into using maintenance as both a state *and* a process. Thus, we arrive again at our paradoxical juncture: If maintenance is used to refer to a process, the question which follows is The process *of what?* The "logical" answer, of course, is the process of maintaining.

The Term *Maintenance*

The second reason for difficulty in unifying the literature concerns the debate surrounding the use of the term *maintenance* itself. Various terms are scattered across these chapters. For example, in addition to the term maintenance, labels such as *sustaining* (Rawlins) and *rejuvenation* (Wilmot) are found. The terms invoked appear to be somewhat unimportant to some (e.g., Wilmot), whereas the precise terms appear to be of critical importance to others (e.g., Rawlins). Maintenance is both condemned and supported as a useful metaphor (Rawlins; Canary and Stafford, respectively).

Rawlins has taken marked disagreement with the term maintenance, primarily because of the mechanistic imagery potentially invoked involving the notion of a steady state or stability. Baxter argues that previous conceptions of maintenance as "preventative efforts to preserve or sustain . . . presupposes that a condition of stability is both desirable for personal relationships. . . . From a dialogic perspective, both 'maintenance' and 'repair' are neither possible nor desirable; a healthy relationship is a changing relationship in which a stable state is nonexistent" (Baxter, this volume).

Much of the concern may arise because of simple cross-understandings or uses of the term *stable*. Concern has been expressed by Rawlins and Baxter,

among others, that "a healthy relationship is a changing relationship in which
a stable state is nonexistent" (Baxter, this volume). Yet, generally when the
term stable is used by maintenance researchers, it is used in the tradition of
family studies, and simply means "intact" (e.g., Canary & Stafford; Dindia;
Duck; Gottman). Wilmot notes stability references the question of "Did this
marriage survive?" This most certainly does not preclude, in fact it likely
includes notions of the ebbs and flows or fluctuations within relationships
such as those discussed by Wilmot (within a dialectical frame).

Change is recognized by most writers invoking maintenance, otherwise the
process of maintenance would not be necessary. It is the constant change
inherent within relationships that necessitates the constant maintenance processes to keep the relationship not at a "stable state" in the static sense of the
word, but rather, both stable (as in intact from the family studies usage) and
keeping the ebbs and flows and fluctuations of important relational properties
within a range (i.e., the parameters of a "healthy relationship"; Baxter). Although it is quite likely that what are considered to be the parameters of
"healthy" change across time.

It seems reasonable to suggest that restoring a relationship to a previously
healthy state does not imply that the same exact state is possible nor desirable. Hence, it is much more likely that in the "keeping" or "returning" to
this healthy or positive state the emphasis is not on the state of previous
existence, but rather on the general characteristics of a satisfactory existence
and of the existence of other (positive) relational properties. The relationship
cannot return to its former state, but it can return (or stay) within the given
acceptable boundaries. "The term 'maintenance' implies that the object being maintained exists over a period of time—that it is more than momentary.
Maintaining a relationship suggests [the ability] to hold certain qualities of
that relationship *relatively* constant" [emphasis added] (Vangelisti & Huston,
this volume). This point is captured well by Wilmot, who views the ebbs and
flows as normal occurrences in intact (stable) relationships (also see Wilmot,
1987).

There may not be as much divergence as initially seen. After all, if relationships go beyond these boundaries (whether from a dialectic view or otherwise), they will no longer be maintained, either at all, or at least not in a
"healthy" manner. Keeping a relationship healthy is indeed a constant process. Various authors use various metaphors for maintenance, many arguing
that the term maintenance itself leads to connotations of mechanistic and
steady state entities. Some of these apparent incongruities are not necessarily
in contradiction. For example, nothing within a conception of maintenance
that emphasizes satisfaction and existence fundamentally disagrees with the
notion that relationships are inherently in a state of change.

Discussions of maintenance as efforts to keep relational characteristics at a given desirable level does not contradict the premise that relationships are changing. Indeed, it incorporates such a premise. In other words, if relationships were not in a constant state of flux, maintenance processes to keep the relationship together, satisfied, or its characteristics "in check," maintenance would not be needed. *Because relationships are in a constant state of flux, so too are relationship maintenance behaviors part of an ongoing relational processes.*

In a similar line of thought, Montgomery (1993) changes levels to resolve the stability versus change dialectic:

> Applied to the notion of ongoing relationships, this means that within the very essence of stability resides the basis for change, and vice versa. That is, to be in a stable relationship is to be in one that is continually changing, adapting to, accommodating or transforming the tensions of relational life. (p. 215)

Resolving the Paradox: A Systems View

Despite diverging conceptual backgrounds and theoretical views, regardless of definition or assumptions, a broad, systems frame may be overlaid. All maintenance literature (whether known by that term or another) is fundamentally systemic in nature.

Maintenance is not the mechanistic view of a closed system, but rather in the view of the open system (cf. Rawlins, this volume). Open systems are in a constant state of change, with every component influencing and being influenced by other components. An open systems approach or an approach such as Hinde and Stevenson-Hinde's (1988) relations with relations, reminds us that all relationships are influenced not only by the two relational partners but by all forces impinging on the partners. Ecological systemic approaches (see e.g., Bronfenbrenner, 1989) consider nested levels and systemic relationships within and between these levels. All micro-level interaction takes place within, and is influenced by, sociocultural patterns (Minuchin, 1985). Or as Rawlins would say, the "sociocultural envelope" (Rawlins, this volume).

Moreover, relationships endure over time, through separations, and may be carried out in the forms of memories of and expectations for interactions (Hinde, 1988). This is highly compatible with Rawlins' discussion of friendships for example. Of course, this position is also consistent with Duck's positions on the importance of talk.

When one changes levels of abstraction to solve the problem of conflicting logical types, it becomes possible to frame virtually all the approaches to maintenance expressed herein within an ecological systems approach. A systemic approach can incorporate a dialectical stance. Relationships, like any open system, are in an ongoing process of change; open systems must continually adapt and change, and manage internal and external contingencies in order to survive as relationships.

Watzlawick et al. (1967) point out that models based in pure homeostasis (that is, no change due to the mechanism of negative feedback) are in error. They comment on a complete steady state of homeostasis, "Clearly this is an undesirable type of stability" (p. 31). Positive feedback which promotes change also occurs within relationships: "[T]he manifestations of life are evidently distinguished by both stability and change, negative and positive feedback mechanisims must occur" (Watzlawick et al., 1967, p. 31). Relationships must balance homeostasis (as in complete stability via negative feedback), and the positive feedback of change. This does not imply a return to the same steady state, but rather a new or different level is achieved as relationships cannot repeat themselves.

Relationships must change. Relationships are composed of people who themselves change developmentally across their life spans. Both individual and relational change must be considered (see Sillars & Wilmot, 1989). What might be satisfying, or enhance a given relational property (e.g., trust), at one point in a "stable" relationship, may be an entirely dysfunctional way to enhance the same characteristic at another point in the same "stable" relationship.

Conclusions

As Canary and Stafford note, the knowledge gained from considering divergent standpoints is, at least for the moment, well worth the cost of a lack of one unified stance. Certainly, there can be no complete agreement as to whether maintenance is a temporal state or a process. Yet, perhaps in order to alleviate this conflict of logical types, to move away from a unidirectional cause-and-effect orientation, one could consider that maintenance is not the process, the state, or both, but rather the *link* between process and state. Perhaps study of this connection (and impinging factors on it) is the study of relational maintenance.

Regarding maintenance as a link allows us to address the systemic nature of relationships without conceptual reliance on exclusively unidirectional forces. Researchers using systems frameworks argue that "we must come to terms with two dialectics—between the characteristics of individuals and interactions on the one hand, and between interactions and relationships on the other, with two-way cause–effect influences in each case" (Hinde & Stevenson-Hinde, 1987, p. 3). In this light, Wilmot's observations of relational "conundrums," Ducks's "shared meaning system," as well as dialectal tensions can be understood.

Despite the overarching systems perspective, there are two important areas in which maintenance research generally lags behind systems concepts. First, systems perspectives have progressed conceptually beyond cause and effect. As Yerby, Buerkel-Rothfuss, and Bochner (1990) note, "from a systems point of view, no one person or thing . . . can realistically be identified as the 'cause'" (p. 63). And although systems frames are highly compatible with maintenance research, most maintenance work falls short because of its hunt for "cause and effect." The alternatives, that relational characteristics may "cause" certain maintenance processes or that both relational activities and outcomes are reflexive and interdependent, are seldom considered in maintenance work—although the possibility has been raised (see Canary & Stafford, 1992; Rusbult et al., this volume).

People maintaining relationships are intricately interwoven, yielding unidirectional orientations that are too simplistic. We really do not know if equity promotes maintenance behavior or vice versa, and the same is true of commitment or virtually any other relational property: which came first? and does it matter? People do indeed tend to punctuate their events (Watzlawick et al., 1967), but to what extent is this punctuation accurate or even meaningful?

Much maintenance research has also generally paid little attention to environmental and contextual factors (however see Rawlins' discussion of the sociocultural envelope and Gottman on societally imposed sex-segregation, both this volume). From an ecological systems view, once we are dealing with relationships that are embedded within other systems, we should consider macro variables impinging on and responsive to the relational subsystem. Then we are no longer dealing with either unidirectional or bidirectional causal links in a chain, but multiple layered and interwoven threads.

Thus, perhaps link is not the best metaphor for this maintenance connection. "One must never forget that the links in a supposed causal chain are in reality spider's webs" (Hinde & Stevenson-Hinde, 1987, p. 10, paraphrasing Hansen, 1955). As we progress in the pursuit to understand maintenance, it is likely that there will be more disentangling to come. In keeping within this encompassing system's view, as students of human relationships attempting to unravel yarn, we must recall we are also fibers in this yarn. Tracing the threads of spider webs requires that we do not forget that we are part of them.

Acknowledgments

I would like to acknowledge Marianne Dainton for coining the title to this essay and to thank both Dainton and Dan Canary for their comments on a draft of this essay.

306   Laura Stafford

References

Bronfenbrenner, U. (1989). Ecological systems theory. In R. Vasta (Ed.), *Annals of child develop-ment* (Vol. 6., pp. 187–250). Greenwich, CT: JAI Press.

Canary, D. J., & Stafford, L. (1992). Relational maintenance strategies and equity in marriage. *Communication Monographs, 59,* 243–267.

Cate, R. M., & Lloyd, S. A. (1992). *Courtship.* Newbury Park, CA: Sage.

Dindia, K., & Canary, D. J. (1993). Definitions and theoretical perspectives on relational mainte-nance. *Journal of Social and Personal Relationships, 10,* 163–173.

Hanson, N. R. (1955). Causal chains. *Mind, 255,* 289–311.

Hinde, R. A. (1988). Introduction. In R. A. Hinde & J. Stevenson-Hinde (Eds.), *Relationships within families: Mutual influences* (pp. 1–4). New York: Oxford University Press.

Hinde, R. A., & Stevenson-Hinde, J. (1987). Interpersonal relationships and child development. *Developmental Review, 7,* 1–21.

Hinde, R. A., & Stevenson-Hinde, J. (Eds.). (1988). *Relationships within families: Mutual influences.* New York: Oxford University Press.

Montgomery, B. M. (1993). Relationship maintenance versus relationship change: A dialectical dilemma. *Journal of Social and Personal Relationships, 10,* 205–223.

Minuchin, P. (1985). Families and individual development: Provocations from the field of family therapy. *Child Development, 56,* 289–302.

Russell, B. (1951). *Introduction to Ludwig Wittgenstein,* Tractacus Logico-Philosophicus. New York: Humanities Press.

Sillars, A., & Wilmot, W. W. (1989). Marital communication across the life span. In J. F. Nussbaum (Ed.), *Life-span communication: Normative processes* (pp. 225–254). Hillsdale, NJ: Lawrence Erlbaum.

Watzlawick, P., Bavelas, J. B., & Jackson, D. (1967). *Pragmatics of human communication: A study of interactional patterns, pathologies, and paradoxes.* New York: Norton.

Wilmot, W. W. (1987). *Dyadic communication* (3rd ed.). New York: Random House.

Yerby, J., Buerkel-Rothfuss, N., & Bochner, A. P. (1990). *Understanding family communication.* Scottsdale, AZ: Gorsuch Scarsbrick.

Index